BOLLINGEN SERIES XXXI

PSYCHOLOGICAL
REFLECTIONS

An Anthology
of the Writings of

C. G. JUNG

SELECTED AND EDITED BY

JOLANDE JACOBI

BOLLINGEN SERIES XXXI

PANTHEON BOOKS

THIS VOLUME IS THE THIRTY-FIRST IN A SERIES OF BOOKS
SPONSORED BY AND PUBLISHED FOR
BOLLINGEN FOUNDATION

Originally published in German as *Psychologische Betrachtungen: Eine Auslese aus
den Schriften von C. G. Jung* by Rascher
Verlag, Zurich, 1945 (second edition, 1949).

Manufactured in the U.S.A.

Library of Congress Catalogue Card No.: 52–10521

TABLE OF CONTENTS

*In the following, a line or two is drawn from the text
to suggest the gist of each page.*

THE NATURE AND ACTIVITY OF THE PSYCHE

RECOGNITION OF THE SOUL

CONTENTS

CONTENTS

DREAMS

MAN IN HIS RELATION TO OTHERS

DOCTOR AND PATIENT

CONTENTS

MAN AND WOMAN

ix

CONTENTS

THE INDIVIDUAL AND THE COMMUNITY

THE WORLD OF VALUES

AWARENESS AND CREATIVE LIVING

PROBLEMS OF SELF-REALIZATION

BETWEEN GOOD AND EVIL

THE LIFE OF THE SPIRIT

ON ULTIMATE THINGS

WESTERN AND EASTERN POINTS OF VIEW

THE DEVELOPMENT OF THE PERSONALITY

FATE, DEATH, AND RENEWAL

NOTE ON SOURCES

The source of each paragraph is indicated by the citation following, which refers to the list of Jung's works in both German and English, at the end of this book. For example, the third paragraph on page 5 is taken from the original *Über die Psychologie des Unbewussten*, p. 206, as translated by H. G. and C. F. Baynes in *Two Essays on Analytical Psychology*, p. 118.

Existing English translations have, in most cases, been incorporated. R. F. C. Hull's new translations prepared for the *Collected Works of C. G. Jung* have been drawn upon in so far as possible—see the Key to Sources, page 329—but this volume was already in press when Mr. Hull's version of *Two Essays on Analytical Psychology* became available. The passages for which no English translation is cited have been translated especially for this anthology by J. Verzar and revised by Elizabeth Welsh. The selections have been made consistent in style.

For permission to use the copyrighted material included in this work, acknowledgement is made as follows: Longmans, Green and Co., New York, for introduction to M. Esther Harding, *The Way of All Women;* Yale University Press for *Psychology and Religion;* Farrar and Rinehart for *The Integration of the Personality*, translated by Stanley M. Dell; Harcourt, Brace and Co. for *The Secret of the Golden Flower*, translated by Cary F. Baynes, *Contributions to Analytical Psychology*, translated by H. G. and Cary F. Baynes, *Psychological Types*, translated by H. G. Baynes, and *Modern Man in Search of a Soul*, translated by W. S. Dell and Cary F. Baynes; Dodd, Mead and Co. for *Collected Papers on Analytical Psychology*, edited by Dr. Constance E. Long, and *Two Essays on Analytical Psychology*, translated by H. G. and C. F. Baynes; Luzac and Co., London, for "On the Psychology of Eastern Meditation," translated by Carol Baumann in *Art and Thought; Transition, an International Quarterly for Creative Experiment*, for "Psychology and Poetry," translated by Eugene Jolas in its number 19–20, June, 1930.

PREFACE

Western man today, engaged in a mighty struggle outwardly and inwardly for a new and universally binding order of life, stands at a point where two worlds meet, amid an almost inconceivable devastation of traditional values. No clear orientation is possible, nothing can as yet point to a way in this whirlwind of spiritual forces striving for form. Human existence itself in all its inadequacy and insecurity must submit to a new revision. The outstanding fateful destruction of enormous material property points more imperatively than ever to the values of the psychic and spiritual world. A general and deep interest is at last turning in this direction. Perhaps—so people hope— psychology, this youngest and still frequently neglected child of science, may be able to help us to some understanding of the incomprehensible factors of life with which man has been more and more relentlessly confronted since the turn of the century, and may thus guide his pathless present towards a more meaningful future. For it is gradually dawning on man that the root of all good and evil lies in his own soul and that the world around him is as he himself has shaped it. It may be he dimly senses that the fate of the world grows out of what is happening in the souls of men. And how can there be law and order in the outer world so long as man does not feel at home in the inner world, in his own soul?

Thus it would seem to be time—indeed, high time, after the countless endeavours made from the most varied standpoints— to say something really substantial about men and the universe, to attempt to draw a wider meaning from the psychological point of view as well. For modern "depth psychology" in particular has the advantage of a position between the natural and the philosophical sciences, bridging the two and committed to both at the same time, and affording besides the possibility— as does no other science—of learning, through the most direct experience of the human being, the reality of all that is created and produced in the psychic and spiritual realm. That the far-reaching and powerful works of the Swiss psychologist C. G. Jung, which probe the remotest depths of the psyche, should be taken as a basis for this purpose hardly needs further explanation. Furthermore the fact that this year* will see Jung's seventieth birthday provides a natural and appropriate occasion. For such an anniversary represents in the life of a man a milestone from which to survey and look back, a pause in which to meditate and take stock. This halt comes in the natural course of things, but it is all the more justified when, as in Jung's case, the stream of creative energy is still a torrent. Therefore the wider, general purpose has quite naturally been associated with a personal one.

This book does not set out to do justice to the personality and work of Jung in any comprehensive way. Nevertheless, his work, as it makes its direct appeal in the following selection of quotations, will also reveal the essence and value of its author. Jung is primarily an empiricist, a practical psychologist; his personal experience forms the premise and the basis of his theory. Whatever he says is always very near the living processes of the soul and he himself is moved by these in his whole personality. He is no friend of the aphoristic, the sententious, the thought out, of all the products of the crystal realm of abstract thinking. Even where his words may sometimes give this impression, they are, actually, always the outcome of a deeply lived experience; they are only, so to speak, the precipitate of the facts experienced during his work on the psyche. But because Jung is not only a scientific empiricist, but at the same time a true artist, who is challenged by the shimmering, mysterious, boundless world of primordial images which is the psyche, everything which he says possesses that unique, compelling force which leaves no one unmoved. All that is experienced in everyday life or in the doctor's consulting-room is permeated with inner vision and becomes a most personal and original world-wide view, encompassing almost all facets of human existence. No one who does not stand aside from real life will be able to avoid a coming to terms with Jung, whether his attitude be one of agreement or disagreement. For Jung, one

* [1945.—Translator.]

who is himself gripped and deeply moved by the mystery of the soul, is capable of moving others as few men can.

The object of compiling the following selection of quotations was not to present Jung's theory in its purely scientific and professional aspect but rather to show by means of a cross-section a few of the more important aspects of existence reflected in humanity in general, when understood and illuminated by psychology; therefore everything which is technical in the narrow sense was excluded from the outset. It was also found necessary to omit the foundations of Jung's theory, the basic lines of his analytical psychology, with its vast number of definitions and its varied weave of concepts and forms, the whole of its case material and the amplifying verifications of the auxiliary sciences—and much more besides. Whoever is particularly interested in this side or is seeking precise information in the field of Jung's analytical psychology should study the series of special investigations in his own books. The present selection is limited to particularly characteristic statements of a more general nature, which can more or less stand by themselves and are capable of providing a true outlook on life from the psychological observatory. To try to see them, however, as moralizing precepts, prescriptions, or warnings would be a complete mistake; it would lead to an absolute misunderstanding of Jung's conceptions at a crucial point and would be a fundamental contradiction of the aims of his psychology. For, owing to his daily encounter with the disastrous results of an unreflecting acceptance of rules and engrafted opinions—sometimes hammered in in early childhood and never properly assimilated, mostly misunderstood or not fully understood—his urgent purpose is to lead people to a responsible attitude towards life and a responsible way of living, suited to the individual peculiarities of each man: to an inner and outer way of behaviour in which it is not the collective standards that rule, but in which the inborn, most personal law of each individual allows him the appropriate space in which to develop.

Many of the chosen passages may therefore at first sight seem unusual, controversial, even alien in contrast to the customary conception of life. But people have so often entirely ignored the psychological point of view in the estimating and judging of things that it is no wonder if a great deal appears in a new and peculiar light when seen from this standpoint. Besides, the fact should not be overlooked that as soon as the realm of the psyche is entered—and thereby the whole of the psyche involved—everything has to be judged according to its structural polarity. Every pronouncement in psychology has to take this into account and every psychological statement bears witness to it. The apparent contradictions which may be found in the following paragraphs chosen from Jung's works are due to this structural antinomy which is peculiar to the psyche as a result of the fundamental tension of the opposites, conscious and unconscious. The recognition and acceptance of this polarity thrusts itself imperatively on everyone in the present period. Upon this hangs the question whether, in future, man will be able to find his way out of the entanglements of fate back to some new kind of order, or whether, in ignorance of his own psychic foundations and those of his fellow men, he will remain at the mercy of the powers of darkness—even as, with horror, we have already known it in this our present age, so puffed up with pride of its cultural and technical progress.

The selected passages are not arranged in chronological order nor in the sequence they may have had within each of Jung's works. The editor's purpose was to relate them to various themes, and they were chosen with regard only to content, in order to do justice to the richness of the psychological outlook as well as to the number and variety of themes encompassed. Nevertheless, care was always taken to give each theme the widest scope; and consequently ideas which lay rather far afield had occasionally to be sacrificed in order, where possible, to devote whole chapters to more significant aspects. A kind of all-round survey of some of the more important spheres of human existence was thus achieved, in which a sharper and more extensive light is thrown on some, a dimmer and more restricted light on others. Paragraphs are not juxtaposed arbitrarily; there is always an inner connection, and where possible a sequence. Thus each quotation is bound to those preceding and following in some continuity of thought, the theme being either developed or presented in a new aspect, and any apparent obscurity can usually be cleared up by reading the next quotation or the next but one. Quotations are taken only from the works so far published in German. To use the many still unpublished manuscripts, works existing only in multigraphed form, or seminar reports (all of which are only for the private use of Jung's pupils) would have enlarged this volume to at least twice its present size, and in these cases comparison with the original text would have been impossible.

Considering the richness of Jung's work, it would have been hopeless to attempt an exhaustive representation—such could not have been the aim of the present selection. It had to be limited to a survey of the general, human aspect of Jung's psychological concepts, free of the restrictions of the purely scientific. The present book is not meant for the expert, but for all who seek knowledge and understanding of the inner forces by which they and the whole world are moved; for all who search for vision to guide them through this life, pulsating between light and darkness; and finally for all who are ready and willing to acknowledge the reality of the soul, to restore to it its true dignity, and to work together for a greater understanding of the new values which every darkness brings to light.

Zurich, Spring, 1945   JOLANDE JACOBI

MOTTO

Little effect have spoken remarks and rejoinders, if many
Join in the talk and each will listen more to his own words
Than to his neighbours' and takes from his neighbours' what he is
    pleased with.
Nearly the same is the case with books; for every one will
Find himself in the book, unless in his strength he decide on
Putting himself into it and amalgamating the substance.
Ever in vain, therefore, you endeavour by writing to change man's
Strong inclination, the form of his thought and his natural bias.
If you achieve success, you strengthen him in his own mind,
Or, if he have none, into a tub you dip and you dye him.

—GOETHE, "First Epistle"

THE NATURE AND ACTIVITY
OF THE PSYCHE

The soul of man
Resembleth water:
From heaven it cometh,
To heaven it soareth,
And then again
To earth descendeth,
Changing ever.

—GOETHE, "Spirit Song
over the Waters"

RECOGNITION OF THE SOUL

"All outer things are also within," as Goethe says: and this "within," which modern rationalism likes to make subsidiary to the "outer," has its own structure which precedes all conscious experience and is in fact an *a priori* of unconscious experience also. For it is impossible to imagine how "experience" in its widest sense, and indeed how anything psychic, can be made up exclusively of outer phenomena. The psyche belongs to the very core of the mystery of life, and like all organic living phenomena, it has its particular characteristic structure and form. Whether the structure of the soul and its elements, the archetypes, ever had a beginning is a metaphysical question and as such not one to be answered. The structure is a given fact, it is that which in every case was already present, the precondition. It is the mother. [XLIII, 436 f

The human psyche is in no way outside nature. It is one of the natural phenomena and its problems are as important as the questions and riddles raised by bodily disease. Furthermore, there is scarcely a disease of the body in which psychic factors do not play a part, just as bodily factors are also involved in so many psychogenic disorders. [XLVIII, 128

A wrong functioning of the psyche can injure the body in important ways, just as conversely a bodily illness can involve the psyche sympathetically, for body and soul are not separate entities but one and the same life. [LI, 206 (D, 118)

Merely to establish the fact that certain people have this or that appearance is of no significance if it does not allow us to infer a psychic correlative. We have learned something only when we have determined what mental attributes go with a given bodily constitution. The body means as little to us without the psyche as the latter without the body. When we try to derive a psychic correlative from a physical characteristic, we

5

are proceeding—as already stated—from the known to the unknown.   [xix, 117 (j, 86 f)

The mind is a series of images in the widest sense, not an accidental juxtaposition or sequence, but a structure that is throughout full of meaning and purpose; it is a picturing of vital activities. And just as the material of the body that is ready for life has need of the psyche in order to be capable of life, so the psyche presupposes the living body in order that its images may live.   [xix, 380 (g, 84 f)

In spite of the materialistic tendency to conceive of the soul mainly as a mere result of physical and chemical processes, there is not a single proof of this hypothesis. On the contrary, innumerable facts show that the soul translates the physical processes into images which frequently bear hardly any recognizable relationship to the objective process. The materialistic hypothesis is much too bold and oversteps the limits of experience with "metaphysical" presumption. There is no reason whatever to picture the soul as a something secondary or as an epiphenomenon; there are indeed sufficient reasons for regarding it, at least hypothetically, as a factor *sui generis,* and for continuing so to regard it until it be adequately proved that psychic processes can also be made in the test tube.   [xxxix, 4

A psychology that treats the mind as an epiphenomenon would do better to call itself brain-physiology, and remain satisfied with the meagre results that such a psychophysiology can yield. The mind deserves to be taken as a phenomenon in its own right; for there are no apparent reasons why it should be regarded as a mere epiphenomenon, dependent though it may be upon the functioning of the brain. One is as little justified in so regarding it as in conceiving life as an epiphenomenon of the chemistry of carbon compounds.   [xiii, 13 ff (g, 6)

Limitation to material reality cuts out from the world as a whole an immeasurably large piece but still only *a piece,* and produces thereby a dark region which we call unreal or supernatural. The Eastern philosophy of life, for instance, has not

6

this limiting barrier, and therefore it needs no philosophical conception of a super-reality. Our arbitrarily circumscribed conception of reality is constantly threatened by such conceptions as "supersensory," "supernatural," "superhuman," etc. Eastern reality quite naturally includes all these conceptions. For the Western mind the point of disturbance begins with our conception of the psychic factor. In our "reality" the psychic factor is nothing else than an indirect effect proceeding from something which has its origin in the physical realm, a "brain secretion" or something equally savoury. And yet this mere appendage of the material world is considered capable not only of over-reaching itself and recognizing the mysteries of the psychic world but also of recognizing itself in the form of "mind," and all this in spite of the fact that it is not accredited with anything more than an indirect reality.   [xxii, 844

Everything which is discovered by valid or apparently valid methods about the nature of the soul automatically and inevitably involves the entire scope of all philosophical sciences; for whatever is thought about the nature of psychic happenings touches the psychic foundations of all philosophical sciences even when the actual decisions fall within the discipline of medical science, which, of course, does not count itself among the philosophical sciences.   [xlv

Like all sciences, psychology has gone through its epoch of scholasticism, and something of the scholastic spirit has lasted on into the present time. Against this kind of philosophical psychology it must be objected that it makes an *ex cathedra* decision as to how the soul shall be constituted and what qualities must belong to it in every possible respect.   [v, 236 (d, 1)

Every natural science becomes descriptive at the point at which it can no longer explore experimentally, but it does not thereby cease to be scientific. An empirical science, however, becomes impossible when it limits its field of action by theoretical conceptions. The psyche does not come to an end where the scope of some physiological or other assumption reaches

7

its limit; that is to say, in every single case which we are considering scientifically, we have to take into account the entire aspect of the psyche. [xxxix, 2

To the dismay of the busy practitioner of the present day, the psyche is completely refractory in the face of any method which attempts to consider it from one point of view only, to the exclusion of all others. [xiii, 151

The psychological investigator is always finding himself obliged to make use of extensive, and in a sense indirect, description for the presentation of the reality he has observed. Only in so far as elementary facts are accessible to number and measure can there be any question of a direct presentation. But how much of the actual psychology of man can be witnessed and observed as mensurable facts? [ix, 587 (i, 518)

I do not find it surprising that psychology should also touch the field of philosophy, for the act of thinking which is the basis of philosophy is a psychic activity and as such an object of psychology. By psychology I always mean the entire scope of the psyche, and this involves philosophy and theology, and a great deal more besides. For over against all philosophies and all religions stand the facts of the human soul, which may perhaps be able in the last resort to decide between truth and error. [xiii, 178

There is no Archimedean point from which to judge, since the psyche is indistinguishable from its manifestation. The psyche is the object of psychology and—fatally enough—at the same time its subject, and there is no getting away from this fact. [xlvi, 91 f (b, 62)

Only that which is psychic has direct reality—indeed, every form of psychic activity, even the so-called "unreal" imaginings and thoughts which have no relation to the outside world. We may call such thoughts imagination or madness, but their power is by no means destroyed thereby, indeed there is no "real" thought which cannot at times be pushed aside by an "unreal" thought which thus proves itself to be of greater strength and effectiveness. The gigantic effects of insane imaginings are greater than all physical dangers, and yet our world-consciousness tries to deny them all reality. Our much prized reasoning power and our boundlessly over-rated will-power prove at times to be powerless against these "unreal" thoughts. The world powers which, for better or worse, govern the whole of humanity are unconscious psychic factors, and they it is that also bring forth consciousness and thereby the *conditio sine qua non* for the very existence of a world. We are overpowered by a world which was created by our psyche. [xxii, 845

Since we do not know everything, practically every experience, fact, or object contains something which is unknown. Hence if we speak of the totality of an experience, the word "totality" can refer only to the conscious part of the experience. As we cannot assume that our experience covers the totality of the object, it is evident that its absolute totality must needs contain the part that has not been experienced. The same holds true, as I have mentioned, of every experience and also of the psyche, whose absolute totality covers a greater surface than consciousness. In other words, the psyche is no exception to the general rule that the universe can be established only in so far as our psychic organism permits. [xlvi, 75 (b, 48 f)

Although common prejudice still believes that the chief foundation of our knowledge comes from outside, and that *nihil esse in intellectu, quod non antea fuerit in sensu,* it is nevertheless true that the atom theory of the ancients Leucippus and Democritus, which should by no means be undervalued, was not based on observation of splitting the atom, but on a "mythological" conception of the smallest possible particles (such as are also known to the paleolithic central Australian aborigines as "soul-atoms," animated smallest particles). Every student of ancient natural history and natural philosophy knows how much of the soul is projected into what is unknown of the outside phenomenon. In fact so much is projected that we are absolutely unable ever to give an account of how the world itself is actually made, since we are forced to translate the physical

9

facts into a psychic process, if we wish to speak at all of knowledge. But how can we guarantee that any sort of adequate "objective" picture of the world is achieved by this transfer?

[xxxix, 3 f

The necessity of a plurality of explanations, however, in the case of a psychological theory is definitely granted, since, unlike any other natural-science theory, the object of psychological explanation is of like nature with the subject: one psychological process has to explain another. This serious difficulty has already driven thinking minds to remarkable subterfuges, as, for instance, the assumption of an "objective mind" which should stand outside psychology and, hence, be able to regard objectively its own psyche; or the similar assumption that the intellect is a faculty which can also stand outside itself and regard itself. With these and similar expedients, that Archimedean, extraterrestrial point is to be created by means of which the intellect shall raise itself from its own hinges. I can understand the profound human need for comfort and ease, but I do not understand why truth should bend to this need. I also understand that, aesthetically, it would be far more satisfactory if, instead of the paradox of mutually contradictory explanations, we could reduce the psychic process to the simplest possible instinctive foundation and be at rest, or if we could credit it with a metaphysical goal of redemption and find peace in that hope.—But whatever we strive to fathom with our intellect will end in paradox and relativity, if, indeed, it be honest work and not a mere *petitio principii* in the service of comfort and convenience.   [ix, 702 f (i, 627 f)

To the *esse in intellectu,* tangible reality is lacking; to the *esse in re,* the mind. Idea and thing come together, however, in the psyche of man, which holds the balance between them. What would the idea amount to if the psyche did not provide its living value? What would the objective thing be worth if the psyche withheld from it the determining force of the sense impression? What indeed is reality if it is not a reality in ourselves, an *esse in anima?* Living reality is the exclusive product neither of the actual, objective behaviour of things nor of the formulated idea; rather does it come through the gathering up

10

of both in the living psychological process, through the *esse in anima*. Only through the specific vital activity of the psyche does the sense-perception attain that intensity and the idea that effective force, which are the two indispensable constituents of living reality. This peculiar activity of the psyche, which can be explained neither as a reflex to sense-stimuli nor as an executive organ of eternal ideas is, like every vital process, a perpetually creative act.   [IX, 74 f (I, 68 f)

It is a remarkable fact, which we come across again and again, that absolutely everybody, even the most unqualified layman, thinks he knows all about psychology as though the psyche were something that enjoyed the most universal understanding. But anybody who really knows the human psyche will agree with me when I say that it is one of the darkest and most mysterious regions in the whole of our experience. There is no end to what can be learned in this field.   [LVIII, 14 (M, 2)

I am of the opinion that the psyche is the most powerful fact in the human world. It is indeed the mother of all human facts, of culture and of murderous wars. All this is at first psychic and imperceptible. As long as it remains "merely" psychic, it is not perceived by the senses, but it is nevertheless indisputably real.   [XLVII, 405

What is illusion? By what criterion do we judge something to be an illusion? Does there exist for the psyche anything which we may call "illusion"? What we are pleased to call such may be for the psyche a most important factor of life—something as indispensable as oxygen for the organism—a psychic actuality of prime importance. Presumably the psyche does not trouble itself about our categories of reality, and it would therefore be the better part of wisdom for us to say: everything that *acts* is actual. He who would fathom the psyche must not confuse it with consciousness, else he veils from his own sight the object he wishes to explore. On the contrary, even to recognize the psyche, he must learn to see how it differs from consciousness. It is highly probable that what we call illusion is actual for the psyche: for which reason we cannot take psychic actuality to be commensurable with conscious actuality.

[xix, 113 (j, 83 f)

Each new day, reality is created by the psyche. The only expression I can use for this activity is "phantasy." Phantasy is just as much feeling as thought; it is intuitive just as much as sensational. There are no psychic functions which in phantasy are not inextricably inter-related with the other psychic functions. At one time it appears primordial, at another as the latest and most daring product of gathered knowledge. Phantasy, therefore, appears to me as the clearest expression of the specific psychic activity. Before everything it is the creative activity whence issue the solutions to all answerable questions; it is the mother of all possibilities, in which too the inner and the outer worlds, like all psychological antitheses, are joined in living union.   [ix, 75 (i, 69)

Phantasy is simply spontaneous psychic activity; and it wells up whenever the repressive action of the conscious mind relaxes or ceases altogether, as in sleep.   [xix, 6 (j, 36)

The soul, as a reflection of the world and of humanity, is so complex that one can consider it and judge it from innumerable different angles. With the psyche it is the same as with the universe; to work out a system of the world is beyond human grasp, and therefore we have merely technical rules and points of interest. Every man cuts his own slice from the world, and makes his private system to fit his private world, often with air-tight walls, so that after a time it seems to him that he has realized the very sense and structure of the world. The finite can never grasp the infinite. Although the psychic world of phenomena is only a part of the whole world, it would seem that, for this very reason, it could be more easily grasped than the world as a whole. But one does not sufficiently realize that the psyche is the only immediate world phenomenon and therefore also the essential condition for a general experience of the world.

[xix, 144

All activity of the psyche is an image and an imagining; otherwise no consciousness and no phenomenality of the process could exist. Imagining is also a psychic process, and therefore it is totally irrelevant whether a "revelation" is described as "real" or "imagined." He who has, or says he has, a revelation believes in any case that he has been enlightened. What others think about it means nothing to him in regard to his experience. Even if he were lying, his lie would also be a psychic fact.

[XLII, 18

Naturally, no human action is quite simple—like an isolated reaction to a single stimulus—but each of our actions and reactions is influenced by complicated psychic preconditions. Using the military analogy, we might compare these processes with the situation at general headquarters. To the man in the ranks it might seem that the army retreated simply because it was attacked, or that an attack were made because the enemy had been seen in the wood. Our conscious function is ever inclined to play the role of the common soldier, and to believe in the simplicity of its actions. But in reality battle has been given on this spot and at this moment because of a general plan of attack which in its ordered unfolding has for days been marshalling the common soldier to this point. And again this general plan is not a mere reaction to reconnaissance reports; it results from the creative initiative of the leader. Furthermore, it is conditioned by the action of the enemy, and also perhaps by wholly unmilitary, political considerations of which the common soldier is quite unaware. These last factors are of a very complex nature and lie far outside the understanding of the common soldier, though they may be only too clear to the leader of the army. But even to him certain factors are unknown, namely, the preconditions of his own personality, with all their complicated presuppositions. Thus the army stands under a simple and single command, but the latter is the result of the co-ordinated operation of infinitely complex factors.

[XIX, 297 f (G, 142)

The breaking up of the harmonious co-operation of the psychic forces that exists in instinctive life is like an ever-open, a never-healing wound, a veritable Amfortas's wound, since the differentiation of one function among several inevitably leads to overgrowth of the one and to neglect and crippling of the rest. [IX, 101 (I, 90 f)

To recognize the psyche's protean life and constant metamorphoses is to admit a truth less comfortable than a one-sided theory that stands secure in its rigidity. It makes the problems of psychology less simple. Yet we are liberated from the incubus of "nothing but,"* which is the inevitable leitmotiv of each one-sided view.   [XL, 34

It is all part of the banality of its outward aspect that the gold is minted, i.e., shaped into coins, stamped, and valued. Applied psychologically, this is what Nietzsche refuses to do in his *Zarathustra:* to give names to the virtues. By being shaped and named, psychic life is broken down into coined and valued units. But this is only possible because it is intrinsically a great variety of things, an accumulation of unintegrated hereditary factors. Natural man is not a "self"—he is the mass and the particle in the mass, collective to such a degree that he is not even sure of his own ego. That is why since time immemorial he has needed the transformation mysteries to turn him into something and to rescue him from the animal collective psyche, which is nothing but an assortment, a "variety performance."
[LVIII, 122 (M, 104)

So long as one knows nothing of a psychic existence, it is projected if it appears at all. Thus the first knowledge of the laws and rules of the psyche was found in the stars, and further knowledge in unknown matter. From both fields of experience, sciences have branched off; from astrology came astronomy, from alchemy came chemistry. The peculiar relationship between astronomic estimation of time and character is, on the contrary, only recently beginning to form itself into something like scientific empiricism. The really important psychic

* [The following explanatory note is entered from the English edition of *Psychology and Alchemy,* where it has been added by the editors: "The term 'nothing but' (*nichts als*) occurs frequently in Jung, and is used to denote the common habit of explaining something unknown by reducing it to something apparently known and thereby devaluing it. For instance, when a certain illness is said to be 'nothing but psychic,' it is explained away as imaginary and is thus devalued."—TRANSLATOR.]

14

elements cannot be measured with the ruler, or the balance, or the test-tube, or the microscope. They are therefore (supposedly) imperceptible, or, in other words, they must be left to those people who have an inner feeling for them, just as one shows colours to those who can see and not to the blind.

[LII, 148

In mythological research, we have contented ourselves until now with solar, lunar, meteorological, vegetal, and other comparisons. But we have almost completely refused to see that myths are first and foremost psychic manifestations that represent the nature of the psyche. The mind of the primitive is little concerned with an objective explanation of obvious things; it has an imperative need—or, rather, his unconscious psyche has an irresistible urge—to assimilate all experience through the outer senses into inner, psychic happening. The primitive is not content to see the sun rise and set: this external observation must at the same time be a psychic event—that is, the sun in its course must represent the fate of a god or hero who dwells, in the last analysis, nowhere else than in the psyche of man. All the mythologized occurrences of nature, such as summer and winter, the phases of the moon, the rainy seasons, and so forth, are anything but allegories of these same objective experiences, nor are they to be understood as "explanations" of sunrise, sunset, and the rest of the natural phenomena. They are, rather, symbolic expressions for the inner and unconscious psychic drama that becomes accessible to human consciousness by way of projection—that is, by being mirrored in the events of nature.

[XXXI, 182 (F, 54)

It was reserved to modern natural science with its objective knowledge of the material world to despiritualize nature. All anthropomorphic projections were withdrawn one by one from their objects: on the one hand the mystic identity of man with nature was reduced to an unheard-of degree, while on the other hand the withdrawal of such projections into the psyche caused such a stimulation of the unconscious that the modern age could no longer possibly avoid the postulation of an unconscious psyche. The first signs of this can be seen in Leibniz and Kant, and then in rapidly increasing degree in Schelling, Carus, and von Hartmann, until modern psychology also discarded the last metaphysical claims of the philosophical psychologists and reduced the idea of psychic existence to the psychological assertions, i.e., to the psychological phenomenology. Instead of the lost Olympian gods, there was disclosed the inner wealth of the soul which lies in every man's heart.   [L, 120 f

In a sense, the old alchemists were nearer to the central truth of the psyche than Faust when they strove to redeem the fiery spirit from the chemical elements, and treated the mystery as though it lay in the dark and silent womb of nature. It was still outside them. But the upward thrust of evolving consciousness was bound sooner or later to put an end to the projection and to restore to the psyche what had been psychic from the beginning. Yet, ever since the Age of Enlightenment, and in the epoch of scientific rationalism, what indeed was the psyche? It had become synonymous with consciousness. The psyche was "what I know." There was no psyche outside the ego. Inevitably, then, the ego identified itself with the contents accruing from the withdrawal of projection. Gone were the days when the psyche was still for the most part "outside the body" and when it imagined "those greater things" which the body could not grasp. The contents that were formerly projected were now bound to appear as personal possessions, as chimerical phantasms of the ego-consciousness. The fire chilled to air, and the air became the great wind of Zarathustra and caused an inflation of consciousness which, it seems, can only be mitigated by the most terrible catastrophe to civilization, another deluge let loose by the gods upon inhospitable humanity.

[LVIII, 642 (M, 562)

But if the historical process of the despiritualization of the world—the withdrawal of projections—is going on as hitherto, then everything of a divine or daemonic character must return to the soul, to the inside of the unknown man, from where it apparently sprang originally.   [XLVI, 153 f (B, 102 f)

It is not only primitive man whose psychic processes are archaic. The civilized man of today shows these archaic processes as well, and not merely in the form of sporadic throw-backs from the level of modern social life. On the contrary, every

16

civilized human being, whatever his conscious development, is an archaic man at the deeper levels of his psyche. Just as the human body links us with the mammals and displays numerous relics of earlier evolutionary stages back even to the reptilian age, so the human psyche is likewise a product of evolution which, followed up to its origins, shows countless archaic traits.

[XIX, 212 (J, 144)

The psychology of the individual can never be exhaustively explained from himself alone: a clear recognition is also needed of the way in which his individual psychology is conditioned by contemporary history and circumstances. It is not merely a physiological, biological, or personal problem, but also a question of contemporary history. [IX, 653 (I, 578)

No psychological fact can ever be exhaustively explained from its causality alone, since, as a living phenomenon, it is always indissolubly bound up with the continuity of the vital process, so that it is always something that on the one side is and on the other is becoming and therefore always creative. The psychological moment is Janus-faced—it looks both backwards and forwards. Because it is becoming, it also prepares for the future event. Were this not so, intentions, aims, the setting up of goals, the forecasting or divining of the future, would be psychological impossibilities. [IX, 653 f (I, 578)

Being that has soul is living being. Soul is the *living* in man, that which lives of itself and causes life: God breathed into Adam a living breath so that he should live. With cunning and playful deception the soul lures into life the inertia of matter that does not want to live. It creates belief in incredible things, in order that life should live. It is full of snares and traps in order that man should fall, should reach the earth, entangle himself there, and stay caught, in order that life should live. Were it not for the motion and the colour-play of the soul, man would suffocate and rot away in his greatest passion, idleness.

[XXXI, 207 (F, 75 f)

The soul holds as many riddles as the world with its starry systems, before whose sublime display only a mind devoid of imagination can fail to feel its own inadequacy. In face of this extreme uncertainty of human comprehension, all effort at enlightening and theorizing is not only laughable but also sadly lacking in spiritual understanding. [xxvII, 229

It is true that our religious teaching speaks of an immortal soul; but it has very few kind words for the actual human psyche, which would go straight to eternal damnation if it were not for a special act of divine grace. [XLVI, 30 f (B, 19)

The immortality of the soul insisted upon by dogma exalts it above the transitoriness of mortal man and causes it to partake of some supernatural quality. It thus infinitely surpasses the perishable, conscious individual in significance, so that logically the Christian is forbidden to regard the soul as a "nothing but." As the eye to the sun, so the soul corresponds to God. Since our conscious mind does not comprehend the soul it is ridiculous to speak of the things of the soul in a patronizing or depreciatory manner. Even the believing Christian does not know God's hidden ways and must leave it to Him whether He will work on man from the outside or from within, through the soul. [LVIII, 22 f (M, 11)

Metaphysical theories are assertions of the psyche and therefore they are psychological. But to the Western mind, this obvious truth appears either too obvious, since owing to a certain resentment our mind enjoys its slavery to rationalism, or else an inadmissible denial of metaphysical "truth." To the Westerner, the word "psychological" always sounds like "only psychological." The psyche appears to him as something very small, unimportant, personal, and subjective. Therefore one prefers to use the word "mind" whereby one always gives the unspoken impression that perhaps a really very subjective assertion of the "mind" has been made, but of course always of the "general" or, if possible, the "absolute" mind. This somewhat ridiculous arrogance is a compensation for the lamentable smallness of the soul. It seems almost as if Anatole France had spoken a compelling truth for the whole Western world when he makes Catherine of Alexandria in *L' Île des pingouins* advise God: *"Donnez leur une âme mais une petite!"*   [xxxii, 18 f

---

It would be blasphemy to assert that God can manifest himself everywhere save only in the human soul. Indeed the very intimacy of the relationship between God and the soul automatically precludes any devaluation of the latter. It would be going perhaps too far to speak of an affinity; but at all events the soul must contain in itself the faculty of relation to God, i.e., a correspondence, otherwise a connection could never come about.   [lviii, 23 (m, 11)

However we may picture the relationship between God and soul, one thing is certain: that the soul cannot be a "nothing but"; on the contrary it has the dignity of a creature endowed with and conscious of a relationship to Deity. Even if this were only the relationship of a drop of water to the sea, that sea would not exist but for the multitude of drops.

     [lviii, 22 (m, 11)

I did not attribute a religious function to the soul, I merely produced the facts which prove that the soul is *naturaliter religiosa*, i.e., possesses a religious function. I did not invent or interpret this function, it produces itself of its own accord without being prompted thereto by any opinions or suggestions of mine. With a truly tragic delusion these theologians fail to see that it is not a matter of proving the existence of the light, but of blind people who do not know that their eyes can see. It is high time we realized that it is pointless to praise the light and preach it if nobody can see it. It is much more needful to teach people the art of seeing. For it is obvious that far too many people are incapable of establishing a connection between the sacred figures and their own psyche; that is to say they cannot see to what extent the equivalent images are lying dormant in their own unconscious. In order to facilitate this inner vision we must first clear the way for the faculty of seeing. How this is to be done without psychology, that is, without making contact with the psyche, is, frankly, beyond my comprehension. [LVIII, 26 f (M, 14)

It is always only the few who reach the rim of the world, where its mirage begins. For the man who stands always upon the normal path the soul has a human, and not a dubious, daemonic character; neither do his fellow men appear to him in the least problematical. Only complete abandonment either to one world or to the other evokes their duality. [IX, 244 (I, 212)

The doctrine that all evil thoughts come from the heart and that the human soul is a sink of iniquity must lie deep in the marrow of their bones. Were it so, then God had made a sorry job of creation, and it were high time for us to go over to Marcion the Gnostic and depose the incompetent demiurge. Ethically, of course, it is infinitely more convenient to leave God the sole responsibility for such a Home for Idiot Children—as they conceive the world to be—where no one is capable of putting a spoon into his own mouth. But man is worth the pains he takes with himself, and he has something in his own soul that can grow. It is rewarding to watch patiently the silent happenings in the soul, and the most and the best happens when it is not regulated from outside and from above.

[LVIII, 148 f (M, 126)

People will do anything, no matter how absurd, in order to avoid facing their own souls. They will practise Indian yoga and all its exercises, observe a strict regimen of diet, learn theosophy by heart, or mechanically repeat mystic texts from the literature of the whole world—all because they cannot get on with themselves and have not the slightest faith that anything useful could ever come out of their own souls. Thus the soul has gradually turned into a Nazareth from which nothing good can come. Therefore let us fetch it from the four corners of the earth—the more far-fetched and bizarre it is the better!

[LVIII, 148 (M, 126)

Whoever speaks of the reality of the soul or psyche is accused of "psychologism." Psychology is spoken of as if it were "only" psychology and nothing else. The notion that there can be psychic factors which correspond to the divine figures is re-

garded as a devaluation of the latter. It smacks of blasphemy
to think that a religious experience is a psychic process; for, so
it is argued, a religious experience "is not *only* psychological."
Anything psychic is *only* Nature and therefore, people think,
nothing religious can come out of it. At the same time such
critics never hesitate to derive all religions—with the exception
of their own—from the nature of the psyche.   [LVIII, 21 (M, 9)

Were it not a fact of experience that supreme values reside
in the soul (quite apart from the *antimimon pneuma* who is
also there), psychology would not interest me in the least, for
the soul would then be nothing but a miserable vapour. I know,
however, from hundredfold experience, that it is nothing of the
sort, but on the contrary contains the equivalents of everything
that has been formulated in dogma and a good deal more,
which is just what enables it to be an eye destined to behold
the light. This requires limitless range and unfathomable depth
of vision. I have been accused of "deifying the soul." Not I but
God himself has deified it!   [LVIII, 26 (M, 14)

To have soul is the risk of life, for the soul is a life-bestowing
demon who plays his elfin game beneath and above human existence, for which reason—in the realm of dogma—he is threatened and propitiated with superhuman punishments and blessings that go far beyond the possible deserts of human beings.
Heaven and hell are the fate of the soul and not of civil man,
who, in his God-created nakedness and imbecility, would have
no idea what to do with himself in a heavenly Jerusalem.
                                  [XXXI, 207 (F, 76)

CONSCIOUSNESS AND THE UNCONSCIOUS

Our consciousness does not create itself—it arises from un-known depths. In childhood it awakens gradually, and all through life it wakes each morning out of the depths of sleep, i.e., out of an unconscious condition.   [LIV, 47 (L, 176)

The world begins to exist when the individual discovers it. He discovers it when he sacrifices the "mother," when he has freed himself from the mists of his unconscious condition within the mother.   [IV, 392

If one reflects upon what consciousness really is, one is deeply impressed by the extremely wonderful fact that an event which occurs within the cosmos produces simultaneously an inner image; thus it also occurs within, so to speak: in other words, it becomes conscious.   [XXXIV, 1

How could man have conceived the idea of dividing the cosmos into a bright day-world and a dark world filled with fabulous beings—as, for instance, the simile of night and day, or summer and rainy winter—if he had not found the model within himself both in his conscious mind and in his active but invisible and unknowable unconscious? The comprehension of an object is only partly determined by the objective behaviour of the thing observed; it is also determined—and often to a greater extent—by intrapsychic elements which are only re-lated to the things observed by means of projection. This is due simply to the fact that primitive man has not yet experienced the mental asceticism of a critical attitude towards his own dis-cernment, but knows the world as a general phenomenon only dimly amidst the stream of visions which fill him and in which the subjective and the objective are not distinguished but merge one into the other.   [XLIII, 436

The primitive cannot assert that he thinks; it is rather that

"something thinks in him." The spontaneity of the act of thinking does not lie, causally, in his conscious mind, but in his unconscious. Moreover, he is incapable of any conscious effort of
will; he must put himself beforehand into the "mood of willing,"
or let himself be put—hence his *rites d'entrée et de sortie*. His
conscious mind is menaced by an almighty unconscious: hence
his fear of magical influences which may cross his path at any
moment; and for this reason, too, he is surrounded by unknown
forces and must adjust himself to them as best he can. Owing to
the chronic twilight state of his consciousness, it is often next to
impossible to find out whether he merely dreamed something
or whether he really experienced it. The spontaneous manifestation of the unconscious and its archetypes intrudes everywhere
into his conscious mind, and the mythical world of his ancestors
—for instance, the *aljira* or *bugari* of the Australian aborigines—
is a reality equal if not superior to the material world. It is not
the world as we know it that speaks out of his unconscious, but
the unknown world of the psyche, of which we know that it
mirrors our empirical world only in part, and that, for the other
part, it moulds this empirical world in accordance with its own
psychic assumptions. The archetype does not proceed from
physical facts; it describes how the psyche experiences the
physical fact, and in so doing the psyche often behaves so auto-
cratically that it denies tangible reality or makes statements
that fly in the face of it.   [XLIX, 108 f (o, 100 f)

The world is as it ever has been, but our consciousness under-
goes peculiar changes. First, in remote times (though it can,
however, still be observed with living primitives), the main
body of psychical life was apparently in human and in non-human objects: as we should say now, it was projected. Consciousness can hardly exist in a state of complete projection. (At most
it would be nothing but a heap of emotions.) Through the withdrawal of projections, conscious knowledge slowly developed.
Science, curiously enough, practically began with the discovery
of astronomical laws, which was a first stage in the despiritualization of the world. One step slowly followed another. In antiquity they removed the gods from mountains and rivers, from
trees and animals. Our science has subtilized its projections to

an almost unrecognizable degree. But our ordinary psychological life is still swarming with projections. You can find them spread out in the newspapers, books, rumours, and ordinary social gossip. All gaps in actual knowledge are still filled with projections. We are still almost certain we know what other people think or what their true character is.

[XLVI, 149 f (B, 100 f)

However one may designate the depths of the soul, the fact remains that the existence and nature of consciousness are influenced by them to the highest degree; and the more so the less one is conscious of it. The layman can hardly conceive to what extent he is influenced in his preferences, moods, and decisions by the dark facts of his soul, and how dangerous or how helpful is their fateful power. Our intellectual consciousness is like an actor who has forgotten that he is playing a part. But when the play is over, he must be able to recollect his subjective reality, for he cannot continue to live as Julius Caesar or Othello, but only as his own particular self, from which a temporary deception of consciousness had separated him. He must realize once again that he was merely a figure on a stage where a play of Shakespeare was being played, and that a producer and a director had an important say in his playing both before and after the performance.   [XXVII, 66 f

Since the stars have fallen from heaven, and our highest symbols have paled, a secret life holds sway in the unconscious. It is for this reason that we have a psychology today, and for this reason that we speak of the unconscious. All this discussion would be superfluous in an age or culture that possessed symbols. For these are spirit from above; and at such a time, also, spirit is above. It would be a foolish and senseless undertaking for such people to wish to experience or investigate an unconscious that contains nothing but the silent, undisturbed sway of nature. But our unconscious conceals natural spirit, which is to say, spirit turned to water; and this spirit disturbs it. Heaven has become empty space to us, a fair memory of things that once were. But our heart glows, and secret unrest gnaws at the roots of our being.   [XXXI, 203 (F, 72)

24

Until recently psychological empiricism was fond of explaining the "unconscious" (as indeed the term itself implies) as the mere absence of consciousness, as shade is absence of light. But it is recognized not only by all the ages before us but also by present-day exact observation of unconscious processes that the unconscious has a certain creative autonomy which could never belong to a mere shadow nature.   [XLVI, 152 f

He who would penetrate into the unconscious with biological presuppositions remains stuck in the sphere of the instincts and can get no further but only back again into the physical existence.   [XXXII, 24

Never, nor in any place, has man governed matter, unless it be when he has exactly observed its behaviour and followed its laws with great attention. And only in so far as he has done this can he govern it and only just to this extent. And so it is also with that spirit which nowadays is called the unconscious: it is as refractory as matter, as mysterious and evasive, and it follows laws which in their unhuman and superhuman character mostly appear to us as a *crimen laesae majestatis humanae*. When man lays his hand to this work, he repeats, as the alchemists say, the creative work of God. For to challenge the unformed chaotic Tiamat world is in fact the primordial experience.   [LII, 150

We know that the mask of the unconscious is not rigid—it reflects the face we turn towards it. Hostility lends it a threatening aspect, friendliness softens its features. It is not a question of mere optical reflection but of an autonomous answer which reveals the self-sufficing nature of that which answers.
                                                              [LVIII, 44 (M, 29)
The unconscious is not a demonic monster but a thing of nature that is perfectly neutral as far as moral sense, aesthetic taste, and intellectual judgment go. It is dangerous only when our conscious attitude towards it becomes hopelessly false. And this danger grows in the measure that we practise repressions.   [XXVII, 89 f (J, 19 f)

Its nursery-tales about the terrible old man of the tribe and its teachings about the "infantile-perverse-criminal" unconscious have led people to make a dangerous monster out of the unconscious, that really very natural thing. As if all that is good, reasonable, beautiful, and worth living for had taken up its abode in consciousness! Have the horrors of the World War really not opened our eyes? Are we still unable to see that man's conscious mind is even more devilish and perverse than the unconscious? [xxvii, 89 (j, 19)

The conscious mind allows itself to be trained like a parrot, but the unconscious does not—which is why St. Augustine thanked God for not making him responsible for his dreams. The unconscious is a psychic fact; any efforts to drill it are only apparently successful, and moreover harmful to consciousness. It is and remains beyond the reach of subjective arbitrary control, a realm where nature and her secrets can be neither improved upon nor perverted, where we can listen but may not meddle. [lviii, 75 (m, 51)

It is typical of the modern hypertrophy of the conscious mind —in other words a hubris—to ignore the dangerous autonomy of the unconscious and to explain it purely negatively as absence of consciousness. The assumption of unseen gods and demons would be psychologically a much more suitable description of the unconscious, although this would be an anthropomorphic projection. But since the development of consciousness demands the withdrawal of all possible projections, no theory of gods in the sense that they exist outside the psyche can be maintained. [xlvi, 153

But the mind is exceeding its limits when it asserts the metaphysical existence of the gods. Such a statement is just as presumptuous as the opinion that they could be invented, for undoubtedly they are personifications of psychic forces. Not that "psychic forces" have anything to do with the conscious mind, though we are very fond of playing with the idea that the conscious mind and the psyche are identical. This is mere intellectual presumption, but we are afraid of the "metaphysical" and therefore have developed a mania for rational explanation. The two were always hostile brothers and it is only natural that we should fear this conflict. "Psychic forces" really belong to the unconscious. Everything that approaches us from this dark realm either comes from outside—and then we are sure that it is real—or is considered a hallucination and therefore not true. The idea that anything can be true which does not come from outside has hardly yet dawned on mankind.

[xxxvi, 662 (k, 7 f)

As the State tries to "comprehend" the individual, so the individual imagines that he can "comprehend" his soul. He even makes a science of it in the absurd assumption that the intellect, which is only a part and function of the psyche, is capable of comprehending the much greater totality of the soul. In reality the psyche is the mother, the subject, and even the possibility for consciousness itself. The psyche reaches so far beyond the boundary line of consciousness that the latter could easily be compared to an island in the ocean. While the island is small and narrow, the ocean is immensely wide and deep and contains a life which is far greater in every way than that of the island. One can lodge the criticism against this conception that there is no proof that consciousness is but a small island in the ocean. But such a proof is *a priori* impossible, for opposed to the known limits of consciousness is the unknown extension of the unconscious, of which we only know that it exists, and, by virtue of its existence, influences consciousness and its freedom in a limiting sense. [xlvi, 152

Man has managed to build up the structure of the world from the little which he can imagine clearly at any one time. What a godly aspect would meet his eyes if he were able to imagine much and at the same time clearly! This question can only apply to the conceptions of which we are capable. Could we add to these the unconscious—that is, the not-yet- or no-longer-knowable contents—and then try to imagine the whole, even the boldest imagination must fail. [xlii, 27

The reason why consciousness exists and why there is an urge to widen and deepen it is a very simple one. Without consciousness things go worse. This is obviously the reason why

27

Mother Nature has allowed consciousness, that most remarkable of all nature's curiosities, to be produced. The well-nigh unconscious primitive can adapt and can make his power felt, but only in his primitive world. Accordingly he falls victim to countless dangers which we on a higher level of consciousness escape without effort. True, a higher consciousness is exposed to dangers undreamed of by the primitive; but the fact remains that conscious and not unconscious man has conquered the earth. Whether in the last analysis, and from a superhuman point of view, this is an advantage or otherwise we are not in a position to decide.   [xix, 301 (g, 144)

The Book of Genesis represents the act of becoming conscious as the breaking of a taboo, as though the gaining of knowledge meant that a sacred barrier had been impiously overstepped. Genesis is surely right, inasmuch as each step to a greater consciousness is a kind of Promethean guilt. Through the realization, the gods are in a certain sense robbed of their fire. That is to say, something belonging to the unconscious powers has been torn out of its natural connections and has been subordinated to conscious choice. The man who has usurped the new knowledge suffers, however, a transformation or enlargement of consciousness, which no longer resembles that of his fellow men. He has certainly raised himself above the human level of his time ("ye will become like God"), but in doing so, he has also alienated himself from humanity. The pain of this loneliness is the gods' revenge, for he can never again return to men. He is, as the myth says, chained to the lonely cliffs of the Caucasus, forsaken of God and man.

[xi, 62 (d, 164)

The man whom we can with justice call "modern" is solitary. He is so of necessity and at all times, for every step towards a fuller consciousness of the present removes him further from his original *participation mystique* with the mass of men—from submersion in a common unconsciousness. Every step forward means an act of tearing himself loose from that all-embracing, pristine unconsciousness which claims the bulk of mankind almost entirely.   [xix, 402 (j, 227)

Every step forward, even the smallest, along the path of consciousness, adds to the world, to the visible and tangible God. There is no consciousness without the distinguishing of opposites. That is the father principle of the Logos, engaged in an unending fight to free itself from the primeval warmth and darkness of the maternal womb which is unconsciousness. Shrinking from no conflict, no suffering, and no crime, the godly sense of curiosity strives for birth, for, as St. Paul says: "The Spirit searcheth all things, yea, the deep things of God." Unconsciousness is the one primary sin, the absolute crime— for the Logos. But the latter's world-creating act of deliverance is matricide, and the spirit which ventured into every height and every depth must, as Synesius says, also suffer the punishment of the gods to be bound on the rock of the Caucasus. Neither can exist without the other, for in the beginning both were one and in the end they must again be one. Consciousness can only exist through constant subjection to the unconscious, just as all living things must pass through many deaths.

[XLIII, 430 f

It is just man's turning away from instinct—his opposing himself to instinct—that creates consciousness. Instinct is nature and seeks to perpetuate nature; while consciousness can only seek culture or its denial. Even when we turn back to nature, inspired by a Rousseauesque longing, we "cultivate" nature. As long as we are still submerged in nature we are unconscious, and we live in the security of instinct that knows no problems. Everything in us that still belongs to nature shrinks away from a problem; for its name is doubt, and wherever doubt holds sway, there is uncertainty and the possibility of divergent ways. And where several ways seem possible, there we have turned away from the certain guidance of instinct and are handed over to fear. For consciousness is now called upon to do that which nature has always done for her children—namely, to give a certain, unquestionable, and unequivocal decision. And here we are beset by an all-too-human fear that consciousness—our Promethean conquest—may in the end not be able to serve us in the place of nature. Problems thus draw us into an orphaned and isolated state where we are abandoned by nature and are driven to consciousness. [XIX, 249 f (J, 110)

When we must deal with problems, we instinctively refuse to try the way that leads through darkness and obscurity. We wish to hear only of unequivocal results, and completely forget that these results can only be brought about when we have ventured into and emerged again from the darkness. But to penetrate the darkness we must summon all the powers of enlightenment that consciousness can offer.　　[xix, 251 (j, 111)

In studying the history of the human mind one is impressed again and again by the fact that the growth of the mind is the widening of the range of consciousness, and that each step forward has been a most painful and laborious achievement. One could almost say that nothing is more hateful to man than to give up even a particle of his unconsciousness. Ask those who have tried to introduce a new idea!　　[xl, 25 f (g, 340)

Every forward step in culture is psychologically an extension of consciousness, a coming to consciousness that can take place only through discrimination. An advance, therefore, always begins with individuation, that is to say, through the fact that an individual, conscious of his uniqueness, cuts a new way through hitherto untrodden country. To do this he must first return to the fundamental facts of his own being, quite irrespective of all authority and tradition, and allow himself to become conscious of his distinctiveness. In so far as he succeeds in giving collective validity to his widened consciousness, he creates a tension of the opposites that provides the stimulation needed by culture for its further advance.　　[xiii, 100 f (g, 68)

If psychic life consisted only of overt happenings—which on a primitive level is still the case—we could content ourselves with a sturdy empiricism. The psychic life of civilized man, however, is full of problems; we cannot even think of it except in terms of problems. Our psychic processes are made up to a large extent of reflections, doubts, and experiments, all of which are almost completely foreign to the unconscious, instinctive mind of primitive man. It is the growth of consciousness which we must thank for the existence of problems; they are the dubious gift of civilization.　　[xix, 248 f (j, 109 f)

Reflection is a provision of human freedom over against the compulsion of natural laws. As the word *reflexio*, i.e., bending back, indicates, it is a mental act in opposition to the natural processes; it is a pausing, a thinking over, a forming of images, and an establishing of an inner connection with that which is seen while making an effort to come to terms with it. Reflection is thus to be understood as an act of becoming conscious.

[L, 46

There is no other way open to us; we are forced to resort to decisions and solutions where we formerly trusted ourselves to natural happenings. Every problem, therefore, brings the possibility of a widening of consciousness—but also the necessity of saying good-bye to childlike unconsciousness and trust in nature. This necessity is a psychic fact of such importance that it constitutes one of the essential symbolic teachings of the Christian religion. It is the sacrifice of the merely natural man— of the unconscious, ingenuous being whose tragic career began with the eating of the apple in Paradise. The biblical fall of man presents the dawn of consciousness as a curse. And as a matter of fact it is in this light that we first look upon every problem that forces us to greater consciousness and separates us even further from the paradise of unconscious childhood.

[XIX, 250 (J, 110 f)

Since we cannot imagine—unless we have lost our critical powers altogether—that mankind today has attained the highest possible degree of consciousness, there must be some potential unconscious psyche left over whose development would result in a further extension and a higher differentiation of consciousness. No one can say how great or small this "remnant" might be, for we have no means of measuring the possible extent of conscious development, let alone the extent of the unconscious.

[LX, 44 f (N, 362)

There are many people who are only partially conscious. Even among absolutely civilized Europeans there is a disproportionately high number of abnormally unconscious individuals who spend a great part of their lives in an unconscious state. They know what happens to them, but they do not know what they do or say. They cannot judge of the consequences of

31

their actions. These are people who are abnormally unconscious, that is, in a primitive state. What then finally makes
them conscious? If they get a slap in the face, then they become conscious; something really happens, and that makes
them conscious. They meet with something fatal and then they
suddenly realize what they are doing.   [xxxiv, 6

An inflated consciousness is always egocentric and conscious
of nothing but its own presence. It is incapable of learning
from the past, incapable of understanding contemporary events,
and incapable of drawing right conclusions about the future.
It is hypnotized by itself and therefore cannot be argued with.
It inevitably dooms itself to calamities that must strike it dead.
                                        [LVIII, 642 f (M, 563)
Everything that man should, and yet cannot, be or do—be it
in a positive or negative sense—lives on as a mythological figure
or an anticipation beside his consciousness, either as a religious
projection or—what is still more dangerous—as unconscious
contents which then project themselves spontaneously into in-
congruous objects, e.g., hygienic and other "salvationist" doc-
trines or practices. All these are so many rationalized substitutes
for mythology, and their unnaturalness does more harm than
good.   [xlix, 129 (o, 121 f)

The stirring up of conflict is a Luciferian quality in the true
sense of the word. Conflict creates the fire of affects and emotions, and like every fire it has two aspects: that of burning and
that of giving light. Emotion is on the one hand the alchemical
fire whose heat brings everything to light and whose intensity
omnes superfluitates comburit (burns up all superfluities), but
on the other hand emotion is the moment where steel meets
rock and a spark is thrown off. Emotion is the chief source of
all becoming-conscious. There can be no transforming of darkness into light and of apathy into movement without emotion.
                                                      [xliii, 431
Since the differentiated consciousness of civilized man has
been granted an effective instrument for the practical realization of its contents through the dynamics of his will, there is all
the more danger, the more he trains his will, of his getting lost

in one-sidedness and deviating further and further from the
laws and roots of his being.   [XLIX, 120 f (o, 113)

Instincts suffice only for a nature which, on the whole, remains on one level. An individual who is more guided by unconscious choice than by the conscious one tends therefore
toward outspoken psychic conservatism. This is the reason the
primitive does not change in the course of thousands of years,
and it is also the cause of his fearing everything strange and
unusual. Were he less conservative, it might lead to maladapta-
tion and thus to the greatest of psychic dangers, namely a kind
of neurosis. A higher and wider consciousness which only comes
by means of assimilating the unfamiliar tends toward autonomy,
toward revolution against the old gods, who are nothing other
than those powerful, unconscious, primordial images which, up
to this time, have held consciousness in thrall. The more powerful and independent consciousness becomes, and with it the
conscious will, the more is the unconscious forced into the background. When this happens, it becomes easily possible for the
conscious structures to be detached from the unconscious
images. Gaining thus in freedom, they break the chains of mere
instinctiveness, and finally arrive at a state that is deprived of
or contrary to instinct. Consciousness thus torn from its roots
and no longer able to appeal to the authority of the primordial
images possesses a Promethean freedom, it is true, but it also
partakes of the nature of a godless hubris. It soars above the
earth, even above mankind, but the danger of capsizing is
there, not for every individual, to be sure, but collectively for
the weak members of such a society who, again Prometheus-
like, are bound by the unconscious to the Caucasus.
                                           [xv, 535 f (H, 84 f)
When there is a marked change in the individual's state of
consciousness, the unconscious contents which are thereby constellated will also change. And the further the conscious situation moves away from a certain point of equilibrium, the more
forceful and accordingly the more dangerous become the
unconscious contents that are struggling to re-establish the
balance. This leads ultimately to a dissociation: on the one
hand, ego-consciousness makes convulsive efforts to shake off

33

an invisible opponent (if it does not suspect a neighbour of being the devil!) while on the other hand it increasingly falls a victim to the tyrannical will of an internal "Government opposition" which displays all the characteristics of a daemonic subman and superman combined. When a few million people get into this state, it gives rise to the sort of situation which has afforded us such an edifying object-lesson every day for the last ten years. These contemporary events betray their psychological background by their very singularity. The insensate destruction and devastation are a reaction against the deflection of consciousness from the point of equilibrium. For an equilibrium does in fact exist between the pyschic ego and non-ego, and that equilibrium is a *religio*, a "careful consideration" of ever-present unconscious forces which we neglect at our peril. The present crisis has been brewing for centuries because of this shift in the state of man's consciousness.

[LX, 52 f (N, 369 f)

Nothing is so apt to challenge consciousness and awareness as being at war with oneself. One can hardly think of any other or more effective means of waking humanity out of the irresponsible and innocent, semi-slumbering condition of the primordial state of mind and of bringing it to a state of conscious responsibility. [XXXV, 266

It is not without justification that the biblical story of creation put the undivided harmony of plant, animal, man, and God into the symbol of Paradise at the beginning of all psychic being, and described the first act of becoming conscious—"ye shall be as gods, knowing good and evil"—as the fatal sin. For it must appear as a sin to the naïve mind to break the law of the sacred primordial oneness of all-consciousness. It is a luciferian defiance of the individual against the oneness. It is a hostile act of disharmony against harmony, it is separation over against all-embracing unity. And yet the gaining of consciousness was the most precious fruit on the tree of life, and the magic weapon which gave man mastery over the earth, and which we hope will enable him to win the even greater victory of mastery over himself. [XXVII, 41

34

The hero's main feat is to overcome the monster of darkness: the long-hoped-for and expected triumph of consciousness over the unconscious. Day and light are synonyms for consciousness, night and dark for the unconscious. The coming of consciousness was probably the most tremendous experience of primeval times, for with it a world came into being whose existence no one had suspected before. "And God said, Let there be light" is the projection of that immemorial experience of the separation of consciousness from the unconscious.　　　[XLIX, 126 (o, 119)

"But why the deuce"—you will certainly ask—"*should* one at all costs reach a higher state of consciousness?" This question strikes at the core of the problem, and I cannot easily answer it. It is a confession of faith. I believe that finally someone had to know that this wonderful universe of mountains, seas, suns and moons, milky ways, and fixed stars exists. Standing on a little hill on the East African plains, I saw herds of thousands of wild beasts grazing in soundless peace, beneath the breath of the primeval world, as they had done for unimaginable ages of time, and I had the feeling of being the first man, the first being to know that all this *is*. The whole world around me was still in the primeval silence and knew not that it was. In this very moment in which I knew it the world came into existence, and without this moment it would never have been. All nature seeks this purpose and finds it fulfilled in man and only in the most differentiated, most conscious man.　　　[XLIII, 429 f

THE PRIMORDIAL IMAGES

It is a great mistake to believe that the psyche of a new-born child is a *tabula rasa* in the sense that there is absolutely nothing in it. Inasmuch as the child comes into the world with a differentiated brain, predetermined by heredity and therefore also individualized, its reactions to outside sense stimuli are not just any reactions but are specific, as a particular (individual) selection and form of apperception necessarily involves. These faculties can be proved to be inherited instincts and even pre-formations conditioned by the family. The latter are the *a priori*, formal conditions of apperception based on instincts. They set their anthropomorphic stamp upon the world of the child and of the dreamer. They are the archetypes, which blaze a definite trail for all imagination and produce astonishing mythological parallels in the images of a child's dreams and in the schizophrenic's delusions and even to a lesser degree in the dreams of both normal and neurotic persons. It is not a question of inherited ideas but of inherited possibilities for these.   [xxxix, 10

The original structural conditions of the psyche are of the same astonishing uniformity as those of the visible body. The archetypes are something like the organs of the pre-rational psyche. They are eternally inherited identical forms and ideas,* at first without specific content. The specific content appears during the individual life span when personal experience is absorbed in just these forms.   [xxxii, 26

Archetypes resemble the beds of rivers: dried up because the water has deserted them, though it may return at any time. An archetype is something like an old watercourse along which the water of life flowed for a time, digging a deep channel for itself. The longer it flowed the deeper the channel, and the more likely it is that sooner or later the water will return.
[xxxvi, 666 f (k, 12)

* [Here Platonic ideas are meant, which are patterns, not ideas in our sense of a specific thought-content.—Translator.]

It is always rather a doubtful business to draw conclusions from the modern civilized frame of mind regarding the totally different primitive state. Experience shows primitive consciousness to differ in very important ways from that of the modern white man. For instance, "to invent" is a very different thing in primitive society from what it is in ours, where one novelty succeeds another. In the primitive state nothing changes for long periods of time, except perhaps the language, which may change without the "invention" of a new one. The language of the primitive "lives" can therefore change of itself, a fact which has proved an unpleasant discovery for many a lexicographer of primitive language. The picturesque slang of America is also never "invented" but arises in inexhaustible richness out of the dark maternal womb of colloquial language. In the same sort of way, rites and their symbolic contents have also developed from indefinable beginnings, and not only in one place but in many places at once or at different times. They have developed spontaneously from those *a priori* facts which are never invented but are everywhere present, and which are peculiar to human nature.   [L, 94

In the psychological sense the soul brings to birth images which the general rational consciousness assumes to be worthless. Such images are certainly worthless in the sense that they cannot immediately be turned to account in the objective world. The artistic is the foremost possibility for their application, in so far as such a means of expression lies in one's power; a second possibility is philosophical speculation; a third is the quasi-religious, which leads to heresies and the founding of sects; there remains the fourth possibility of employing the forces contained in the images in every form of licentiousness.   [IX, 352

Archetypes were, and still are, psychic forces that demand to be taken seriously, and they have a strange way of making sure of their effect. Always they were the bringers of protection and salvation, and their violation has as its consequence the "perils of the soul" known to us from the psychology of primitives. Moreover, they are the infallible causes of neurotic and even psychotic disorders, behaving exactly like neglected or maltreated physical organs or organic functional systems.

[XLIX, 112 (O, 105)

I can only stand in deepest awe and admiration before the depths and heights of the soul whose world beyond space hides an immeasurable richness of images, which millions of years of living have stored up and condensed into organic material. My conscious mind is like an eye which perceives the furthermost spaces; but the psychic non-ego is that which fills this space in a sense beyond space. These images are not pale shadows, but powerful and effective conditions of the soul which we can only misunderstand but can never rob of their power by denying them. For comparison I can think only of the wonder of the starry night sky, for the equivalent of the inner world can only be in the outer world; and just as I experience this world through the medium of the body, so I experience that other world through the medium of the soul. [XVII, 15

The organism confronts light with a new formation, the eye, and the psyche meets the process of nature with a symbolical image, which apprehends the nature-process just as the eye catches the light. And in the same way as the eye bears witness to the peculiar and independent creative activity of living matter, the primordial image expresses the unique and unconditioned creative power of the mind. The primordial image, therefore, is a recapitulatory expression of the living process.

[IX, 600 (I, 557)

The great problems of life are always related to the primordial images of the collective unconscious. These images are really balancing or compensating factors which correspond with the problems life presents in actuality. This is not to be marvelled at, since these images are deposits representing the accumulated experience of thousands of years of struggle for adaptation and existence. Every great experience in life, every profound conflict, evokes the treasured wealth of these images and brings them to inner perception; as such, they become accessible to consciousness only in the presence of that degree of self-awareness and power of understanding which enables a man also to think what he experiences instead of just living it blindly. In the latter case he actually lives the myth and the symbol without knowing it.   [IX, 311 (I, 271 f)

The things of the soul are processes of experience, i.e., transformations, which can never be clearly defined without changing the living thing into something static. The indefinite yet definite mythological theme and the iridescent symbol express the processes of the soul more aptly, more completely, and therefore infinitely more clearly than the clearest definition: for the symbol gives not only a picture of the process but also—what is perhaps just as important—the possibility of simultaneously experiencing or re-experiencing the process, whose twilight character can only be understood through a sympathetic approach and never by the brutal attack of clear intellectual definition.   [XLVIII, 135

The symbol is thus a living body, *corpus et anima;* hence the "child" is such an admirable formula for the symbol. The uniqueness of the psyche is a magnitude that can never be made wholly real, it can only be realized approximately, though it still remains the absolute basis of all consciousness. The deeper "layers" of the psyche lose their individual uniqueness as they retreat farther and farther into darkness. "Lower down" —that is to say, as they approach the autonomous functional systems—they become increasingly collective until they are universalized and extinguished in the body's materiality, i.e., in the chemical bodies. The body's carbon is simply carbon. Hence "at bottom" the psyche is simply "world." In this sense I hold Kerényi to be absolutely right when he says that in the symbol the world itself is speaking. The more archaic and "deeper"—that is, the more physiological—the symbol is, the more collective and universal, the more "material," it is. The more abstract, differentiated, and specific it is, the more its nature approximates to conscious uniqueness and individuality, the more it sloughs off its universal character. Having finally attained full consciousness, it runs the risk of becoming a mere *allegory* which nowhere oversteps the bounds of conscious comprehension, and is then exposed to all sorts of attempts at rationalistic and therefore inadequate explanation.

[XLIX, 134 (o, 127 f)

Not for a moment dare we succumb to the illusion that an archetype can be finally explained and disposed of. Even the best attempts at explanation are only more or less successful translations into another metaphorical language. (Indeed, language itself is only a metaphor.) The most we can do is to dream the myth onwards and give it a modern dress. And whatever explanation or interpretation does to it, we do to our own soul as well, with corresponding results for our own well-being. The archetype—let us never forget this—is a psychic organ present in all of us. [XLIX, 117 (o, 109)

In reality we can never legitimately cut loose from our archetypal foundations unless we are prepared to pay the price of a neurosis, any more than we can rid ourselves of our body and its organs without committing suicide. If we cannot deny the archetypes or otherwise neutralize them, we are confronted, at every new stage in the differentiation of consciousness to which civilization attains, with the task of finding a new *interpretation* appropriate to this stage, in order to connect the life of the past that still exists in us with the life of the present, which threatens to slip away from it. If this link-up does not take place, a kind of rootless consciousness comes into being no longer oriented to the past, a consciousness which succumbs helplessly to all manner of suggestions and, practically speaking, is susceptible to psychic epidemics. With the loss of the past, now become "insignificant," devalued, and incapable of revaluation, the saviour is lost too, for the saviour either is the insignificant thing itself or else rises out of it. Over and over again in the *Gestaltwandel der Götter* (Ziegler), he rises up as the prophet or first-born of a new generation and appears unexpectedly in the most unlikely places (sprung from a stone, tree, furrow, water, etc.) and in ambiguous form (Tom Thumb, dwarf, child, animal, and so on). [XLIX, 113 (o, 105 f)

Mankind cannot stand a total loss of archetypes. Hence the

colossal "uneasiness of civilization," in which one no longer feels at home, is due to the lack of "father" and "mother." We all know how religion always supplied these needs. But there are unfortunately very many people of limited intelligence who always thoughtlessly pose the question of truth where it is really a matter of a psychological need. "Reasonable" explanations do not help at all in this case, and in the meanwhile the piling up of "uneasiness" has dangerous consequences.

[xxxix, 13

In reality all psychic events are to such an extent based on the archetypes and interwoven with them that in every case it requires a considerable critical effort to separate with certainty that which is individual from the type. In the final count, every individual life is at the same time also the life of the eons of the species. The individual is always "historical," because he is strictly bound to time; but the relation of the type to time is immaterial. In so far as the life of Christ is to a great extent archetypal, it represents to that degree the life of the archetype. But since the latter is the unconscious presupposition of every human life, through Christ's revealed life, the secret unconscious basic life of every individual is also revealed; i.e., that which happens in the life of Christ occurs always and everywhere. In other words, in the Christ-archetype all life of this nature is exemplified, and ever again or once for all time given expression.

[xlvi, 160 f

A symbol loses its magical or, if one prefers it, its redeeming power, as soon as its dissolubility is recognized. An effective symbol, therefore, must have a nature that is unimpeachable. It must be the best possible expression of the existing world philosophy, a container of meaning which cannot be surpassed; its form must also be sufficiently remote from comprehension as to frustrate every attempt of the critical intellect to give any satisfactory account of it; and, finally, its aesthetic appearance must have such a convincing appeal to feeling that no sort of argument can be raised against it on that score.

[ix, 331 f (i, 291)

Do we ever understand what we think? We only understand that thinking which is a mere equation, and from which noth-

41

ing comes out but what we have put in. That is the working of the intellect. But beyond that there is a thinking in primordial images—in symbols which are older than historical man, which have been ingrained in him from earliest times, and, eternally living, outlasting all generations, still make up the groundwork of the human psyche. It is only possible to live the fullest life when we are in harmony with these symbols; wisdom is a return to them. [xix, 273 (j, 129 f)

If such a super-individual soul should exist, then all that is translated into the imagery which is its language would be removed from the merely personal; and if this were to become conscious, it would then seem to us *sub specie aeternitatis;* no longer *my* sorrow but the sorrow of the world, no longer a personal isolated pain but a pain without bitterness, relating the individual to all mankind. That this would be salvation does not need to be proved to us. [xix, 161

The vision of the symbol is a significant indication as to the further course of life, an alluring of the libido towards a still distant aim, but which henceforth operates unquenchably within him, so that his life, kindled like a flame, moves steadily onward to the far goal. This is the specific life-promoting significance of the symbol. This is the value and meaning of the religious symbol. I am speaking, of course, not of symbols that are dead and stiffened by dogma, but of living symbols that rise from the creative unconscious of living man. The immense significance of such symbols can be denied only by the man whose history of the world begins at the present day. [ix, 175 (i, 158)

Why, indeed, is psychology the youngest of all the sciences of experience? Why have we not long ago discovered the unconscious and salvaged its treasures of eternal images? Simply because we had a Christian formula for all the things of the psyche—one that is far more beautiful and comprehensive than direct experience. Though for many persons the Christian view of the world has paled in its turn, the symbolic treasure-rooms of the East are still full of wonders that can nourish for a long time to come the passion for show and new clothes. And what is more, these images—be they Christian or Buddhist or anything else—are lovely, mysterious, and full of presentiment. To be sure, the more we are accustomed to them the more has constant usage polished them smooth, so that what remains of them is banal superficiality, clothed in almost senseless paradoxes. [xxxi, 184 (f, 56)

The Catholic way of life is completely unaware of psychological problems in this sense. The whole life of the collective unconscious has been absorbed without remainder, so to speak, in the dogmatic archetypes, and flows like a well-controlled stream in the symbolism of ritual and of the church calendar. This is not a manifestation of the individual psyche. It never was, because the Christian Church was preceded by the Greco-Roman mysteries, and these reach back into the grey mists of neolithic prehistory. Mankind has never lacked powerful images to lend magic aid against the uncanny, living depths of the world and of the psyche. The figures of the unconscious have always been expressed in protecting and healing images and thus expelled from the psyche into cosmic space.

[xxxi, 188 f (f, 60)

The gods of Hellas and Rome perished from the same disease as did our Christian symbols; men discovered then, as they do today, that they had no thoughts whatever on the subject. On the other hand, the gods of the strangers still had unexhausted mana. Their names were curious and unintelligible and their deeds portentously dark—a very different matter from the trite scandalmongery of Olympus. The Asiatic symbols were at least not understandable, and so they were not banal like the long-accustomed gods. That people accepted the new as unreflectively as they had rejected the old did not become a problem at that time. Is it becoming a problem today? Will we be able to clothe ourselves, as though in a new garment, with ready-made symbols grown on foreign soil, saturated with foreign blood, spoken in a foreign language, nourished by a foreign culture, interwoven in a foreign history, and so resemble a beggar who wraps himself in kingly raiment, a king who disguises himself as a beggar? No doubt this is possible. Or are we not commanded, somewhere, to hold no masquerade, but perhaps even to make our own garment ourselves? [xxxi, 191 (f, 62)

It would seem to me far better to confess strong-mindedly to the spiritual poverty of a want of symbols than to feign a possession of which we can in no case be the spiritual heirs. We are, indeed, the rightful heirs of Christian symbolism, but this inheritance we have somehow squandered. We have let the house that our fathers built fall to pieces, and now we try to break into Oriental palaces that our fathers never knew. Why do we not rather say "We are poor" and for once deal earnestly with our famous belief in God that people are always talking about? But whenever it comes to a pinch, we stop the dear Lord halfway and wish to do it ourselves, not only as though we were afraid, but because we actually have a terrible fear that things would then go wrong. [xxxi, 192 f (f, 63)

All ages before ours believed in gods in some form or other. Only an unparalleled impoverishment in symbolism could enable us to rediscover the gods as psychic factors, which is to say, as archetypes of the unconscious. No doubt this discovery is hardly credible as yet. [xxxi, 202 f (f, 72)

To *understand* religious things, we have nowadays only the psychological approach; and therefore I try to melt down the historically fixed forms of thinking and to remodel them in terms of direct experience. It is certainly a difficult task to find the bridge connecting the standpoint of dogma with the direct experience of psychological archetypes; but the investigation of the natural symbols of the unconscious gives us the necessary building stones. [xlvi, 161 f

Veneration for the great natural mysteries, which religious language endeavours to express in symbols consecrated by their antiquity, significance, and beauty, will suffer no injury from the extension of psychology upon this terrain, to which science has hitherto found no access. We only shift the symbols back a little, thus shedding light upon a portion of their realm, but without embracing the error that by so doing we have created anything more than a new symbol for that same enigma which confronted all the ages before us. Our science is also a language of metaphor, but from the practical standpoint it succeeds better than the old mythological hypothesis, which expresses itself by concrete presentations instead of, as we do, by conceptions. [IX, 355 (I, 314)

Eternal truth needs a human language that alters with the spirit of the times. The primordial images undergo ceaseless transformation and yet ever remain the same, but only in a new form can they be understood anew. Always they require a new interpretation if, as each formulation becomes obsolete, they are not to lose their spellbinding power over that *fugax Mercurius* and allow that useful though dangerous enemy to escape. Where is the new wine for the old bottles? Where are the answers to the spiritual needs and troubles of a new epoch? And where the knowledge to deal with the psychological problems raised by the development of modern consciousness? Never before has "eternal" truth been faced with such a hubris of will and power. [LX, 53 (N, 371)

DREAMS

The dream is the small hidden door in the deepest and most intimate sanctum of the soul, which opens into that primeval cosmic night that was soul long before there was a conscious ego and will be soul far beyond what a conscious ego could ever reach. For all ego-consciousness is individualized and recognizes the single unit in that it separates and distinguishes, and only that which can be related to the ego is seen. This ego-consciousness consists purely of restrictions, even when it stretches to the most distant stars. All consciousness divides; but in dreams we pass into that deeper and more universal, truer and more eternal man who still stands in the dusk of original night, in which he himself was still the whole and the whole was in him, in blind, undifferentiated, pure nature, free from the shackles of the ego. From these all-uniting depths rises the dream, however childish, grotesque, or immoral.   [xxvii, 49

No amount of scepticism and critical reserve has ever enabled me to regard dreams as negligible occurrences. Often enough they appear senseless, but it is obviously ourselves who lack the sense and the ingenuity to read the enigmatical message from the nocturnal realm of the psyche. When we see that at least a half of man's life is passed in this realm, that consciousness has its roots there, and that the unconscious operates in and out of waking existence, it would seem incumbent upon medical psychology to sharpen its perceptions by a systematic study of dreams. No one doubts the importance of conscious experience; why then should we doubt the importance of unconscious happenings? They also belong to human life, and they are sometimes more truly a part of it for weal or woe than any events of the day.   [xxvii, 87 f (j, 18)

The dream has for the primitive an incomparably higher value than it has for the civilized man. The primitive is usually a good deal taken up with his dreams; he talks much about them and attributes an extraordinary importance to them. When he talks of his dreams he is frequently unable to discriminate between them and actual facts. They are quite real to him. A competent explorer of primitive psychology says, "*Le rêve est le vrai dieu des primitifs.*" To the civilized man dreams as a rule appear valueless; yet there are some individuals who attribute a high importance to them, at least to particularly weird or impressive dreams. Such impressive dreams make one understand why the primitive should conceive them as inspirations.

[XIII, 204 (G, 253)

The psychology of dreams opens the way to a general comparative psychology, from which we expect to gain an understanding of the development and structure of the human psyche similar to what comparative anatomy has provided with regard to the human body. [XIII, 130

Dreams are products of the whole of the psyche, as is every piece of the psychic structure. Therefore we may expect to find in dreams all that has been of significance in the life of man since time immemorial. Just as human life as such is not limited to this or that basic instinct but is built up on a multiplicity of instincts, needs, necessities, and physical and psychic conditionalities, so dreams cannot be explained from this or that element, however attractively simple such an explanation may seem. We may be sure that it is wrong, for no simple theory of instincts will ever be capable of comprehending that powerful and mysterious thing, the human psyche, nor yet the dream which is its expression. To do any justice to dreams, we shall need to be armed with weapons painstakingly collected from every field of the philosophical sciences. The problem of dreams is not to be solved with a few cheap jokes or with evidence of certain repressions. [XIII, 179

The dream is apparently occupied with extremely silly details. The general impression it produces upon us is consequently absurd, or it is on the surface so unintelligible as to leave us thoroughly perplexed. Hence we have always to overcome a certain resistance before we can seriously set about disentangling the intricate web. But when at last we penetrate to

47

its real meaning, we find ourselves deep in the dreamer's secrets and discover with astonishment that an apparently quite senseless dream is in the highest degree significant, and that it speaks only of extraordinarily important and serious things. This discovery compels more respect for the so-called superstition of dream-interpretation, to which the rationalistic temper of our age has hitherto given short shrift.　　　　[LI, 44 f (D, 21 f)

Dreams are impartial, spontaneous products of the unconscious psyche, far removed from the arbitrariness of the conscious mind. They are pure nature, and therefore of an unspoilt, natural truth, and thus more apt than anything else to bring us back to the primary essence of humanity when our consciousness has moved on too far from its foundations and reached a deadlock in some impossible situation.　　　　[XXVII, 56

As in our waking state things and human beings enter our field of vision, so in the dream psychic contents, images of different kinds, enter the field of consciousness of the dream-ego. We do not feel as if we were producing the dreams, but rather as if they came to us. They do not submit to our direction but obey their own laws. Obviously they are autonomous complexes, which form themselves by their own methods. Their motivation is unconscious. We may therefore say that they come from the unconscious. Thus, we must admit the existence of independent psychic complexes, escaping the control of our consciousness and appearing and disappearing according to their own laws.　　　　[XIII, 208 (G, 255 f)

In sleep, phantasy shows itself in the form of dreams. And we continue to dream in waking life beneath the threshold of consciousness, especially when this activity is conditioned by a repressed or otherwise unconscious complex.　　　[XIX, 6 f (J, 36)

The dream is specifically the utterance of the unconscious. We may call consciousness the daylight realm of the human psyche, and contrast it with the nocturnal realm of unconscious psychic activity, which we apprehend as dreamlike phantasy.
　　　　[XXVII, 81 f (J, 13)

Dreams are psychic structures which seem, in contrast to the other contents of consciousness, not to lie within the continuity of development of conscious contents as regards form and significance. In any case, dreams appear as a rule not as an integral part of the conscious life of the psyche but rather as a more external and apparently accidental experience. The reason for this exceptional position of dreams lies in their peculiar mode of genesis; for unlike the other contents of consciousness, they do not originate in a clearly manifest, logical, and emotional continuity of experience but are a survival of a peculiar psychic activity which takes place during sleep. This mode of genesis in itself suffices to isolate dreams from the other contents of consciousness; but still more so does their peculiar contents, which is in marked contrast to conscious thought.   [xⅢ, 112

It is certain that consciousness consists not only of wishes and fears, but of vastly more than these, and it is highly probable that the unconscious psyche contains a wealth of contents and living forms equal to or even greater than does consciousness, which is characterized by concentration, limitation, and exclusion.   [xxvⅡ, 82 (J, 13)

Dreams contain images and thought-associations that we cannot create with conscious intention. They develop spontaneously without our assistance; hence they represent a mental activity that is withdrawn from voluntary direction. Essentially therefore the dream is a highly objective and, in a sense, natural product of the psyche. Accordingly we might with reason expect from it some indications, or suggestions at least, about the fundamental tendencies of the psychic process. Now, since the psyche is a vital process, hence not merely a final orientation, we might expect that the dream (which presents a kind of self-portrait of the total psychic process) would give us indications about objective causality as well as about objective tendencies.   [xI, 18 f (D, 130 f)

The dream rectifies the situation. It supplies that which is lacking and thereby improves the attitude. This is the reason why we need dream analysis for our therapy.   [xiii, 133

The dream gives a true picture of the subjective state, while the conscious mind denies that this state exists or recognizes it only grudgingly.   [xxvii, 73 (j, 5)

The unconscious is the unknown of a given moment, therefore it is not surprising that all those aspects that are essential for a totally different point of view should be added by dreams to the conscious psychological factors of a given moment. It is evident that this function of dreams signifies a psychological adjustment, a compensation essential for properly balanced action. In the conscious process of reflection it is indispensable that, so far as possible, we should realize all the aspects and consequences of a problem in order to find the right solution. This process is continued automatically in the more or less unconscious state of sleep, where—as our previous experience seems to show—all those other points of view occur to the dreamer (at least by way of allusion) that during the day were underestimated or even totally ignored—in other words, were comparatively unconscious.   [xiii, 125 (c, 307 f)

The dream, as the expression of an involuntary psychic process not controlled by the conscious outlook, presents the subjective state as it really is. It has no respect for my conjectures or for the patient's views as to how things should be, but simply tells *how the matter stands.*   [xxvii, 74 (j, 6)

The more one-sided the conscious attitude is and the more it deviates from the optimum possibilities of life, the more probable is the occurrence of lively dreams, with strongly contrasting but purposefully compensating contents, as the expression of the individual's psychological self-guidance.

[xiii, 138

The primitive peoples of East Africa whom I have studied believed that "great" dreams were only dreamed by "great" persons—that is, by witch-doctors and chieftains. This may be true at the primitive stage. With us such dreams occur to simple

people also, namely, when they are suffering from too narrow a
spiritual outlook. [xxvii, 61 f

Dreams, as children of nature, have certainly no moralizing
intention; they merely demonstrate the universal law according to which no tree grows up to reach the heavens. [xxvii, 60

The psyche is a self-regulating system that maintains itself in
equilibrium as the body does. Every process that goes too far
immediately and inevitably calls forth a compensatory activity.
Without such adjustments a normal metabolism would not
exist, nor would the normal psyche. We can take the idea of
compensation, so understood, as a law of psychic happening.
Too little on one side results in too much on the other.
[xxvii, 90 (j, 20)
It is not easy to make special rules for the different kinds of
dream compensation. The nature of the compensation is always
intimately bound up with the entire being of the individual.
The possibilities of compensation are innumerable and inexhaustible. [xiii, 140

Although dreams contribute to psychological self-guidance
by supplying automatically all that is repressed and ignored or
unknown, their compensatory significance is often by no means
clear at first sight, because we still have a very imperfect understanding of the nature and the needs of the human soul.
There are psychological compensations which seem to be very
remote. In these cases, it must always be remembered that
every human being is in a certain sense representative of the
whole of humanity and its history. What was possible on a big
scale in human history is possible on a small scale in every individual human being. What humanity needed in the past the
single human being may need under certain circumstances.
Therefore it is not surprising that religious compensations play
a big part in dreams; and that this is perhaps especially so in
our present age is a natural consequence of the immanent realism of our present attitude to life. [xiii, 134

I would not deny the possibility of "parallel" dreams, i.e.,

51

dreams whose meaning coincides with or supports the conscious attitude, but in my experience, at least, these are rather
rare.   [LVIII, 74 (M, 48)

Just as the body reacts in a purposeful way to wounds or
infections or an abnormal way of living, so the psychic functions react to unnatural or injurious disturbances with appropriate means of defence. One of these purposeful reactions is
the dream, in which the unconscious material constellated
round a given conscious position is presented to the conscious
mind in symbolic form. In this unconscious material are all
those associations which have remained in the unconscious because they were only weakly emphasized but which nevertheless have sufficient energy to make themselves felt during sleep.
Naturally the purposeful character of the dream-content cannot be directly seen from the manifest dream-content; it requires an analysis of this manifest content to reach the actual
compensatory factors of the latent dream-content. But most
physical defensive reactions are of the same scarcely recognizable and, so to speak, indirect nature, and their purposeful
character also has only been recognized through deep investigation and exact observation. I might recall, for instance, the
meaning of fever and of the processes of suppuration in an infected wound.   [XIII, 138 f

---

Much may be said for Freud's view as a scientific explanation
of dream psychology. But I must dispute its completeness, for
the psyche cannot be conceived merely from the causal aspect
but necessitates also a final viewpoint. Only a combination of
both points of view—which has not yet been attained to the
satisfaction of the scientific mind, owing to great difficulties
both of a practical and theoretical nature—can give us a more
complete conception of the essence of dreams.
                                              [XIII, 128 (C, 309 f)
A purely causalistic approach is too narrow to do justice to
the true significance either of the dream or of the neurosis. A
person is biased who turns to dreams for the sole purpose of
discovering the hidden cause of the neurosis, for he leaves aside

the larger part of the dream's actual contribution.

[xxvii, 75 f (j, 7)

Dreams can be anticipatory and, in that case, must lose their particular meaning if they are treated in a purely causalistic way. Such dreams give clear information about the analytical situation, and for the purposes of therapy it is extremely important that this be rightly understood.   [xxvii, 77 (j, 9)

The view that dreams are merely imaginary fulfilments of suppressed wishes has long ago been superseded. It is certainly true that there are dreams which embody suppressed wishes and fears, but what is there which the dream cannot on occasion embody? Dreams may give expression to ineluctable truths, to philosophical pronouncements, illusions, wild fantasies, memories, plans, anticipations, irrational experiences, even telepathic visions, and heaven knows what besides.   [xxvii, 81 (j, 12 f)

The causal point of view tends by its very nature towards uniformity of meaning, that is, towards a fixed significance of symbols. On the other hand, the final viewpoint perceives in an altered dream picture the expression of an altered psychological situation. It recognizes no fixed meaning of symbols. From this standpoint all the dream pictures are important in themselves, each one having a special significance of its own, to which it owes its inclusion in the dream. From the standpoint of finality the symbol in the dream is approximately equivalent to a parable; it does not conceal, but it teaches.

[xiii, 126 f (c, 308 f)

In my opinion, the somatic stimuli have a determinative significance only in exceptional cases. Generally they become totally submerged in the symbolic expression of the unconscious dream content; that is, they are used with it as means of expression. Not infrequently dreams show a remarkable inner symbolic connection between an undoubtedly physical illness and a certain psychic problem, whereby the physical disorder seems a mimicking of the psychical situation.   [xiii, 153

Reviewing the dream from the standpoint of finality, which

I contrast with that of Freud, does not—as I wish to establish explicitly—involve a denial of the dream's *causae*, but rather a different interpretation of the associative material collected around the dream. The material facts remain the same, but the standard by which they are measured is altered. The question may be formulated simply as: What is this dream's purpose? What should it effect? These questions are not arbitrary, inasmuch as they may be applied to every psychic activity. Everywhere the question of the "why" and "wherefore" may be raised; for every organic structure consists of a complicated synthesis of purposeful functions and every function can be resolved into a series of purposefully orientated single facts.

[xiii, 121 f (c, 305 f)]

I wish to make a distinction between the prospective function of the dream and its compensatory function. The latter means in the first place that the unconscious, considered in relation to consciousness, adds to the conscious situation all those elements which had remained below the threshold of consciousness on the previous day, by reason of repression and also by reason of the fact that they were too weak to penetrate through to consciousness. This compensation, in the sense of the self-guidance of the psychic organism, must be regarded as purposeful. The prospective function, on the other hand, is an anticipation of future conscious achievements arising in the unconscious, somewhat like a preparatory exercise or the sketching of a plan thought out in advance. [xiii, 142

The fact that the prospective function of the dream is sometimes considerably superior to the conscious plan designed in advance is not surprising when one considers that the dream arises from a mingling of elements below the threshold of consciousness and is therefore a combination of all those perceptions, thoughts, and feelings which have escaped consciousness because of their weaker emphasis. Furthermore the dream has also the help of those traces of remembrances which lie below the conscious threshold and which are no longer capable of influencing consciousness effectively. Therefore, where the prognosis is concerned, the dream is sometimes in a much more favourable position than consciousness. [xiii, 143

As a further determinant of the dream, I must recognize the telepathic phenomenon. The general fact of this phenomenon can no longer be doubted nowadays. Of course it is very simple to deny the existence of this phenomenon without examining the existing evidence, but this is unscientific behaviour unworthy of consideration. I have experienced the fact that the telepathic phenomenon also influences dreams, as has been believed since earliest times. Certain people are especially sensitive in this respect and very often have dreams which are telepathically influenced. By this recognition of the telepathic phenomenon I do not mean an unconditional acceptance of the common theory of the nature of *actio in distans*. The phenomenon undoubtedly exists, but the theory seems to me to be extremely complicated.   [xiii, 154

Dream-analysis stands or falls with the hypothesis of the unconscious. Without it the dream appears to be merely a freak of nature, a meaningless conglomerate of memory-fragments left over from the happenings of the day.   [xxvii, 69

He who would interpret a dream must himself be, so to speak, on a level with the dream, for in no single thing can one ever hope to see beyond what one is oneself.   [xxvii, 62

On paper a dream interpretation may perhaps look arbitrary, unclear, and artificial; but it can in reality be a little drama of incomparable realism. To experience a dream and its interpretation is quite different from being shown a lukewarm exposition on paper. Everything in this psychology is fundamentally a living experience; even the theory itself, at its most abstract, arises directly out of the living experience.   [li, 209

The art of interpreting dreams cannot be learned from books. Methods and rules are only good if one can get on without them. Only he who can do the thing can be said to have true ability; and only he who really understands is the expert.

[xxvii, 62

It is at once clear that mere intuitive guesswork will not be successful when interpreting the so-called "great" dreams. This requires extensive knowledge, such as the specialist should possess. But with knowledge alone one cannot interpret dreams. Such knowledge must not be dry memorized material; it must have the quality of a living experience in him who uses it. What use, for instance, is philosophical knowledge in the head of one who is not at heart a philosopher? [xxvii, 62

It is best to treat a dream as one would treat a totally unknown object: one looks at it from all sides, one takes it in one's hand, carries it about, has all sorts of ideas and fantasies about it, and talks of it to other people. Primitives always relate their impressive dreams if possible in a public gathering, a custom which was still used in late antiquity, for all the ancient peoples believed dreams to have great significance. During this process, all sorts of things occur to one as regards the dream and bring one near to its meaning. The question of its meaning is, of course, if one may say so, a thoroughly arbitrary thing, for here in the interpretation begins the risk. According to experience, temperament, and personal taste, one sets the limits of its meaning either nearer or further. Some are content with little, others cannot have enough. Furthermore, the meaning, i.e., the interpretation of the dream, is to a great extent dependent on the purpose of the interpreter or his expectations, or his demands upon the meaning. The significance such as it has emerged will necessarily be shaped by certain presuppositions, and it will depend largely on the conscientiousness and honesty of the investigator whether he can gain anything from the explanation of the dream or whether he becomes still more deeply entangled in his own mistaken notions. [xxvii, 58 f

The psychological context of dream-contents consists in the web of associations in which the dream is naturally embedded. Theoretically we can never know anything in advance about this web, but in practice it is sometimes possible, granted long enough experience. Even so, careful analysis will never rely too much on technical rules; the danger of deception and suggestion is too great. In the analysis of isolated dreams above all, this kind of knowing in advance and making assumptions on the grounds of practical expectation or general probability is positively wrong. It should therefore be an absolute rule to assume that every dream and every part of a dream is unknown at the outset, and to attempt an interpretation only after carefully taking up the context. We can then apply the meaning we have thus discovered to the text of the dream itself and see whether this yields a working solution, or rather whether a satisfying meaning emerges. [LVIII, 73 (M, 48)

Anyone who analyses the dreams of others should always be conscious that there is no simple and generally known theory of psychic phenomena, either as regards their nature, their cause, or their purpose. We have therefore no general standard of judgment. We know that there are conscious and unconscious, sexual and intuitive, intellectual, moral, aesthetic, and religious phenomena, phenomena associated with the will, etc. But of their nature we know nothing definite. We only know that a careful consideration of the psyche from any one separate standpoint may indeed give us quite valuable details, but never a complete theory from which we could make deductions. Neither have we any theory of the unconscious which determines the contents of the unconscious qualitatively and which would thereby enable us to interpret dream-images corresponding to the actual facts. Both the sexual theory and that of desire as well as the will-to-power theory are valuable points of view, but they cannot in any way do justice to the depth and richness of the human soul. If we had such a theory, then it would be enough to learn the method mechanically, for then it would be necessary only to read certain signs which would represent the well-established contents, for which purpose the mere memorizing of certain semiotic rules would suffice. A deeper knowledge and true judgment of the conscious situation would then be as superfluous as it is for a lumbar puncture. [XIII, 150 f

One must never forget that one dreams primarily, and, so to speak, exclusively, about oneself and out of oneself. [XXVII, 59 f

I call every interpretation in which the dream-symbols are

treated as representations of real objects an interpretation on the objective plane. In contrast to this is the interpretation which refers back to the dreamer himself every part of the dream, as, for instance, all the personalities who take part in it. This is interpretation on the subjective plane. Objective interpretation is analytic, because it dissects the dream contents into complexes of reminiscence which refer to actual conditions. Subjective interpretation is synthetic in that it detaches the underlying complexes of reminiscence from their actual causes, and presents them as tendencies or parts of the subject, reintegrating them with the subject. In this case, therefore, all the dream-contents are considered as symbols for subjective contents.   [LI, 152 f (D, 87 f)

When our dreams produce certain conceptions, these are primarily our own conceptions, and in the forming of these the whole of our being is interwoven. They are subjective factors which are grouped in such or such a way in the dream, to express such or such a meaning, not for external reasons, but due to the most intimate impulses of our soul. This whole creation is essentially subjective, and the dream is the theatre where the dreamer is at once scene, actor, prompter, stage manager, author, audience, and critic.   [XIII, 162

It is impossible to interpret a dream with any degree of certainty unless we know what the conscious situation is. For it is only in the light of this knowledge that we can make out whether the unconscious content carries a plus or minus sign. The dream is not an isolated psychic event completely cut off from daily life. If it seems so to us, that is only an illusion that arises from our lack of understanding. In reality, the relation between consciousness and the dream is strictly causal, and they interact in the subtlest of ways.   [XXVII, 92 (J, 21 f)

The relation between conscious and unconscious is compensatory. This fact, which is easily verifiable, affords a rule for dream interpretation. It is always helpful, when we set out to interpret a dream, to ask: What conscious attitude does it compensate?   [XXVII, 90 f (J, 20)

If we wish to interpret a dream correctly, we need a thorough knowledge of the conscious situation at that moment, for the dream contains its unconscious completion, that is, the material which is constellated in the unconscious owing to the conscious situation at that moment. Without such knowledge, it is impossible to interpret a dream sufficiently correctly, apart, of course, from lucky guesses. [XIII, 131

But in no circumstances may we anticipate that this meaning will fit in with any of our subjective expectations; for quite possibly, indeed, very frequently, the dream is saying something surprisingly different from what we would expect. As a matter of fact, if the meaning we find in the dream happens to coincide with our expectations, that is a reason for suspicion; for as a rule the standpoint of the unconscious is complementary or compensatory to consciousness and thus unexpectedly "different." [LVIII, 73 f (M, 48)

If anyone should set out to replace his conscious outlook by the dictates of the unconscious—and this is the prospect which my critics find so alarming—he would only succeed in repressing the former, and it would reappear as an unconscious compensation. The unconscious would thus have changed its face and completely reversed its position. It would have become timidly reasonable, in striking contrast to its former tone. It is not generally believed that the unconscious operates in this way, yet such reversals constantly take place and constitute its essential function. This is why every dream is a source of information and a means of self-regulation, and why dreams are our most effective aids in the task of building up the personality. [XXVII, 91 (J, 21)

The real difficulty begins when dreams, as is often the case, do not point to anything tangible—especially when they show a kind of foreknowledge of the future. I do not mean that such dreams are necessarily prophetic, but that they anticipate or "reconnoitre." Such dreams contain inklings of possibilities, and so can never be made plausible to an outsider. [XIX, 99 (J, 73)

But any one keenly interested in the dream problem cannot

have failed to observe that a dream has also a *progressive* continuity—if such an expression be permitted—since dreams occasionally exert a remarkable influence upon the conscious mental life, even of persons who cannot be considered superstitious or particularly abnormal. [XIII, 113 (C, 299)

It is not denied in medieval ecclesiastical writings, for instance, that a divine influx could take place in dreams, but this view is not exactly encouraged, and the Church reserves the right to decide whether a revelation is to be considered authentic or not. In spite of the fact that the Church recognizes the undeniable emanation of certain dreams from God, it is disinclined, even positively averse, to any serious concern with dreams, while admitting that some might contain an immediate revelation. Thus the change in mental attitudes which has taken place in recent centuries is, from this point of view at least, not wholly unwelcome to the Church, because it has effectively discouraged the former introspective attitude which was favourable to a serious consideration of dreams and inner experiences. [XLVI, 34 f (B, 22)

Being both subject and individual, we are also not entirely unique, but like all other human beings. Therefore a dream with a collective meaning applies primarily to the dreamer, but at the same time it expresses the fact that his momentary problem is also that of other human beings. Such conclusions are often of great practical significance, for there are many people who are inwardly isolated from humanity as a whole and who labour under the impression that other people do not have such problems as they have. Or sometimes it is a case of overmodest persons who, on account of their exaggerated modesty, have kept their claim on the collective effort too low. Furthermore, every individual problem is somehow connected with the problems of the age, so that every subjective difficulty can also be seen from the angle of the entire human situation. This is in practice only admissible when the dream actually uses a mythological, i.e., a collective, symbolism. [XXVII, 61

Immediate life is always individual, since the carrier of life is the individual, and whatever emanates from the individual is in a way unique, transitory, and imperfect, particularly so when it is a matter of involuntary mental products such as dreams and the like. No one else will have the same dreams, although many have the same problem. But just as there is no individual differentiated to a condition of absolute uniqueness, so also are there no individual products of an absolutely unique quality.   [XLVI, 92 f (B, 63)

If we realize that everything which is lacking in the conscious mind is present to excess in the unconscious, and that the unconscious has therefore a compensatory tendency, then we can draw some conclusions from the dream, provided that it does not arise from very great depths of the psyche. Such a dream usually contains what one calls mythological motifs, that is, conceptions or images such as one finds in the mythology of one's own race or of foreign nations. In this case the dream contains a so-called collective meaning which applies to all humanity.   [XXVII, 60 f

---

Just as the interpretation of dreams requires exact knowledge of the conscious status quo, so the treatment of dream symbolism demands that we take into account the dreamer's philosophical, religious, and moral convictions. It is far wiser in practice not to regard the dream-symbols as signs or symptoms of a fixed character. We should rather take them as true symbols—that is to say, as expressions of something not yet consciously recognized or conceptually formulated. In addition to this, they must be considered in relation to the dreamer's immediate state of consciousness.   [XXVII, 95 (J, 24 f)

But it is characteristic that a dream never expresses itself in a logically abstract way, but always in the language of parable or simile. This peculiarity is also a characteristic feature of primitive languages, whose flowery idioms always strike us. If you call to mind the writings of ancient literature—e.g., the language of simile in the Bible—you will find that what nowadays is expressed by means of abstract expression could then be expressed only by means of simile. Even such a philosopher as Plato did not disdain to express certain fundamental ideas by means of concrete simile.   [xiii, 129 f (c, 310 f)]

The comparison of the typical themes of dreams with those of mythology obviously suggests the idea (already put forward by Nietzsche) that from a phylogenetic point of view dream-thought should be conceived as an older form of thought.
[xiii, 129 (c, 310)]
Just as the body bears traces of its phylogenetic development, so also does the human mind. There is therefore nothing surprising in the possibility that the allegories of our dreams might be a survival of archaic modes of thought.   [xiii, 130 (c, 311)]

My researches have clearly shown that the sexual language of dreams is by no means always to be misunderstood in a concrete way—that is to say, that it is an archaic language which is naturally full of all the nearest analogies without necessarily referring to any recent sexual incident. It is therefore not justifiable to take the sexual language of dreams absolutely concretely, while other dream-contents are explained symbolically. As soon as one conceives the sexual forms of dream language as symbols for more complicated things, the whole attitude towards the nature of dreams becomes at once more profound.
[xiii, 157 f]
I take the dream for granted. The dream is such a difficult and intricate subject that I do not dare to make any assumptions about its possible cunning. The dream is a natural event and there is no reason under the sun why we should assume that it is a crafty device to lead us astray. The dream occurs when consciousness and will are to a great extent extinguished. It seems to be a natural product which is also to be found in people who are not neurotic. Moreover, we know so little about the psychology of the dream process that we must be more than careful when we introduce elements foreign to the dream itself into its explanation.   [xlvi, 48 f (b, 31)]

There is no justification for suspecting the dream of being a sort of intentional deceptive manoeuvre. Nature is often dark

and impenetrable, but not crafty like a human being. Therefore one must assume that the dream is just what it should be,
no more and no less. If it presents something in a negative aspect, there is no reason to suppose that a positive aspect is intended, and so on.   [LI, 180

We cannot, of course, dispense with theory entirely, for it is
needed to make things intelligible. It is on the basis of theory,
for instance, that I expect dreams to have a meaning. I cannot
prove in every case that dreams are meaningful, for there are
dreams that neither doctor nor patient understands. But I must
regard them as hypothetically meaningful in order to find
courage to deal with them at all.   [xxvii, 82 f (j, 13 f)

I never, if I can help it, interpret one dream by itself. As a rule
a dream belongs in a series. As there is a continuity in consciousness, despite the fact that it is regularly interrupted by sleep,
there is probably also a continuity of unconscious processes
and perhaps even more so than with the events of consciousness. In any case my experience is in favour of the probability
that dreams are the visible links in a chain of unconscious
events.   [xlvi, 60 (b, 38)

Every interpretation is hypothetical, for it is a mere attempt
to read an unfamiliar text. An obscure dream, taken by itself,
can rarely be interpreted with any certainty, so that I attach
little importance to the interpretation of single dreams. With
a series of dreams we can have more confidence in our inter-
pretations, for the later dreams correct the mistakes we have
made in handling those that went before. We are also better
able, in a dream-series, to recognize the important contents and
basic themes.   [xxvii, 85 f (j, 16)

Looked at from the side of theory, this dream-image can
mean anything or nothing. For that matter, does a thing or a
fact ever mean anything in and of itself? We can only be sure
that it is always the human being who interprets—that is, gives
meaning to—a fact. And that is the gist of the matter for psychology.   [xix, 101 (j, 74)

The analyst who wishes to rule out conscious suggestion must consider any dream interpretation invalid that does not win the assent of the patient, and he must search until he finds a formulation that does. [xxvii, 81 (j, 12)

It is relatively unimportant whether the doctor understands or not, but everything hangs on the patient's doing so. What is really needed is a mutual agreement which is the fruit of joint reflection. It is one-sided and therefore dangerous understanding for the doctor to prejudge the dream from the standpoint of a certain doctrine and to make a pronouncement which may be theoretically sound, but does not win the patient's assent. In so far as the pronouncement fails in this respect, it is incorrect in the practical sense; and it may also be incorrect in the sense that it anticipates and thereby cripples the actual development of the patient. We appeal only to the patient's brain if we try to inculcate a truth; but if we help him to grow up to this truth in the course of his own development, we have reached his heart, and this appeal goes deeper and acts with greater force. [xxvii, 79 (j, 10 f)

But when, one might reasonably ask, can one be certain that the interpretation is right? Is there any criterion even approaching reliability for the correctness of an interpretation? Happily this question can be answered in the affirmative, for if we have missed the meaning or found it only incompletely, this will become evident, possibly in the very next dream. For instance, the earlier motif may be repeated in still more definite form, or our interpretation may be undermined by an ironical paraphrase or a direct and vigorous opposition may arise. Let us suppose that this second interpretation also misses the mark, then the general lack of results, the futility of our whole investigation, makes itself felt soon enough in the desolation, fruitlessness, and senselessness of the undertaking, so that both patient and doctor are stifled in boredom or in doubt. Just as the right interpretation is rewarded by its animating effect, so the wrong one condemns itself by stagnation, opposition, and doubt and above all by a silting up on both sides. [li, 199 f

As long as I help the patient to discover the effective elements in his dream, and as long as I try to show him the general meaning of his symbols, he is still, psychologically speaking, in a state of childhood. For the time being he depends on his dreams and is always asking himself whether the subsequent dream will give him new light or not. Moreover, he is dependent on my having ideas about his dreams and on my ability to increase his insight through my knowledge. Thus he is still in an undesirably passive condition in which everything is uncertain and questionable; neither he nor I know the journey's end. Often it is not much more than a groping about in Egyptian darkness. In this condition we must not expect any very marked effects, for the uncertainty is too great. Moreover we constantly run the risk that what we have woven by day the night will unravel. The danger is that nothing comes to pass; that nothing keeps its shape. [xix, 105 (j, 77 f)

I need not try to prove that my dream interpretation is correct—that would be a somewhat hopeless undertaking—but must simply help the patient to find what it is that activates him (I was almost betrayed into saying what is actual).
[xix, 102 (j, 75)

I have no theory about dreams; I do not know how dreams arise. I am altogether in doubt as to whether my way of handling dreams even deserves the name of "method." I share all my readers' prejudices against dream-interpretation as being the quintessence of uncertainty and arbitrariness. But, on the other hand, I know that if we meditate on a dream sufficiently long and thoroughly—if we take it about with us and turn it over and over—something almost always comes of it. This something is of course not of such a kind that we can boast of its scientific nature or rationalize it, but it is a practical and important hint which shows the patient in what direction the unconscious is leading him. I even *may* not give first importance to the question whether our study of the dream gives a scientifically verifiable result; if I do this, I am following an exclusively personal aim, and one which is therefore autoerotic. I must content myself with the fact that the result means something to the patient and sets his life into motion again. I may allow myself only *one* criterion for the validity of my interpretation of the dream: Does it work? As for my scientific hobby—my desire to know why it is that the dream works—this I must reserve for my spare time.   [XIX, 98 (J, 71 f)

It is difficult to imagine how there could ever be a method, i.e., a technically controlled way, of obtaining absolutely reliable results, if one tries to realize the endless variability of dreams. Indeed, it is a good thing that there is no definitely valid method, otherwise the meaning of the dream would be limited in advance and would forfeit that very virtue which makes it so especially valuable for psychological purposes, namely its capacity for presenting a new point of view.
[XXVII, 58

Even though in the twentieth century we are somewhat more free-thinking in this respect, the idea of dream-interpretation is nevertheless burdened by too much historical prejudice for us to accept it readily. But—one will ask—does such a thing as a reliable method of dream-interpretation really exist? One cannot trust mere speculation. I share these doubts to the fullest extent, and I am even convinced that there is no absolutely reliable method of interpretation. Absolute reliability of interpretation of any given facts of nature can only exist within the narrowest limits, where nothing more ever comes out than is put in. Our whole explanation of nature is a presumption.
[XXVII, 57

The use of dream-analysis in psychotherapy is still a much-debated question. Many practitioners find it indispensable in the treatment of neuroses, and ascribe as much importance to the psychic activity manifested in dreams as to consciousness itself. Others, on the contrary, dispute the value of dream-analysis, and regard dreams as a negligible by-product of the psyche. Obviously, if a person holds the view that the unconscious plays a leading role in the formation of neuroses, he will attribute practical significance to dreams as direct expressions of the unconscious. If, on the other hand, he denies the unconscious or thinks that it has no part in the development of neuroses, he will minimize the importance of dream-analysis.

[xxvII, 68 (J, 1)

The evolutionary stages through which the human psyche has passed are more clearly discernible in the dream than in consciousness. The dream speaks in images, and gives expression to instincts, that are derived from the most primitive levels of nature. Consciousness all too easily departs from the law of nature, but it can be brought again into harmony with it by the assimilation of unconscious contents. By fostering this process we lead the patient to the rediscovery of the law of his own being. [xxvII, 102 (J, 30)

In many cases dreams point directly to the past and bring to mind what is forgotten and lost to the personality. It is from these very losses that one-sidedness results, and this causes the standstill and consequent disorientation. In psychological terms, one-sidedness may lead to a sudden loss of libido. All our previous activities become uninteresting, even senseless, and the goals towards which we strove lose their value. What in one person is merely a passing mood may in another become a chronic condition. In these cases it often happens that other possibilities of development of the personality lie somewhere or other in the past, and no one, not even the patient, knows about them. But the dream may reveal the clue.

[xIx, 98 f (J, 72)

Within each one of us there is another whom we do not know. He speaks to us in dreams and tells us how differently *he* sees us from how *we* see ourselves. When we find ourselves in an insolubly difficult situation, this stranger in us can sometimes show us a light which is more suited than anything else to change our attitude fundamentally, namely just that attitude which had led us into the difficult situation. [xxvII, 62 f

Where must we lead our patient to give him at least the glimmer of a notion of something other than his everyday world, which he knows only too well? We must lead him, by long detours, to a dark and absurdly unimpressive, totally unimportant, and worthless place in his soul, by a long-disused path to an illusion which has long been recognized as such, of which the whole world knows that it is nothing. . . . That place is the dream, that fleeting, grotesque thing of the night, and the path is the understanding of dreams. [xxvii, 48

To be concerned with dreams is a form of self-realization. This, however, does not mean that the ego-consciousness is concerned with itself. It considers the objective data of the dream as a report or message from the unconscious "all-one" soul of humanity. True, one meditates on the Self but not on the ego; that is, one meditates on that strange Self which is our primary Self and origin from which the ego has grown, and which is foreign to us because we have become estranged from it through the illusions of the conscious mind. [xxvii, 56 f

A dream is nothing else than a message from the all-uniting dark soul. What then could be more natural, when we have lost ourselves in the endless details and separate units of the surface of the earth, than that we should look to the dream to find a point of view which would bring us nearer again to the basic facts of human existence? But we are met with the obstinate prejudice—"dreams are shadows" not reality, they lie, they are mere wish-fulfilments. These are mere excuses not to have to take dreams seriously, for that would be troublesome. This isolating individualization is dear to the intellectual pride of consciousness in spite of all its disadvantages, and therefore one is not ready to accept as reality the truth of dreams. There are saints who have very ugly dreams, and what would happen to their saintliness, which raises them so high above the common mass, if the obscenities of dreams had true reality? But just the most unpleasant dreams can best bring us near to the blood-relationship of humanity and can most effectively reduce the arrogance which goes with lack of instinct. Even if a whole world is out of joint, the all-embracingness of the dark soul can never break to pieces; and the wider and the more numerous become the cracks in the surface, the greater grows the strength of the one in the depths. [xxvii, 50 f

MAN IN HIS RELATION TO OTHERS

How many a heart floats lost in generalness;
The noblest is devoted to the One.
         —GOETHE, "Urworte. Orphisch"

DOCTOR AND PATIENT

The man who would learn the human mind will gain almost nothing from experimental psychology. Far better for him to put away his academic gown, to say good-bye to the study, and to wander with human heart through the world. There, in the horrors of the prison, the asylum, and the hospital, in the drinking-shops, brothels, and gambling hells, in the salons of the elegant, in the exchanges, socialist meetings, churches, religious revivals, and sectarian ecstasies, through love and hate, through the experience of passion in every form in his own body, he would reap richer store of knowledge than text-books a foot thick could give him. Then would he know to doctor the sick with real knowledge of the human soul.   [v, 238 (D, 2 f)

The research worker has a scientific need to find rules and regulations with which to catch the most vitally alive of all living things. But the doctor and observer must be free from every formula to allow the living reality to work upon him in its entire lawless richness.   [vi, 113

It is a terrible misfortune that practical psychology can offer no generally valid recipes and norms. There are only individual cases, whose needs and demands are totally different—so different that we really cannot foresee what course a given case will follow. It is therefore wise of the physician to renounce all premature assumptions. This does not mean that he should throw all his assumptions overboard, but that he should regard them in any given case as hypothetical.   [xix, 31 (J, 56)

An ancient Chinese adept has said: But if the wrong man uses the right means, the right means work in the wrong way. This saying, unfortunately all too true, stands in sharp contrast to our belief in the "right" method irrespective of the man who applies it. In reality, when it comes to things like these, everything depends on the man and little or nothing on the method.

71

The latter is only the way and direction laid down by a man in order that his action may be the true expression of his nature. If it fails to be this, then the method is nothing more than an affectation, something artificially pieced on, rootless and sapless, serving only the illegitimate goal of self-deception. It becomes a means of fooling oneself and of evading what is perhaps the implacable law of one's being.   [xv, 531 f (h, 79)

Because the treatment of every serious case leads into a supreme conflict beyond the efficacy of any technique whatever, nobody should play with analysis as with an easy tool. Those who write superficial and cheap books about the subject are either unconscious of the far-reaching effects of analytical treatment or else ignorant of the real nature of the human soul.
[xl, 30 (g, 343)

When we are dealing with the human soul, we can only meet it on its own ground, and this is what we have to do when we are faced with the real and overpowering problems of life.
[xviii, 14

The remarkable strength of the unconscious contents, therefore, always indicates a corresponding weakness in the conscious mind and its functions. It is as though the latter were threatened with impotence. For primitive man this danger is one of the most terrifying instances of "magic." So we can understand why this secret fear is also to be found among civilized people. In serious cases it is the secret fear of madness; in less serious, the fear of the unconscious—a fear which even the normal person reveals in his resistance to psychological views and explanations. This resistance borders on the grotesque when it comes to scouting all psychological explanations of art, philosophy, and religion, as though the human psyche had, or should have, absolutely nothing to do with these things. The doctor knows these well defended zones from his consulting hours: they are reminiscent of island fortresses from which the neurotic tries to ward off the octopus. ("Happy neurosis island," as one of my patients called his conscious state!) The doctor is well aware that the patient needs an island and would be lost without it. It serves as a refuge for his consciousness and as the last stronghold against the threatening embrace of the unconscious. The same is true of the normal person's taboo regions which psychology must not touch. But since no war was ever won on the defensive, one must, in order to terminate hostilities, open negotiations with the enemy and see what his terms really are. Such is the intention of the doctor who volunteers to act as a mediator. He is far from wishing to disturb the somewhat precarious island idyll or pull down the fortifications. On the contrary, he is thankful that somewhere there is a firm foothold that does not first have to be fished up out of the chaos, always a desperately difficult task. He knows that the island is a bit cramped and that life on it is pretty meagre and plagued with all sorts of imaginary wants because too much life has been left outside. [LX, 27 f (N, 349)

Practical medicine is and has always been an art, and the same is true of practical analysis. True art is creation, and creation is beyond all theories. That is why I say to any beginner: Learn your theories as well as you can, but put them aside when you touch the miracle of the living soul. Not theories but your own creative individuality alone must decide.

[XL, 60 (G, 361)

Although in illnesses of the body there is no remedy and no treatment that can be said to be infallible in all circumstances, there are still a great many which will probably have the desired effect without either doctor's or patient's having the slightest need to insert a *Deo concedente.* But we are not dealing with the body—we are dealing with the psyche. Consequently we cannot speak the language of the body—cells and bacteria; we need another language adapted to the nature of the psyche, and equally we must have an attitude which measures the danger and can meet it. And all this must be genuine or it will have no effect, for if it is hollow, it will damage both doctor and patient. The *Deo concedente* is not just a rhetorical flourish; it expresses the firm attitude of the man who does not imagine that he knows better on every occasion and who is fully aware that the unconscious material before him is something *alive,* a paradoxical Mercurius of whom an old master says: "And he is that on whom nature has worked but a little and whom she hath wrought into metallic form yet left unfinished"

—a natural being, therefore, that longs for integration within the wholeness of a man. It is like a fragment of primeval psyche into which no consciousness has as yet penetrated to create division and order, a "united dual nature," as Goethe says, an abyss of ambiguities. [LX, 43 f (N, 361)

Neither our modern medical training nor academic psychology and philosophy give the doctor the necessary knowledge or means to deal effectively and understandingly with the often very urgent demands of psychotherapeutic practice. We must therefore not be deterred by the fear of being inadequate amateurs in history, but must see whether we cannot learn something from the medical philosophers of a remote past when body and soul had not yet been torn asunder and handed over to separate faculties. Although we are specialists par excellence, our specialized field, strangely enough, forces us to universalism and requires us completely to overcome our specialist attitude. We have to do this if the totality of body and soul is not to be a mere matter of words. [LV, 163 (K, 44)

Even the so-called highly scientific suggestion-therapy employs the wares of the medicine-man and the exorcising shaman. And please, why should it not? The public is not even now much more advanced, and it continues to expect miracles from the doctor. And truly those doctors should be deemed clever—worldly-wise in every respect—who understand the art of investing themselves with the halo of the medicine-man. Not only have they the biggest practices, they have also the best results. This is simply because countless physical maladies (leaving out the neuroses) are complicated and burdened with psychic elements to an extent scarcely yet suspected. The medical exorcist's whole behaviour betrays his full valuation of the psychic element when he gives the patient the opportunity of fixing his faith firmly upon the doctor's mysterious personality. Thus does he win the sick man's mind, which henceforth helps him indeed to restore his body also to health. The cure works best when the doctor really believes in his own formulae, otherwise he may be overcome by scientific doubt and so lose the correct, convincing tone. [VII, 3 f (C, 238 f)

I regard the conscience-searching question of the doctor's remaining true to his scientific convictions as rather unimportant in comparison with the incomparably weightier question as to how he can best help his patient. The doctor *must*, on occasion, be able to play the augur. *Mundus vult decipi*—but the cure is no deception. It is true there is a conflict between ideal conviction and concrete possibility. But we should ill prepare the ground for the seed of the future were we to forget the tasks of the present and seek only to cultivate ideals. That is but idle dreaming. Do not forget that Kepler cast horoscopes for money, and that countless artists have been condemned to work for wages. [vii, 19 (c, 251 f)

As a doctor it is my task to help the patient to cope with life. I cannot presume to pass judgment on his final decisions, because I know from experience that all coercion—be it suggestion, insinuation, or any other method of persuasion—ultimately proves to be nothing but an obstacle to the highest and most decisive experience of all, which is to be alone with his own self, or whatever else one chooses to call the objectivity of the psyche. The patient must be alone if he is to find out what it is that supports him when he can no longer support himself. Only this experience can give him an indestructible foundation.
[lviii, 48 (m, 32)

Since man is not only an individual but also a member of society, these two inherent tendencies of human nature can never be separated nor the one overruled by the other without serious harm to the whole being. At best, the patient should come out of the analysis as he actually is, in harmony with himself, neither good nor bad, but as man truly is, a natural being. [vi, 106

It is incredible how people can allow themselves to be bewitched by words. They always imagine that a name can actually create a thing; as if, for instance, we had dealt the devil a serious blow by calling him neurosis. [xxvii, 52

Neurosis is integrally bound up with the problem of our

time, and actually demonstrates the unsuccessful effort of the individual to solve in himself what is essentially a universal problem. Neurosis is division with the self.　　　　[v, 261 f (D, 19)

People whose own temperaments offer problems are often neurotic, but it would be a serious misunderstanding to confuse the existence of problems with neurosis. There is a marked distinction between the two in that the neurotic is ill because he is unconscious of his problems, while the man with a difficult temperament suffers from his conscious problems without being ill.　　　　　　　　　　　　　　　　[XIX, 256 (J, 116)

The greatest mistake which an analyst can occasionally make is to assume that the patient's psychology is similar to his own.
　　　　　　　　　　　　　　　　　　　　　　[XIII, 150
Medicine in the hands of a fool has always been poison and death. Just as we must demand from a surgeon a skilful hand, courage, presence of mind, and power of decision, in addition to his specialized knowledge, so must we even more expect the psychoanalyst to have had a thoroughly earnest psychoanalytical education of his own personality if we are to entrust a patient to him. I would even say that the practice of psychoanalysis requires not only psychological skill but above all a serious effort on the part of the doctor to develop his own character.　　　　　　　　　　　　　　　　　　　　[VI, 109 f

Each new case that requires thorough treatment is pioneer work, and every trace of routine then proves to be a blind alley. Consequently the higher psychotherapy is a most exacting business, and sometimes it sets tasks which challenge not only our understanding or our sympathy, but the whole man. The doctor is inclined to demand this total effort from his patients, yet he must realize that this same demand only works if he is aware that it also applies to himself.　　　　　　　　[LX, 22 (N, 342)

There are doctors who believe that it is enough to analyse themselves. This is the Munchausen psychology, with which they are certain to get stuck. They forget that one of the most important therapeutic conditions is precisely submission to the objective judgment of another. Towards ourselves it is well known that we are blind in spite of everything.   [vi, 109

It has been believed for too long that psychotherapy can be used "technically" like a recipe or an operational method or a dyeing process. The general practitioner can use all sorts of techniques without hesitation, whether or not he has this or that personal opinion about his patient, or this or that psychological theory or philosophical or religious conviction. But psychotherapy cannot be used in such a way. *Nolens volens* the doctor himself is just as much there with all his preconceptions as the patient. Indeed it is to a great extent immaterial which technique he uses, for it does not depend on "technique" but primarily on the personality who uses this method. The object of the method is neither a dead anatomical preparation, nor an abscess, nor a chemical body, but the whole of a suffering personality. It is not the neurosis which is the object of the therapy but the person who has the neurosis. A heart neurosis, for instance, as we have known for some time, does not arise from the heart, as the ancient mythology of medicine would have it, but from the soul of the sufferer. It arises not from some dark corner of the unconscious, as many psychotherapists still try to believe, but from a whole person's years and tens of years of living and experiencing, and finally not only from this single life but also from the psychic experience of the family or even of the social group.   [xxvi, 2 f

The personality of the patient demands the personality of the doctor and not artificial technical procedures.   [xxvi, 3

Psychotherapy is in reality a dialectic relationship between doctor and patient, a discussion between two psychic entities in which all knowledge is a mere tool. The aim is a transformation which is not predetermined, but much more an indeterminable change, of which the only criterion is the disappearance of the rule of the ego. No effort made by the doctor can provoke the experience. He can at best only smooth the way towards achieving an attitude which will oppose the minimum of resistance to the decisive experience. [XLII, 32

The psychotherapist should not harbour the illusion that the treatment of neuroses requires nothing more than knowledge of the technique. He must be absolutely clear that the treatment of the soul of a patient is a *relationship* in which the doctor is just as much involved as the patient. A real treatment of the soul can only be *individual,* and therefore even the best technique is of purely relative value. But the general attitude of the doctor is all the more important, and he must know enough about himself to ensure that he will not destroy the particular qualities—whatever these may be—of the patient entrusted to him. [XXVI, 7 f

Most people need a vis-à-vis, otherwise the basis of experience is not sufficiently real. Otherwise the individual cannot "hear" himself and has no opportunity of contrasting himself with what is different from himself in order to ascertain what he himself really is. In such a case everything remains unclear and without shape and is answered only by oneself and not by another, a different, being. It makes an enormous difference whether I admit my guilt only to myself or to another. [LVI, 17

The process of psychological differentiation is no light work, it needs tenacity and patience. . . . As alchemical symbolism shows, a radical understanding of this kind is impossible without a human partner. A general and merely academic "insight into one's mistakes" is ineffectual, for then the mistakes are not really seen at all, only the idea of them. They show up acutely when a human relationship brings them to the fore and when they are noticed by the other person as well as by oneself. Then and then only can they really be felt and their true nature recognized. Similarly, confessions made to one's secret self generally have little or no effect, whereas confessions made to another are much more promising. [LX, 212 f (N, 478)

Nobody can meddle with fire or poison without being affected in some way in some vulnerable spot: for the true physician never stands outside his work but is always in the thick of it.

[LVIII, 17 (M, 5)

The task of coming to terms with his philosophy of life is one which psychotherapy inevitably sets itself, even though not every patient probes to the deepest levels. The question of the measuring rod with which to measure, and that of the ethical criteria which are to determine our actions, must be answered somehow, for it may happen that the patient expects us to account for our judgments and decisions. Not all patients will allow themselves to be condemned to a position of infantile inferiority because we refuse to render such an account, quite apart from the fact that such an error in therapeutical technique would cut the ground from under our own feet. In other words, the art of psychotherapy requires that the therapist should be in possession of an ultimate conviction which can be stated, which is credible and defensible, and which has proved its validity by the fact that it either has resolved any neurotic dissociations of his own or has never let them develop. A therapist who has a neurosis does not deserve the name, for it is not possible to bring the patient to a more advanced stage than one has reached oneself. [LV, 159 (K, 38 f)

If, however, the therapist is not prepared to allow his own convictions to be called in question for the sake of his patient, then there is justified ground to doubt whether his fundamental attitude is really firmly established. He may perhaps be unable to give way because he needs to protect his own security, which lays him open to the danger of rigidity. The limits of psychic elasticity, however, differ very greatly, both individually and collectively, and often the degree of elasticity at a person's disposal is so small that he really cannot get beyond a certain degree of rigidity. *Ultra posse nemo obligatur.* [LV, 161 (K, 41)

If the doctor wants to offer guidance to another, or even to accompany him a step of the way, he must be in touch with this other person's psychic life. He is never in touch when he passes judgment. Whether he puts his judgments into words, or keeps them to himself, makes not the slightest difference.

[XXI, 18 (J, 270)

Unfortunately, we are too inclined to talk of man as it would be desirable for him to be rather than as he really is. But a doctor has always to do with the real man, who remains obstinately himself until the nature of his reality is recognized in its completeness. True education can proceed only from naked reality, not from any ideal illusion about man, however attractive.

[LI, 113 (D, 63)

We cannot change anything unless we accept it. Condemnation does not liberate, it oppresses. I am the oppressor of the person I condemn, not his friend and fellow sufferer. I do not in the least mean to say that we must never pass judgment in the cases of persons whom we desire to help and improve. But if the doctor wishes to help a human being he must be able to accept him as he is. And he can do this in reality only when he has already seen and accepted himself as he is.

[XXI, 18 f (J, 271)

As long as you feel the human contact, the atmosphere of mutual confidence, there is no danger; even if you have to face the terror of insanity, or the menace of death, there is still that sphere of human trust, that certainty of understanding and of being understood, that belief that both will persist, no matter how dark the way.   [XL, 48 (G, 354)

The little word "ought" in itself proves the helplessness of the therapist, and is a confession that he has come to the end of his resources.   [LV, 158 (K, 38)

We can wax indignant over man's notorious lack of spirituality, but when one is a doctor one does not invariably think that the disease is intractable or the patient morally inferior; instead, one supposes that the negative results may possibly be due to the remedy applied.   [LX, 51 (N, 368)

At any rate the doctor cannot afford to point, with a gesture of facile moral superiority, to the tablets of the law and say, "Thou shalt not." He has to examine things objectively and weigh up possibilities, for he knows, less from religious training and education than from instinct and experience, that there is something very like a *felix culpa*. He knows that one can miss not only one's happiness but also one's final guilt, without which a man will never reach his wholeness. Wholeness is in fact a charisma which one can manufacture neither by art nor by cunning, which we can only grow into and whose reign we must simply endure.   [LVIII, 51 f (M, 36)

What do people want nowadays? In any case they do not want moralizing lectures, for all that can be said in that direction most of them have known long ago. Therefore they go to the doctor, hoping to find a little understanding and knowledge of life. This is comprehensible, for they hope to be understood at least to the extent that they are justified in holding that there is really something the matter, something which cannot be moralized away; for, alas, they have tried to do this long ago to their own cost and have nearly destroyed themselves in the process. Such conflicts cannot be solved by reason; this can only happen in a highly mysterious way through symbolic growth. But this is something which we absolutely cannot understand. If we were Chinese, we would understand it easily. But we think so differently, so much only in the "upper story," that we are incapable of anything like symbolic growth, which is a gradual transformation. For us the conscious mind is paramount, for the conscious mind with its reasoning powers has helped us to conquer the universe and bring the world under our domination. But it has not helped us to understand our own being and that world of things infinitely small within us. That is the mystery which the "lower man" in us knows well, while it is unknown to the conscious mind.   [XXXIV, 85 f

The psyche cannot be treated without taking into account man as a whole, including the ultimate and deepest aspects, any more than the sick body can be treated without taking into account the totality of its functions—or rather, as a few representatives of modern medicine have maintained—the totality of the sick man himself. The more "psychic" a condition is, the greater is its complexity, and the more closely is it related to the whole of man's being.   [LV, 157 (K, 37)

It is impossible to treat the soul, and the human personality in general, sectionally. In all disturbances of the psyche it is apparent—perhaps even more so than in the case of physical illness—that the psyche is a whole in which everything is connected with everything else. When the patient comes to us with a neurosis, it is not a specialism he brings but a whole psyche, and with it a whole piece of the world on which that psyche is dependent, and without which it can never be properly understood. [LIX, 3 f (K, 18)

A conscientious doctor must be capable of doubting all his arts and theories, otherwise he falls a victim to a mere abstract plan, which means narrow-mindedness and inhumanity. There can no longer be any doubt that, whatever else a neurosis may be, it most certainly cannot be classed as a "nothing but." Neurosis is the suffering of a human soul in its whole, worldwide complexity, and this is so enormous that any theory of neurosis may well be described straight away as a worthless *aperçu,* unless it is a gigantic image of the soul to estimate which even a hundredfold *Faust* would not suffice. [XXVI, 11

The neurotic is ill not because he has lost his old faith, but because he has not yet found a new form for his finest aspirations. [VII, 51 (C, 277)

We need not be neurotic to feel "the need of healing"; this also exists in those who deny with full conviction the possibility of such a healing. Even such people cannot avoid, in a weak moment, a curious glance into a psychological book, perhaps merely to find a recipe for bringing a refractory wife (or husband) to reason. [XVII, 4 f

Every illness is at the same time an unsuccessful attempt at healing. Instead of regarding the sick person as the secret evildoer or accomplice of morally inadmissible desires, he might just as well be considered the unwitting victim of problems of instinct which have not been understood and which no one has helped him to solve. His dreams might also be understood as the prophesies of nature, far beyond all human and all-too-human manoeuvres of self-deception. [XLV

Neurotic symbolism is ambiguous: it points both forward and backward, downward and upward. Generally the forward aspects are more important than the backward, because the future comes while the past goes. Only those who are preparing a retreat do better to look backward. But even the neurotic person need not consider himself defeated; he has merely misjudged his inevitable foe and has thought to escape from him by cheap means. But just in that which he seeks to avoid lies the challenge to his personality. A doctor who deceives him into dismissing the problem does him a bad turn. The sick man has not to learn how to get rid of his neurosis but how to bear it. For the illness is not a superfluous and senseless burden, it is himself, he himself is that "other" which we were always trying to shut out, from childish indolence, or fear, or some other reason. In this way, as Freud rightly says, we make the "ego" into an "abode of fear," which it would never be if we did not defend ourselves neurotically against ourselves.

[xxvi, 12 f

We do our neurotic patients a grievous wrong if we try to force them all into the category of the unfree. Among neurotics, there are not a few who do not require any reminders of their social duties and obligations; rather are they born or destined to become the bearers of new social ideals. They are neurotic so long as they bow down to authority and refuse the freedom to which they are destined. While we look at life only retrospectively, as is the case in the Viennese psychoanalytic writings, we shall never do justice to this type of case and never bring the longed-for deliverance. For in that fashion we can only educate them to become obedient children, and thereby strengthen the very forces that have made them ill—their conservative retardation and their submissiveness to authority.

[vi, 43 f (c, 271)

The little world of childhood with its familiar surroundings is a model of the greater world. The more intensively the family has stamped its character upon the child, the more it will tend

to feel and see its earlier miniature world again in the bigger
world of adult life. Naturally this is not a conscious, intellectual
process. On the contrary, the neurotic person feels and sees
the contrast between then and now, and tries to adapt himself
as well as he can. Perhaps he thinks he has quite adapted himself in that he has an intellectual grasp of the situation, but that
does not alter the fact that his feelings drag far behind his intellectual realization.   [vi, 49

In the neurosis, there is in reality a piece of undeveloped
personality, a precious piece of the soul, without which the individual is damned to resignation and bitterness and other feelings of hostility towards life. A psychology of neurosis which
only sees the negative side throws away the vital part by
neglecting the sense and worth of the "infantile"—i.e., creative
—imagination.   [xxvi, 10

Where the ego has been made into an "abode of fear," someone is running away from himself and will not admit it.
                                                          [xxvi, 12 f
"Infantile" is something which is not unequivocal. First, it
can be genuine or merely symptomatic, and second, it can be
merely retarded or germinal. There is an enormous difference
between something which has remained infantile and something which is in the process of coming into life. Both may have
an infantile or embryonic form, and it is often, or indeed generally, impossible to recognize at first glance whether it is a
surviving piece of childhood which is to be deplored or an important creative beginning. Only a fool would laugh at these
possibilities, not realizing that the future is more important
than the past.   [xxvi, 5

Neurosis is by no means only negative; it is also positive. Only
a soulless rationalism could and does overlook this fact, supported by the narrowness of a purely materialistic philosophy
of life. In reality, the neurosis contains the soul of the sick person, or at least a considerable part of it, and if the neurosis
could be taken out like a decayed tooth, in the rationalistic way,
then the patient would have gained nothing and lost something

very important, as much as a thinker who loses his doubt of the truth of his conclusions, or a moral man who loses his temptations, or a courageous man who loses fear. For the neurotic to lose his neurosis is tantamount to losing his object in life, whereby life is robbed of its zest and its meaning.   [xxvi, 10

The thing that cures a neurosis must be as convincing as the neurosis; and since the latter is only too real, the helpful experience must be of equal reality. It must be a very real illusion, if you want to put it pessimistically. But what is the difference between a real illusion and a healing religious experience? It is merely a difference in words. You can say, for instance, that life is a disease with a very bad prognosis, it lingers on for years to end with death; or that normality is a generally prevailing constitutional defect; or that man is an animal with a fatally overgrown brain. This kind of thinking is the prerogative of habitual grumblers with bad digestions.

[xlvi, 189 f (b, 114)

Healing may be called a religious problem. In the sphere of social or national relations, the state of suffering may be civil war, and this state is to be cured by the Christian virtue of forgiveness of those who hate us. That which we try with the conviction of good Christians to apply to external situations we must also, in the treatment of neurosis, apply to the inner state. This is why modern man has heard enough about guilt and sin. He is sorely enough beset by his own bad conscience, and wants rather to learn how he is to reconcile himself with his own nature—how he is to love the enemy in his own heart and call the wolf his brother.   [xxi, 21 (j, 273 f)

A neurosis has really come to an end when it has overcome the wrongly oriented ego. The neurosis itself is not healed; it heals us. The man is ill, but the illness is an attempt of nature to heal him. We can therefore learn a great deal for the good of our health from the illness itself, and that which appears to the neurotic person as absolutely to be rejected is just the part which contains the true gold which we should otherwise never have found.   [xxvi, 13

The labours of the doctor as well as the quest of the patient are directed towards that hidden and as yet unmanifest "whole" man, who is at once the greater and the future man. But the right way to wholeness is made up, unfortunately, of fateful detours and wrong turnings. It is a *longissima via*, not straight but snake-like, a path that unites the opposites, reminding us of the guiding caduceus, a path whose labyrinthine twists and turns are not lacking in terrors. It is on this *longissima via* that we meet with those experiences which are said to be "barely accessible." Their inaccessibility consists in the fact that they demand a great expenditure of effort: they demand the very thing that men fear most, namely the wholeness they are always prating about and which lends itself to endless theorizing, though in actual life they give it the widest possible berth. Infinitely to be preferred is the cultivation of that popular "compartment psychology" where the left-hand pigeonhole does not know what is in the right.   [LVIII, 17 f (M, 6)

If this purpose of achieving wholeness and realizing the originally intended personality should happen to grow in a natural way within the patient, then we should help it along with great understanding. If it does not grow of itself, then it cannot be planted there without always remaining a foreign body. We therefore deny ourselves such tricks, unless nature itself is obviously working in this direction. As a medical art, armed with weapons of human ability, my psychology does not venture to preach a cure or to recommend a path of healing, for that does not lie within its power.   [LVI, 18

MAN AND WOMAN

Where love rules, there is no will to power; and where power predominates, there love is lacking. The one is the shadow of the other. [LI, 97

It is, I think, characteristic of our psychology that the present epoch was, as it were, ushered in by two minds who were destined to have immense influence upon the hearts and minds of the younger generation: Wagner, the advocate of love, who in his music sounds the whole scale of feeling from Tristan down to incestuous passion, and from Tristan up to the loftiest spirituality of the Grail; and Nietzsche, the advocate of power and of the victorious will of the individuality. In his last and loftiest utterance Wagner took hold of the Grail legend, as Goethe selected Dante, while Nietzsche chose the image of a lordly caste and a lordly morality, an image which had found its embodiment in many a fair-haired heroic and knightly figure of the Middle Ages. Wagner breaks the bonds that stifle love, while Nietzsche shatters the "tables of value" that cramp the individuality. They both strive after similar goals, at the same time creating irremediable discord, for where love is individual power can never prevail, while the dominating power of the individual precludes the reign of love. [IX, 338 (I, 297 f)

It is difficult to imagine that this rich world should be too poor to offer the human atom an object for its love. That reproach against the world cannot be made; for it offers infinite opportunity for everyone. It is much more the inability to love which robs man of his possibilities. The world is only empty to him who does not understand how to direct his libido on to outside things, to make them living and beautiful to him. The beauty lies not in the things themselves but in the feeling which we give to those things. What compels us to find a substitute in ourselves is not the lack of outside objects, but our own inability to comprehend with love an object outside of ourselves.

Certainly the difficulties of life and the hardships of the struggle for existence oppress us, but even a difficult external situation should not prevent us from giving out our libido; on the contrary it should inspire us to greater effort, thus enabling us to bring our whole libido into touch with reality. [IV, 166 f

Our present humbug of sentimentality has reached quite indecent proportions. We need only think of the positively disastrous role of popular sentiment in time of war! Or of our so-called humanity! How much each individual is the helpless victim of his own sentiments, unworthy of pity, the psychiatrist could best tell us. Sentimentality is a superstructure covering brutality. Lack of feeling is the inevitable counterpart of sentimentality, which inevitably suffers from the same deficiencies.
[XXVII, 154

Unfortunately, it is almost a collective ideal to be as negligent and unconscious of love matters as possible. Behind the mask of respectability and decency the power of neglected love poisons the children. Of course you cannot blame the average man, as he receives no guidance in solving the great problem of love from current ideals and conventions. These, unfortunately, are all in favour of negligence and repression.
[XL, 83 (G, 375)

The further away and the more unreal the personal mother is, the deeper the son's longing plunges into the depths of his soul to awaken that original and eternal image of the mother, through which everything comprehensive, sheltering, nourishing, and helpful assumes for us the maternal figure, from the *alma mater* of the university to the personification of towns, countries, sciences, and ideals. [XLVIII, 45

A mother-complex can never be dissolved by reducing the mother in a one-sided way to human proportions and in this manner, so to speak, "correcting" the conception. This would entail the risk of splitting up into atoms the living experience of "mother" and thereby destroying one of the highest values, in fact throwing away the golden key which the good fairy had laid in our cradle. Therefore man has always instinctively added to the natural parents the pre-existing godparents as "godfather" and "godmother" of the new-born child, so that the child should never so far forget himself in sinful rationalism as to burden his parents with godliness.   [XLIII, 426

The positive aspect of the glorification of the mother-instinct is that image of the mother which has been sung and praised at all times and in all tongues. It is that mother-love which is among the most touching and most unforgettable memories of the adult human being; it is the secret root of all birth and of all transformation; it means for us the home-coming and the in-coming, and is the silent primordial source of every beginning and every end. Intimately known and as strange as nature, lovingly tender and fatefully cruel—a joyful, never-tiring giver of life, a *mater dolorosa* and the silent, unanswering gateway which shuts behind the dead. Mother is mother-love; it is *my* experience and *my* secret. What all should we say about that particular human being who was called mother, of whom we might even say that she was the accidental bearer of that ex-perience which includes me and all humanity, and even all living creatures that come and go, the very experience of life whose children we are? Whatever we say will always be too much, too false, too inadequate, and even too misleading. Yet we have always done this and we shall always do it; but one who understands can no longer put such an enormous load of significance, of responsibility and duty, the weight of all heaven and hell, upon the weak and erring human being in need of love, care, understanding, and forgiveness, who was our mother. He knows that the mother is the bearer of that image inborn in us of *mater natura* and *mater spiritualis,* that image of the whole scope of life to which we are entrusted and at the same time delivered over as helpless children.   [XLIII, 425 f

In spite of all vehement protestations to the contrary, the fact remains that love (here used in the wider meaning which belongs to the word by right, a meaning including more than sexuality), its problems and its conflicts, is of fundamental sig-nificance for human life, and, as careful inquiry consistently shows, is of far greater importance than the individual suspects.
                                              [v, 254 (D, 14)

The love problem is part of mankind's heavy toll of suffering, and nobody should be ashamed that he must pay his tribute.

[xl, 84 (g, 375)

It is difficult to gauge the spirit of one's own time, but let us observe the way in which the arts are developing, the kind of sensibility in vogue, the tendencies of popular taste. Let us observe what men read, what they write, the societies they found, the "questions" that are the order of the day. Note also against what the Philistines are up in arms. We shall then find that in the long array of our present social questions by no means the last is the so-called "sexual question." Its discussion is carried on by men who challenge the recognized sexual morality and who seek to throw off the burden of guilt which past centuries have heaped on Eros. The existence of these movements cannot be simply denied, nor can they be condemned as indefensible. They exist, and have sufficient ground for their existence. It is more interesting and more useful to probe attentively the underlying causes of these characteristic movements of our age than to join in the lamentations of the professional mourners of morality who prophesy the moral downfall of humanity.

[v, 257 (d, 16)

It is self-evident, we all agree, that murder, stealing, and ruthlessness of every sort are inadmissible; yet we speak of a sexual question, not of a murder question nor of a rage problem. Social reform is never invoked in favour of those who wreak their bad tempers on their fellow men. All these things are examples of instinctive behaviour, yet the necessity for their suppression seems to us self-evident. Only after sexuality do we put the mark of interrogation. This points to a doubt. We begin to wonder whether our present moral concepts and the legal institutions based upon them are really adequate or suitable for their ends. No discerning person would contest the fact that in this field there are sharply divided opinions. No problem of this kind could exist if public opinion were united about it. Manifestly a reaction is taking place against a too rigorous morality. It is not just an outbreak of primitive instinct; such outbreaks, we know, are never concerned with restrictive laws and moral problems. In this reaction, however, the question is seriously raised whether our present moral conceptions have dealt fairly with the nature of sexuality. Out of this doubt there springs a legitimate interest in the attempt to understand sexuality more truly and deeply. [xiii, 94 f (G, 64)

It is doubtless true that instinct in the field of sexuality collides most frequently and most conspicuously with moral views. The collision between infantile instinctiveness and the ethical order can never be avoided. It is, as I believe, the *conditio sine qua non* of psychic energy. [xiii, 94 (G, 63 f)

We must learn to understand that psychoanalytical thinking, in contrast to the habitual way of thinking hitherto, goes back to just those symbolic forms which had become increasingly complicated through innumerable modifications. This means that a simplification is taking place which, were it a case of something else, would be intellectually welcome, but which here seems to be not only aesthetically but also ethically distasteful, for the repressions which have to be overcome are the result of our best intentions. We must begin by overcoming our virtuousness, with the justifiable fear of falling into vice on the other side. This danger certainly exists, for the greatest virtuousness is always compensated inwardly by a strong tendency to vice, and how many vicious characters treasure inside themselves sugary virtues and a moral megalomania? [iv, 221 f

Surely I cannot be suspected of being so thoughtless as, so to speak, to try through analytical reduction to put back the libido to a primitive stage which has almost been overcome, and to forget quite what terrible misery would then spread over humanity. Doubtless a few individuals here and there will allow themselves to be swept away by the ancient orgies of a sexuality freed from the burden of guilt, to their own dire injury, but these are types which would have gone under prematurely in any case, though in a different way—nevertheless I know the most effective and merciless regulator of human sexuality: it is stern necessity. [iv, 222 f

It is a favourite neurotic misconception that a true adaptation to the world can be found by giving full rein to sexuality.

[VI, 105

On the one hand, our civilization enormously underestimates the importance of sexuality, and, on the other, just because of the oppressive repressions imposed upon it, sexuality breaks into all possible fields which do not belong to it, and uses such an indirect mode of expression that we can expect suddenly to detect it practically everywhere. Thus even the idea of the intimate understanding of a human soul, which is actually something very beautiful and pure, becomes besmirched and perversely distorted by the intrusion of an indirect sexual meaning. A direct and spontaneous expression of sexuality is a natural happening and, as such, never unpleasant or ugly. It is "moral" repression which makes sexuality on the one hand dirty and hypocritical, and on the other impudent and pushing. This fact—that the denied and repressed sexuality misuses the highest functions of the soul—gives certain of our opponents the opportunity to scent out indecent confessional romances in psychoanalysis.

[IV, 295

Today we have no real sexual morality, only a legal attitude towards sexuality; just as the early Middle Ages had no genuine morality for financial transactions, but only prejudices and a legal standpoint. We are not yet sufficiently advanced in the domain of free sexual activity to distinguish between a moral and an immoral relationship. We have a clear expression of this in the customary treatment, or rather ill-treatment, of unmarried motherhood. For a great deal of sickening hypocrisy, for the high tide of prostitution, and for the prevalence of sexual diseases, we may thank both our barbarous, undifferentiated legal judgments about the sexual situation and our inability to develop a finer moral perception of the immense psychologic differences that may exist in free sexual activity.

[VII, 49 (c, 276)

The conflict between the ethical and the sexual is today not just a direct collision between the instincts and morality; it is a struggle to give to an instinct its proper place in existence. We have to recognize in this instinct a power which seeks expression and which apparently may not be trifled with; accordingly it cannot be just made to fit in with our well-meaning moral laws. Sexuality is not merely instinctiveness, but an indisputable creative power that is not only the fundamental cause in our individual lives but also an increasingly serious factor in our psychic life. Today we know all too well the grave results that sexual disorders can bring in their train.

[xiii, 96 (g, 65)

Eros is in reality an all-powerful force which, like nature, allows itself to be overcome and used as if it were powerless. But a triumph over nature is heavily paid for. Nature needs no basic explanations, she is content with patience and wise moderation. "Eros is a great demon," as wise Diotima said to Socrates. We can never quite get the better of him, or rather we overcome him only to our own cost. He is not the whole of nature within us, but he is at least one of her chief aspects. [li, 51

The conflict between "love" and "duty" must be solved upon that particular plane of character where "love" and "duty" are no longer in opposition, for indeed they really are not so. The familiar conflict between "instinct" and "conventional morality" must be solved in such a way that both factors are taken satisfactorily into account, and this is only possible through a change of character. This change psychoanalysis can bring about. In such cases external solutions are worse than none at all.   [vii, 19 (c, 251)

The erotic instinct is something questionable, and will always be so whatever a future set of laws may have to say on the matter. It belongs, on the one hand, to the original animal nature of man, which will exist as long as man has an animal body. On the other hand, it is connected with the highest forms of the spirit. But it blooms only when spirit and instinct are in true harmony. If one or the other aspect is missing, then an injury occurs, or at least there is a one-sided lack of balance which easily slips into the pathological. Too much of the animal disfigures the civilized human being, too much culture makes a sick animal.   [li, 51

Normal sexuality as a common and apparently similarly directed experience strengthens the feeling of unity and of identity. This condition is described as one of complete harmony, and is extolled as a great happiness ("one heart and one soul"), and with reason, because the return to the original condition of unconscious unity is like a return to childhood. Hence the childish gestures of all lovers. Even more is it like a return into the mother's womb—into the teeming depths of a still unconscious fertility. It is indeed a true and undeniable experience of divinity, the transcending power of which blots out and consumes everything individual; it is a real communion with life and with impersonal fate. The individual will holding to its own integrity is broken; the woman becomes a mother, the man a father, and thus both are robbed of freedom and made instruments of onward-striving life.   [xix, 280 (g, 192 f)

As far as we know, consciousness is always ego-consciousness. In order to be conscious of myself, I must be able to differentiate myself from others. Relationship can only take place where this differentiation exists.   [xix, 276 (g, 189 f)

Although man and woman unite, they nevertheless represent irreconcilable opposites which, when activated, degenerate into deadly hostility. This primordial pair of opposites symbolizes every conceivable pair of opposites that may occur: hot and cold, light and dark, north and south, dry and damp, good and bad, conscious and unconscious.   [lviii, 212 f (m, 192)

The meeting of two personalities is like the contact of two chemical substances: if there is any reaction, both are transformed.   [xix, 32 (j, 57)

All that pertains to the opposite sex has a mysterious attraction coupled with bashfulness and perhaps even with a certain feeling of aversion; and just therefore, the attraction is especially strong and fascinating, even if it does not come from outside in the form of a woman but from inside as a psychic activity, such as the temptation to give way to a mood or an affect.   [x, 17

It is true that a youth of marriageable age possesses an ego-consciousness (as a rule a girl has more than a man), but since he has only recently emerged as it were from the mists of the original unconsciousness, he necessarily has wide regions which still lie in the shadows of that state. In so far as these regions extend, they do not admit the formation of a psychological relationship. The practical outcome of this is that the young man (or woman) can have only an incomplete understanding of himself or others and therefore is informed only imperfectly as to the motives of others and of himself. As a rule he acts almost entirely from unconscious motives. Naturally it appears to him subjectively as though he were very conscious, for one constantly overestimates the conscious content. It is and remains a great and surprising discovery, when we find out that what we had supposed to be a final peak is in reality nothing but the lowest step of a very long approach.   [xix, 276 f (g, 190)

We live in a time when there dawns upon us a realization that the people living on the other side of the mountain are not made up exclusively of red-headed devils responsible for all the evil on this side of the mountain. A sign of this dim intuition has also penetrated the relation between the sexes; we do not all of us say to ourselves, "Everything good dwells within me, everything evil within thee." Today there already exist super-moderns who ask themselves in all seriousness if something or other is not out of joint? If we are not perhaps somewhat too unconscious, somewhat antiquated? And whether this may not be the reason why, when confronted with difficulties in relationship between the sexes, we continue to apply with disastrous results methods of the Middle Ages if not those of the cave-man?   [xxxiii, 11 (a, xi)

In so far as the soul-relation to woman was expressed in the collective Virgin-worship, the image of woman lost a value to which human nature has a certain natural claim. This value, for which only individual choice can provide a natural expres-

sion, relapses into the unconscious when the individual is replaced by a collective expression. In the unconscious the image
of woman now receives an energic value which in its turn activates certain infantile archaic dominants. The relative depreciation of the real woman is thus compensated by dæmonic
impulses.   [IX, 332 f (I, 292)

In a certain sense man loves woman less as a result of her
relative depreciation—hence she appears as a persecutor, i.e.,
a witch. Thus the delusion about witches, that ineradicable
blot upon the later Middle Ages, developed along with, and indeed as a result of, the intensified worship of the Virgin.
                                                            [IX, 333 (I, 293)

Although we are far from having overcome our prehistoric
mentality, and although it is just in the field of sexuality that
man becomes most vividly aware of his mammalian nature and
also experiences its most signal triumphs, none the less, certain
ethical refinements have entered in which permit the man who
has behind him from ten to fifteen centuries of Christian education to progress toward a somewhat higher level. On this level,
spirit—from the biological point of view, an incomprehensible
psychic phenomenon—plays no small psychological role. Spirit
had an important word to say in the idea of Christian marriage
itself, and in the modern questioning and depreciation of marriage the question of spirit enters vigorously into the discussion. It appears in a negative way as counsel for the instincts
and in a positive way as defender of human dignity. Small wonder then that a wild and confusing conflict arises between man
as an instinctual creature of nature and as a spiritually conditioned, cultural being. The worst thing about it is that the one
is forever trying to do violence to the other, in order to bring
about a so-called harmonious and unified solution of the conflict. Unfortunately, too many persons still believe in this method
which continues to be all-powerful in the world of politics;
there are only a few here and there who condemn it as barbaric,
and who would rather set up in its place a just compromise
whereby each side would receive a hearing.   [XXXIII, 11 (A, xii)

How is a man to write about woman, his exact opposite? I

mean of course something accurate, that is outside the sexual programme, not contaminated by resentment, and beyond illusion and theory. Where is the man to be found capable of such superiority? For woman stands just where man's shadow falls. So that he is only too liable to confuse her with his own shadow. Then, when he wishes to repair this misunderstanding, he tends to overvalue the woman and believe in her desiderata.

[x, 7 f (G, 164)

The elementary fact that a man always presupposes another's psychology as being identical with his own aggravates the difficulty and hinders a correct understanding of the feminine psyche. [x, 14 (G, 168)

———————

Unhappily, in the problem between the sexes, no one can bring about a compromise by himself alone; it can only be brought about in relation to the other sex. Therefore the necessity of psychology! On this level, psychology becomes a kind of special pleading or, rather, a method of relationship. Psychology guarantees real knowledge of the other sex and thus supplants arbitrary opinions which are the source of the uncurable misunderstandings now undermining in increasing numbers the marriages of our time. [xxxiii, 11 f (A, xii)

The discussion of the sexual problem is, of course, only the somewhat crude beginning of a far deeper question, namely, that of the psychic or human relationship between the sexes. Before this latter question the sexual problem pales in significance, and with it we enter the real domain of woman. Her psychology is founded on the principle of Eros, the great binder and deliverer; while age-old wisdom has ascribed Logos to man as his ruling principle. [x, 26 (G, 175)

Whereas logic and objective reality commonly prevail in the outer attitude of man, or are at least regarded as an ideal, in the case of woman it is feeling. But in the soul the relations are reversed: inwardly it is the man who feels, the woman who reflects. Hence man's greater liability to total despair, while a woman can always find comfort and hope; hence man is more liable to put an end to himself than woman. However prone a woman may be to fall a victim to social circumstances, as for instance in prostitution, a man is equally delivered over to impulses from the unconscious in the form of alcoholism and other vices. [IX, 668 (I, 595)

The struggle of the opposites, which in the world of the European man takes place in the province of applied mind, finding expression in battlefields and bank balances, is a psychic conflict in the woman. [x, 9 (G, 165)

The woman is increasingly aware that love alone can give her her full stature, just as the man begins to discern that spirit alone can endow his life with its highest meaning. Fundamentally, therefore, both seek a psychic relation one to the other, because love needs the spirit, and the spirit love, for their fulfilment. [x, 41 (G, 185)

The modern woman has become aware of the undeniable fact that only in the estate of love can she attain her highest and best, and this consciousness brings her to the other realization, that love is beyond and above law; and against this her personal respectability revolts. [x, 39 (G, 184)

The love of woman claims the whole man, not mere masculinity as such, but also just that in him which implies the negation of it. The love of woman is not sentiment—that is only man's way—but a life-will that at times is terrifyingly unsentimental and can even force her to self-sacrifice. A man who is loved in this way cannot escape his inferior side, for he can only answer this reality with his own. [x, 34 f (G, 180 f)

But as long as a woman is content to be a *femme á homme*, she has no feminine individuality. She is empty and merely glitters—a welcome vessel for masculine projections. Woman as a personality, however, is a very different thing: here illusion no longer works. So that when the question of personality arises, which is as a rule the painful fact of the second half of life, the childish form of the self disappears too. [XLIX, 236 (o, 239)

A woman who is at war with her father has still the possibility of the instinctive female life, for she merely rejects that which is foreign to her. But if she is at war with her mother, she may reach a higher consciousness at the risk of damage to her instincts, for in denying the mother she denies all the darkness, the instinctive urge, the ambiguity, and the unconsciousness of her own being. [XLIII, 435

It is a woman's outstanding characteristic that she can do everything for the love of a man. But those women who can achieve something important for the love of a thing are most exceptional, because this does not really agree with their nature. The love of a thing is a man's prerogative. But, since the nature of the human being unites masculine and feminine elements, a man can live the feminine in himself, and a woman the masculine in herself. None the less, in man the feminine is in the background, as is the masculine in woman. If one lives out the opposite sex in oneself, one is living in one's own background, and that restricts too much the essential individuality. A man should live as a man, a woman as a woman.

[x, 16 f (G, 169 f)

The emotional nature of man, not his "mind," corresponds to the conscious nature of woman. Mind makes up the "soul," or better, the "animus" of woman, and, just as the anima of the man consists of inferior relatedness, full of resentment, so the animus of woman consists of inferior judgments or, better said, opinions. [XIV, 53 (H, 117)

Unconscious assumptions or opinions are the worst enemies of woman; they can even grow into a downright demonic passion that irritates and disgusts men, and that does the woman herself the greatest injury by gradually smothering the charm and meaning of femininity and driving it into the background. Such a development naturally ends in a deep, psychological division, in short, a neurosis. [x, 18 f (G, 171)

No man is throughout so masculine that he possesses no feminine qualities at all. The facts are rather the reverse. For it is just these very masculine men who reveal, albeit in a very

99

guarded form, a very sensitive feeling-life (often incorrectly described as "womanish"). A man regards it almost as a virtue to repress his feminine traits as much as possible, just as a woman, until quite recently, considered it unbecoming to be a man-woman. The repression of feminine traits and dispositions leads naturally to a heaping up of these tendencies in the unconscious. But just as naturally, the imago of woman (the soul) becomes the receptacle of these demands. And this explains the fact that, in his love choice, a man is strongly tempted to win the woman who best corresponds to his own unconscious femininity, a woman, in short, who can unhesitatingly receive the projection of his soul. Despite the fact that such a choice may seem to be as ideal as he feels it to be, it is perfectly possible in the long run that he finds he has married his own worst weakness.   [XI, 118 f (D, 203)

Every man carries within himself an eternal image of woman, not the image of this or that definite woman, but rather a definite feminine image. This image is fundamentally an unconscious, hereditary factor of primordial origin, and is engraven in the living system of man, a "type" ("archetype") of all the experiences with feminine beings in the age-long ancestry of man, a deposit, as it were, of all the impressions made by woman; in short, an inherited psychical system of adaptation. Even if there were no women, it would be possible at any time to deduce from this unconscious image how a woman must be constituted psychically. The same is true of the woman; that is, she also possesses an innate image of man.   [XIX, 289 (G, 199)

The persona, the ideal picture of the man as he should be, is inwardly compensated by feminine weakness, and as the individual plays the strong man in his outer role, he becomes inwardly a woman, the anima, because the anima is the opposite function to the persona. But because the inner world is dark and invisible to the extroverted consciousness and because, in addition to this, a man is just so much less capable of reflecting on his weaknesses the more he is identified with the persona, the counterpole to the persona—namely, the anima—remains completely in the dark, and hence is immediately projected, whereby the hero is brought under the slippered heel of his wife. Even though her increase of power be considerable she may suffer it none too well. She becomes inferior, thus providing the husband with the welcome proof that it is not he, the hero, who is inferior in "private life" but his wife. In return the wife may cherish the illusion, so attractive to many, that at least she is married to a hero; accordingly she remains unperturbed by her own useless life. This play of illusion is often made to serve for the real content of life.   [XI, 128 f (D, 210 f)

It does not help in any way to learn a list of the archetypes by heart. Archetypes are complexes of experience that come upon us fatefully, their effects being in our most personal life. The anima no longer confronts us as a sublime goddess, but rather, under certain conditions, as our most personal and bitter misunderstanding. When, for instance, a highly honoured scholar in his seventies deserts his family and marries a twenty-year-old red-haired actress, then we know that the gods have claimed another victim.   [XXXI, 211 f (F, 79 f)

What man has found to say about feminine eroticism, and especially about the feeling-life of women, is derived for the most part from the projection of his own anima and is accordingly distorted.   [XIX, 290 (G, 200)

A great feminine indefiniteness is the longed-for counterpart to a male definiteness and unequivocalness, which latter can only in a measure be satisfactorily established if a man can manage to get rid of all that is doubtful, ambiguous, uncertain, and unclear in himself by projecting it on to a charming feminine innocence. Owing to the characteristic inner indifference and the feeling of inferiority which constantly masquerades as offended innocence, the man finds himself in the favourable role of being able to bear the well-known feminine inadequacies in a superior but yet indulgent way, quasi with knightly chivalry.   [XLIII, 422

Emptiness is a great feminine mystery. It represents to man the absolutely "strange," the yawning hollow, the unfathom-

101

able "other," the Yin. The pitiful wretchedness of this nothingness (I speak here as a man) is—I might almost say unfortunately
—the powerful mystery of the incomprehensibility of femininity. Such a woman is sheer fate. Whatever a man may say about
it, in its favour or against it, everything or nothing or both, in
the end he will throw himself in blissful ecstasy into this chasm,
or else he will have missed the one and only chance to experience his manliness. In the former case, it is impossible to explain away his ridiculous happiness; in the latter, one cannot
make his misfortune evident to him. "The mothers, the mothers,
it sounds so strange!"   [XLIII, 433

The proverbial helplessness of the young girl is especially
attractive. She is so very much a part of the mother that she
positively does not know what is happening to her if a man
comes anywhere near her. She is so helpless, and so very much
in need of help, and so completely ignorant of anything that
even the mildest shepherd boy will soon find himself in the role
of a bold ravisher and treacherously steal the daughter from
her loving mother. This marvellous chance to be for once a
hundred-per-cent he-man does not happen every day, and
therefore exerts no small motivating power. Thus Pluto carried
off Persephone from the inconsolable Demeter, but, by the
decision of the gods, he had always to return his wife to his
mother-in-law for the summer season.   [XLIII, 422 f

In contrast to objective understanding and agreement as to
facts, human relationship leads into the psychic world, that
middle kingdom which reaches from the world of sense and
affect to that of the spirit. Something of both is contained in it,
yet it never loses its own unique, individual character. Into
this territory man has to venture, if he means to respond adequately to woman. Circumstances have forced her to master a
part of masculinity, which alone could save her from remaining embedded in an antiquated, purely instinctive femininity,
like a spiritual baby, alien and forlorn in the world of men.
Similarly, man will find himself forced to develop within himself some feminine characters, namely, to become observant
both psychologically and erotically. It is a task he cannot avoid,

unless he prefers to go trailing after woman, in a hopeless boy-
ish fashion, always in danger of finding himself put away in her
pocket.   [x, 31 (G, 178 f)

The masculinity of the woman and the femininity of the man
are inferior, and it is regrettable that their full value should be
contaminated by something that is less valuable. Yet on the
other hand, to the totality we call personality there is also a
shaded side; the strong man must somewhere be weak, the
clever man somewhere stupid, otherwise he becomes untrustworthy, and into the picture come pose and bluff. Is it not an
ancient truth that woman loves the weaknesses of the strong
man more than his strength, and the stupidity of the clever
more than his cleverness?   [x, 34 (G, 180)

The (other) partner of simpler character may easily lose himself in such a labyrinthine nature, that is to say, he finds in it
such abundant possibilities of experience that his personal interest becomes fully taken up, perhaps not always in an agreeable way, since he becomes preoccupied in tracking the other
through every possible highway and by-way. The more complicated personality often presents such an horizon of possibilities that the simpler personality is surrounded, even caught up
in them; thus he becomes absorbed in his more complex partner
and does not see beyond. It is almost a regular occurrence for
a woman to be wholly contained intellectually by her husband,
he being wholly contained emotionally by his wife. One can
describe this as the problem of the "contained" and the "container."   [xix, 284 (G, 195 f)

If the individual is to be regarded only as an instrument for
maintaining the species, then the purely instinctive choice in
marriage is by far the best. But since the foundations of such a
choice are unconscious, only a kind of impersonal connection
can be founded upon them, connections such as we can observe
very beautifully among primitives. If we can speak here of a
"relationship" at all, it is at best but a pallid and distant connection of a very impersonal character; one that is wholly

regulated by traditional customs and prejudices, a pattern for every conventional marriage. [xix, 279 (g, 192)

The soul of Europe is torn by the hellish barbarism of the war. While all men's hands are full in repairing the outer damage, the woman begins—unconsciously as ever—to heal the inner wounds, and to do this she needs, as her most important instrument, the psychic or human relationship. But nothing hinders this more than the exclusiveness of the medieval marriage, because it makes relationship superfluous. Relationship is only possible where there is a certain psychic distance, just as morality must always presuppose freedom. For this reason the unconscious tendency of woman is towards a weakening of marriage, but not towards the destruction of the marriage and family ideal. [x, 44 (g, 187)

For those in love with masculinity or femininity per se the traditional medieval marriage suffices—that thoroughly praiseworthy, practical, and amply-verified institution. The man of today, however, finds it extremely difficult to return to it, and in certain cases the way back is simply impossible, since this sort of marriage can exist only by virtue of the exclusion of present-day problems. [x, 31 f (g, 179)

The question of relationship touches a field which for the man is dark and painful. He is content only when the woman carries the burden of the relationship, that is, when he is contained or, in other words, when she can conceive herself as also having relations with another man, and as a consequence suffering a division within herself. For then it is she who has the painful problem, and he is not obliged to see his own, which is a great relief to him. In this situation he is not unlike a thief who, quite undeservedly, finds himself in the enviable position of having been forestalled by another thief, who has been caught by the police. Suddenly he becomes an honourable, impartial onlooker. In any other situation, however, a man always finds the discussion of personal relations troublesome and tedious, just as the woman would find it boring if her husband examined her on the *Critique of Pure Reason*. For the man, Eros

104

belongs to a shadowland; it entangles him in his feminine unconscious—the "psychical"; while to the woman Logos is a
deadly, boring kind of sophistry, if she is not simply afraid of
and repelled by it. [x, 28 f (G, 177)

In modern speech we could express the concept of Eros as
psychic relationship and that of Logos as objective or factual
interest. Whereas in the conception of the ordinary man love
in its real sense coincides with the institution of marriage, beyond which there is for him only adultery or a strictly proper
friendship, for the woman marriage is not an institution at all,
but a human, erotic relationship. [x, 26 f (G, 176)

To modern woman—let men take note of this—the medieval
marriage is no longer an ideal. She keeps this doubt and her resistance secret, it is true; one woman because she is married
and, therefore, finds it highly inconvenient if the door of the
safe be not hermetically closed; another because she is unmarried, and too virtuous to make herself quite plainly conscious of
her tendencies. But the newly-won masculinity both have
achieved makes it impossible for these women to believe in
marriage in its traditional form: "He shall be thy master." Masculinity means to know one's goal and to do what is necessary
to achieve it. [x, 32 f (G, 179 f)

We deceive ourselves greatly if we suppose that many married women are neurotic only because they are unsatisfied sexually, or because they have not found the right man, or because
they still have a fixation on their infantile sexuality. The real
ground of the neurosis is, in many cases, the inability to recognize the work that is waiting for them of helping to build up a
new civilization. We are all far too much at the standpoint of
the "nothing-but" psychology: we persist in thinking we can
squeeze the new future which is pressing in at the door into the
framework of the old and the known. [vii, 50 f (c, 277)

Most men are blind erotically They commit the unpardon-
able mistake of confusing Eros with sexuality. A man thinks he
possesses a woman if he has her sexually. He never possesses

her less, for to the woman the erotic relation is the only real and determining factor. To her marriage is a relationship with sexuality as an accompaniment. [x, 28 (G, 176)

Traditionally, man is regarded as the disturber of marital peace. This legend comes from times long past, when men still had time to pursue all manner of pastimes. But today life makes such demands on man, that the noble hidalgo Don Juan is to be seen nowhere save in the theatre. More than ever man loves his comfort; for ours is an age of neurasthenia, impotence, and easy chairs. There is no longer a surplus of energy for window-climbing and duellos. If anything is to happen in the way of adultery it must not be too serious. In no respect must it cost too much, hence the adventure can be only of a transitory kind. The man of today is entirely averse to jeopardizing marriage as an institution. [x, 20 (G, 172)

The woman feels that there is no longer real security in marriage; for what does the fidelity of the husband signify when she knows that his feelings and thoughts are running afield and that he is merely too cautious or too cowardly to follow them? What does her own fidelity amount to when she knows that, in holding to the bond, she is merely enthralled by a lust for legal possession, by which she allows her soul to be stunted? There is a higher fidelity which she begins to discern, a fidelity to the spirit and to love that can go beyond human weakness and incompleteness. [x, 41 f (G, 185)

Does the legal paragraph really know what adultery is? Is its definition the final embodiment of eternal truth? From the psychological standpoint, which for the woman is the only one that counts, it is in reality an extremely poor piece of bungling, as is everything contrived by man for the purpose of codifying love. For the woman the erotic principle has nothing whatever to do with "genital connections," or some such savoury formulae invented by the erotically blind masculine reason, and which, moreover, the opinionating devil in the woman delights to echo. Neither has it to do with "episodic adultery," nor "extramarital sexual intercourse," nor with "hoodwinking" the husband; but simply with love. Nobody but the absolute believer in the inviolability of traditional marriage could perpetrate such breaches of good taste, just as no one but a believer in God can really blaspheme. But whoever dares to question marriage cannot break it, and for him the legal definition has no validity, because, like St. Paul, he feels himself beyond the law, in the higher estate of love. But, because all those believers in the law so frequently trespass against their own laws, out of stupidity, temptation, or mere viciousness, the modern woman begins finally to wonder whether she too may not belong to the same category. [x, 38 f (G, 183)

Secretaries, stenographers, modistes—all are agents of this process, and by millions of subterranean channels they create the influence that is undermining marriage. For the desire of all these women is not concerned with sexual adventures—only stupidity could believe that—but with the state of marriage. The *beatae possidentes*, the married woman must be driven out; not as a rule by open and forcible means, but by that quiet and obstinate wish that works, as we all know, magically, like the fixed eye of the snake. This has always been the way of woman. [x, 23 f (G, 174)

It is no longer the question of a dozen or so of voluntary or involuntary old maids here and there; it is a matter of millions. Our legal code and our social morality offer no answer to this question. Or can the Church give a satisfactory answer? Should we build gigantic nunneries in order to provide suitable accommodation for these women? Or should police-controlled prostitution be increased? Obviously this is impossible, since we are dealing neither with saints nor with prostitutes, but with normal women who cannot register their spiritual claims with the police. They are decent women who want to marry, and if this is not possible, well—the next best thing. [x, 21 f (G, 172 f)

Unlived life is a destructive and irresistible force working quietly but relentlessly. The result is that the married woman begins to doubt marriage. The unmarried woman believes in it, because she desires marriage. [x, 24

It is a bad sign when physicians begin to write books of advice as to how to achieve a "complete marriage." Healthy people need no doctors. But marriage today has actually become rather unstable. (In America one fourth of the marriages end in divorce!) And what is noticeable in this connection is that the scapegoat is not the man this time, but the woman. She is the one who doubts and is uncertain. That this is the case is not surprising, since in post-war Europe there is such a notable excess of women that it would be inconceivable if there were no reaction from that side.   [x, 21 (G, 172)

Seldom, or perhaps never, does a marriage develop into an individual relationship smoothly and without crises; there is no coming to consciousness without pain.   [xix, 281 (G, 193)

Since the aims of the second half of life are different from those of the first, to linger too long in the youthful attitude means a division of the will. Consciousness still presses forward, in obedience as it were to its own inertia, but the unconscious lags behind because the strength and inner will-power needed for further expansion have been sapped. This lack of unity with oneself begets discontent, and since one is not conscious of the real state of things, the causes of it are ordinarily projected upon the married partner. Thus there grows up a critical atmosphere, the indispensable precondition to becoming conscious. This condition does not usually begin simultaneously for each of the married pair. The best of marriages cannot blot out individual differences so completely that the condition of the partners is absolutely identical. In general one will adapt himself to the marriage more quickly than the other. The one who is grounded on a positive relationship to the parents will find little or no difficulty in adjusting to the partner; the other, on the contrary, may be hindered by a deep-lying unconscious tie to the parents. The latter, therefore, will achieve a complete adaptation only later, and this adaptation, because won with greater difficulty, will perhaps be held longer intact. The difference in tempo on the one hand, and in the degree of development of the personality on the other, are the chief reasons which cause a typical difficulty to appear at a critical moment. [XIX, 282 f (G, 194 f)

Little wonder that by far the greater number of marriages reach their highest psychological limit in the fulfilment of the biological aim, without injury either to spiritual or moral health. Relatively few people fall into deep disharmony with themselves. Where there is much external pressure, from sheer lack of energy the conflict cannot reach a state of dramatic tension. But psychological insecurity increases in proportion to the social security, at first unconsciously, causing neuroses, then consciously, bringing with it separations, discord, divorces, and other marital disorders. On still higher levels possibilities of new psychological development are recognized; these touch the sphere of religion, where critical judgment comes to an end. [XIX, 294 (G, 203)

As to those—and they are many—who are not obliged to live in the present, it is most important that they believe in the ideal of marriage and hold to it. Because nothing is won when an ideal and an undoubted value is merely destroyed, unless something better comes in its place. Therefore, whether married or not, woman hesitates. She cannot go over whole-heartedly to the side of rebellion, but remains suspended in doubt.
[x, 37 (G, 182)

One thing, however, is indubitable—the woman of today is under the same process of transition as man. Whether this transition is a historical turning point or not remains to be seen.
[x, 8 (G, 164)

YOUTH AND AGE

To speak of the morning and spring, of the evening and autumn of life is not mere sentimental jargon. We thus give expression to a psychological truth and even more to physiological facts. [xix, 265 (j, 123)

Our life is like the course of the sun. In the morning the sun gains continually in strength until it blazes forth in the zenith-heat of high noon; then comes the enantiodromia: its continued movement forward does not mean an increase but a decrease in strength. Thus our task in handling young people is different from that presented by people who are getting on in years. In the case of the former, it is enough if we remove all the hindrances that make expansion and the upward way difficult; but for the latter, the older people, we must summon up all that gives support to the downward journey. [li, 134 (d, 77)

It is best not to apply to children the high ideal of education to personality. For what is generally understood by personality —namely, a definitely shaped, psychic abundance, capable of resistance and endowed with energy—is an adult ideal. It is only in an age when the individual is still unconscious of the problem of his so-called adulthood, or—still worse—when he consciously evades it, that people could wish to foist this ideal upon childhood. [xxvii, 183 f (f, 284)

If there is anything that we wish to change in the child, we should first examine it and see whether it is not something that could better be changed in ourselves. As an example, take our enthusiasm for pedagogy. Perhaps we misconstrue the pedagogical need, because it would remind us uncomfortably that we are ourselves still children in some ways and are in urgent want of bringing up. [xxvii, 185 (f, 285)

In general, our approach to education suffers from a one-sided emphasis upon the child who is to be brought up, and from an equally one-sided lack of emphasis upon the deficient upbringing of the adult educator.   [xxvii, 183 (F, 283)

I therefore suspect that the *furor paedogogicus* is a god-sent method of by-passing the central problem touched on by Schiller, namely the education of the educator. Children are educated by what the grown-up *is* and not by his *talk*.

[xlix, 136 (o, 130)

A child certainly allows himself to be impressed by the grand talk of its parents. But is it really imagined that the child is thereby educated? Actually it is the parents' lives that educate the child—what they add thereto by word and gesture at best serves only to confuse him. The same holds good for the teacher. But we have such a belief in method that, if only the method be good, the practice of it seems to hallow the teacher.

[ix, 578 f (i, 512)

An inferior man is never a good teacher. But he can conceal his injurious inferiority, which secretly poisons the pupil, behind an excellent method or an equally brilliant intellectual capacity. Naturally the pupil of riper years desires nothing better than the knowledge of useful methods, because he is already defeated by the general attitude, which believes in the victorious method. He has already learnt that the emptiest head, correctly echoing a method, is the best pupil. His whole environment not only urges but exemplifies the doctrine that all success and happiness are external, and that only the right method is needed to attain the haven of one's desires. Or is the life of his religious instructor likely to demonstrate that happiness which radiates from the treasure of the inner vision?

[ix, 579 (i, 512 f)

We think of our efficient teachers with a sense of recognition, but those who touched our humanity we remember with gratitude. Learning is the essential mineral, but warmth is the life-element for the child's soul, no less than for the growing plant.

[liii, 8

If education is understood as a means whereby a tree can be propped up into a beautifully artificial form, then psychoanalysis is not an educational method. But he who has a higher conception of education will value most that method in which the tree is cultured so that all the possibilities of growth with which it was endowed by nature can come to the fullest perfection.

[VI, 106

Aesthetism* is not fitted to solve the exceedingly serious and difficult problem of the education of man; for it always presupposes the very thing it should create, namely the capacity for the love of beauty. It actually prevents a deeper searching of the problem, since it always looks away from the evil, the ugly, and the difficult, and aims at enjoyment, even though it be of a noble kind. Aesthetism, therefore, lacks all moral motive power, because *au fond* it is still only refined hedonism. [IX, 169 (I, 152)

It is a well-known fact that children are almost uncannily sensitive to the teacher's personal shortcomings. They know intuitively the false from the true. Therefore the teacher should watch his own psychic condition, so that he can be sure of the source of the trouble when things are going wrong with a child in his care. He himself may be the unconscious cause of evil. Of course we should not be naïve about that: there are people, analysts, as well as teachers and parents, who secretly think that they have the right to behave as they like, and that it is up to the child to adapt for better or worse, much as he must adapt to the life of the world when the time comes for him to enter it. Such people are convinced at heart (not openly) that the only thing that matters is material success, and that the only convincing moral limitations are those of the penal code. Where unconditioned adaptation to the tangible powers of the world is accepted as the supreme principle, it would of course be vain to expect the person in authority to exercise psychological introspection as a moral obligation. I myself cannot endorse such a philosophy; but since we are not the judges of the world we cannot call such an attitude "wicked." We should know what our convictions are, and stand for them. Upon one's own philosophy, conscious or unconscious, depends one's ulti-

* I employ the word "aesthetism" [*Aesthetismus*] as an abbreviated expression for "aesthetic world-philosophy." Hence, I do not mean that aesthetism with the evil accompaniment of aesthetic action and sentimentality which might perhaps be described as "aestheticism" [*Aesthetizismus*]. (*Author's note.*)

mate interpretation of facts. Therefore it is wise to be as clear
as possible about one's subjective principles. As the man is, so
will be his ultimate truth.   [xl, 74 f (g, 369 f)

It is certainly right to open the eyes and the ears of the
younger generation to the wide world, but it is the greatest ab-
surdity to suppose that young people are thereby equipped for
life. This type of upbringing can only just help them to adapt
themselves to worldly realities, but no one seems to think of the
adaptation to the Self, to the psychic forces which are infinitely
stronger than any of the great worldly powers. True, there is
still one system of education, and that is the Christian Church.
But it cannot be denied that during the last two centuries
Christianity, just like Confucianism and Buddhism in China,
has lost a great part of its effectiveness as an educating force.
The reason is not the wickedness of man but the gradual and
general change of mentality of which the first symptom, where
we are concerned, was the Reformation. This change severely
shook the educative authority of the Church, and the crumbling
of the actual principle of authority set in. The inevitable result
was the growth in importance of the individual, which has
reached its greatest expression in the modern ideals of humanity, of social welfare, and of democratic equality of rights.
                                              [xxvii, 63 f

The fact that by far the greater part of mankind is not only
in need of leadership but also desires nothing better than to be
shepherded and protected justifies to some extent the moral
emphasis which the Church lays upon confession. The priest,
armed with all the attributes of fatherly power, is the responsible leader and shepherd of his flock. He is the father-confessor
and the members of his congregation are the confessing children. Thus the priest and the Church replace the parents, and
to this extent they free the individual from the narrower bonds
of the family. In so far as the priest is a personality of high
moral standing with a natural nobility of soul and corresponding spiritual culture, the institution of confession is an excellent
method of social guidance and education; and, in actual fact,
for more than fifteen hundred years it has fulfilled a prodigious
educative task. So long as the Christian Church of the Middle

113

Ages understood how to protect the arts and sciences—in which she was successful thanks to the wide tolerance which she showed at times towards worldly things—confession was an admirable method of education. But confession lost its educative value, at least for individuals of higher spiritual level, as soon as the Church proved unable to maintain its leadership in the sphere of the things of the mind, which was the inevitable result of spiritual rigidity.   [vi, 101 f

---

Besides the biological rights there are also spiritual rights which are equally inviolable. It is certainly not a matter of chance that primitive peoples, even in adult life, maintain the most fantastic assertions concerning well-known sexual processes, as for instance that coition has nothing to do with pregnancy. We might be tempted to suppose that these people do not even know the connection between the two processes, but closer investigation has shown that they know very well that in animals mating results in pregnancy. Only where man is concerned is the fact denied: it is not that it is not known, but it is denied because a mythological explanation which is free from concretism is preferred. It is not difficult to see that this phenomenon, which has frequently been found among primitive peoples, is the beginning of abstraction, which is of such importance for our whole culture. There is every reason to believe that the same is true for the psychology of the child.   [ii, 35

Childhood is not only important because it is the starting point for possible cripplings of instinct, but also because this is the time when, terrifying or encouraging, those far-seeing dreams and images come from the soul of the child, which prepare his whole destiny. In childhood, too, those retrospective intuitions first arise, which extend far beyond the limits of childish experience into the life of the ancestors. Thus in the child's soul there is already a "natural" as opposed to a spiritual condition.   [xiii, 88 (g, 59)

Fairy-stories seem to be the myths of childhood, and therefore, among other things, they contain the mythology which

114

the child has woven around sexual processes. The fascination which the poetic charm of the fairy-story has for adults is also perhaps due not least to the fact that some of these old theories are still alive in our unconscious. We experience an especially curious and secret feeling when some piece of our far-off childhood is stimulated, not reaching consciousness, but only sending a reflected ray of its intensity of feeling up into the conscious mind. [II, 24 f

An infantile individual is infantile because he has freed himself only insufficiently or not at all from the environment of childhood, that is to say from the adaptation to his parents; and so he reacts wrongly to the outside world, on the one hand, like a child to its parents, always crying for love and the immediate lavishing of feeling, and, on the other, identifying himself with the parents, because of the too close bond, so that he behaves like the father and like the mother. The infantile individual is not able to live himself and to find the type which belongs to him. [IV, 275

Nothing has a stronger influence psychologically on their environment, and especially on their children, than the unlived life of the parents. [XXVII, 106

As a rule, all of the life that could have been lived by the parents, but in which they were thwarted because of artificial motives, is bequeathed to the children in a perverted form. This means that the latter are unconsciously forced into a line of life that compensates for what was unfulfilled in the lives of the parents. It is because of this that exaggeratedly moral parents have so-called immoral children, that an irresponsible and vagrant father has a son who is afflicted with a pathological amount of ambition, etc. [XIX, 278 (G, 191)

To remain a child too long is childish, but it is just as childish to move away and then assume that childhood no longer exists because we do not see it. But if we return to the "children's land" we succumb to the fear of becoming childish, because we do not realize that everything psychic in origin has a double

115

face. One face looks forwards, the other back. It is ambivalent and therefore symbolic, like all living reality.

[LVIII, 95 f (M, 74)

The human being cannot live too long in the infantile environment, that is, in the bosom of his family, without serious danger to his psychic health. Life demands from him independence, and he who fails to answer the stern call through childish laziness and timidity is threatened with a neurosis. Once the neurosis has broken out, it becomes itself an ever-increasing justification to flee from the struggle with life and to withdraw permanently within the morally pernicious infantile atmosphere. [IV, 293

It is necessary for the health of the individual that, having been during his childhood a mere passive particle in a rotating system, he should, as an adult, himself become the centre of a new system. [IV, 388

If we try to extract the common and essential factors from the almost inexhaustible variety of individual problems found in the period of youth, we meet in nearly all cases with a particular feature: a more or less patent clinging to the childhood level of consciousness—a rebellion against the fateful forces in and around us which tend to involve us in the world. Something in us wishes to remain a child; to be unconscious, or, at most, conscious only of the ego; to reject everything foreign, or at least subject it to our will; to do nothing, or in any case indulge our own craving for pleasure or power. In this leaning we observe something like the inertia of matter; it is persistence in a hitherto existing state whose level of consciousness is smaller, narrower, and more egoistic than that of the dualistic stage. For in the latter the individual finds himself compelled to recognize and to accept what is different and strange as a part of his own life—as a kind of "also-I." [XIX, 257 (J, 116)

Obviously it is the youthful period of life that has most to gain from the thorough-going recognition of the instinctive

116

side. The timely recognition of sexuality, for example, can prevent that neurotic suppression which keeps a man unduly withdrawn from life, or which forces him into a wretched and unsuitable way of living with which he is bound to be in conflict. The proper recognition and evaluation of the normal instincts leads a young man into life and entangles him with fate, thus bringing him to life's necessities and the consequent sacrifices and efforts through which his character is developed and his experience matured. For the adult man, however, the continued extension of life is obviously not the right principle, because the descent towards the afternoon of life demands simplification, limitation, and intensification; that is to say, it demands individual culture.   [xiii, 101 f (g, 69)

It even seems as if young people who have had to struggle hard for their existence are spared inner problems, while those for whom adaptation is for some reason or other made easy run into problems of sex or conflicts growing from the sense of inferiority.   [xix, 256 (j, 116)

That solution of the problems of the period of youth which consists in restricting ourselves to the attainable is only temporarily valid and not lasting in a deeper sense. Of course, to win for oneself a place in society and so to transform one's nature that it is more or less fitted to this existence is in every instance an important achievement. It is a fight waged within oneself as well as outside, comparable to the struggle of the child to defend his ego. This struggle, we must grant, is for the most part unobserved because it happens in the dark; but when we see how stubbornly childish illusions, presuppositions, and egoistic habits are still clung to in later years we are able to realize the energy it took to form them. And so it is also with the ideals, convictions, guiding ideas, and attitudes which in the period of youth lead us out into life—for which we struggle, suffer, and win victories: they grow together with our own beings, we apparently change into them, and we therefore perpetuate them at pleasure and as a matter of course, just as the child asserts its ego in the face of the world and in spite of itself—occasionally even to spite itself.   [xix, 260 (j, 119)

117

Achievement, usefulness, and so forth are the ideals which appear to guide us out of the confusion of crowding problems. They may be our lodestars in the adventure of extending and solidifying our psychic existences—they may help us in striking our roots in the world; but they cannot guide us in the development of that wider consciousness to which we give the name of culture. In the period of youth, at any rate, this course is the normal one and in all circumstances preferable to merely tossing about in the welter of problems.   [xix, 259 (j, 118)

The nearer we approach to the middle of life, and the better we have succeeded in entrenching ourselves in our personal standpoints and social positions, the more it appears as if we had discovered the right course and the right ideals and principles of behaviour. For this reason we suppose them to be eternally valid, and make a virtue of unchangeably clinging to them. We wholly overlook the essential fact that the achievements which society rewards are won at the cost of a diminution of personality. Many—far too many—aspects of life which should also have been experienced lie in the lumber-room among dusty memories. Sometimes, even, they are glowing coals under grey ashes.   [xix, 260 f (j, 119 f)

The discovery of the value of human personality belongs to a riper age. For young people the search for the valuable personality is very often merely a cloak for the evasion of their biological duty. On the other hand, an older person's exaggerated looking back towards the sexual valuation of youth is an undiscerning and often cowardly and convenient retreat from a duty which demands the recognition of personal values and his own enrolment among the ranks of the priesthood of a newer civilization. The young neurotic shrinks back in terror from the extension of his tasks in life, the old from the dwindling and shrinking of the treasures he has attained.
          [vii, 47 (c, 274)

The psyche does not only *react;* it also gives its own individual reply to the influences at work upon it, and at least half the resulting configuration and its existing disposition is due to this. Civilization is never, and again never, to be regarded as merely reaction to environment. That shallow explanation we may abandon peacefully to the past century. It is just these very dispositions which we must regard as imperative in the psychological sphere; it is easy to get convincing proof daily of their compulsive power. What I call "biological duty" is identical with these dispositions.   [vii, 48 (c, 275)

It is highly important for a young person, who is still unadapted and has as yet achieved nothing, to shape the conscious ego as effectively as possible—that is, to educate the will. Unless he is positively a genius he even may not believe in anything active within himself that is not identical with his will. He must feel himself a man of will, and he may safely depreciate everything else within himself or suppose it subject to his will—for without this illusion he can scarcely bring about a social adaptation. It is otherwise with the patient in the second half of life, who no longer needs to educate his conscious will, but who, to understand the meaning of his individual life, must learn to experience his own inner being. Social usefulness is no longer an aim for him, although he does not question its desirability. Fully aware as he is of the social unimportance of his creative activity, he looks upon it as a way of working out his own development and thus benefiting himself. This activity likewise frees him progressively from a morbid dependence, and he thus wins an inner firmness and a new trust in himself.
[xix, 110 (j, 81)

The middle of life is a time of supreme psychological importance. The child begins its psychological life within very narrow limits, within the magic circle of the mother and the family. With developing maturity, the horizon and the spheres of one's own influence are widened; hope and intention are focused upon increasing the domains of personal power and property; desire reaches out to the world with an ever-widening range; the will of the individual becomes more and more identical with the natural goals of the unconscious motivations. Thus to a certain degree man breathes his life into things, until finally they begin to live of themselves and to increase, and imperceptibly he is overgrown by them. Mothers are overtaken by their children, men by their creations, and what was at first brought into being with labour and even the tensest kind of struggle can no longer be held in bounds. First it was a passion, then it became a duty, and finally it is an unbearable burden, a vampire which has sucked the life out of its creator into itself.

[xix, 281 f (G, 193 f)

Middle life is the moment of greatest unfolding, when a man still gives himself to his work with his whole power and his whole will. But in this very moment evening is born, and the second half of life begins. Passion now changes her face, and is called duty; what was voluntary becomes inexorable necessity, and the turnings of the way which formerly brought surprise and discovery become dulled by custom. The wine has fermented and begins to settle and clear. Conservative tendencies develop if all goes well; instead of looking forward one looks backward, for the most part involuntarily, and one begins to take account of the manner in which life has developed up to this point. Thus real motivations are sought and real discoveries made. The critical survey of himself and his fate permits a man to recognize his individuality, but this knowledge does not come to him easily. It is gained only through the severest shocks. [xix, 282 (G, 194)

Imagine the daily course of the sun—but a sun that is endowed with human feeling and man's limited consciousness. In the morning it arises from the nocturnal sea of unconsciousness and looks upon the wide, bright world which lies before it in an expanse that steadily widens the higher it climbs in the firmament. In this extension of its field of action caused by its own rising, the sun will discover its significance; it will see the attainment of the greatest possible height—the widest possible dissemination of its blessings—as its goal. In this conviction the sun pursues its unforeseen course to the zenith: unforeseen, because its career is unique and individual, and its culminating point could not be calculated in advance. At the stroke of noon the descent begins. And the descent means the reversal of all the ideals and values that were cherished in the morning.

[xix, 264 (J, 122)

The transition from morning to afternoon is a revaluation of earlier values. There comes the necessity of examining into the value of the opposites of our previous ideals, of becoming aware of the error in our former convictions, of recognizing the falsehood in what had before been truth, and of feeling how much resistance and even hostility lay in that which we had till now accepted as love. [LI, 136 (D, 78)

The wine of youth does not always clear with advancing years; oftentimes it grows turbid. [XIX, 262 (J, 120)

Wholly unprepared, they embark upon the second half of life. Or are there perhaps colleges for forty-year-olds which prepare them for their coming life and its demands as the ordinary colleges introduce our young people to a knowledge of the world and of life? No, there are none. Thoroughly unprepared we take the step into the afternoon of life; worse still, we take this step with the false presupposition that our truths and ideals will serve us as hitherto. But we cannot live the afternoon of life according to the programme of life's morning—for what was great in the morning will be little at evening, and what in the morning was true will at evening have become a lie.

[XIX, 266 f (J, 124 f)

Concerned solely with the education of youth, we disregard the education of the adult man, of whom it is always assumed —on what grounds who can say?—that he needs no more education. There is an almost total lack of guidance for this extraordinarily important change of attitude with its transformation of energy from the biological to the cultural form. The transformation process is individual and cannot be enforced through general rules and maxims. [XIII, 102 f (G, 70)

An inexperienced youth thinks, indeed, that one can let the old people go, because in any case there is nothing much that can be done with them: life is behind them, and they cannot be considered as much more than petrified pillars of the past. But it is a great error to assume that the meaning of life is exhausted with the period of youth and growth; that, for example, a woman who has passed the menopause is "finished." The afternoon of life is just as full of meaning as the morning, only its meaning and purpose is a wholly different one.   [LI, 134 f (D, 77)

Aging people should know that their lives are not mounting and unfolding but that an inexorable inner process forces the contraction of life. For a young person it is almost a sin—and certainly a danger—to be too much occupied with himself; but for the aging person it is a duty and a necessity to give serious attention to himself. After having lavished its light upon the world, the sun withdraws its rays in order to illumine itself. Instead of doing likewise, many old people prefer to be hypochondriacs, niggards, doctrinaires, applauders of the past, or eternal adolescents—all lamentable substitutes for the illumination of the self, but inevitable consequences of the delusion that the second half of life must be governed by the principles of the first.   [XIX, 267 f (J, 125)

The very frequent neurotic disturbances of adult years have this in common, that they betray the attempt to carry the psychic dispositions of youth beyond the threshold of the so-called years of discretion. Who does not know those touching old gentlemen who must always warm up the dish of their student days, who can fan the flames of life only by reminiscences of their heroic youth—and who for the rest, are stuck in a hopelessly wooden Philistinism? As a rule, to be sure, they have this one merit which it would be wrong to undervalue: they are not neurotic, but only boring or stereotyped. The neurotic is rather a person who can never have things as he would like them in the present and who can therefore never enjoy the past.
[XIX, 262 f (J, 121)
The right soil for the soul is natural life. He who will not follow this road is left hanging in the air and grows rigid. From the middle of life onwards, only those remain alive who are ready to die along with life.   [XXVII, 216

According to my experience there are, among people of mature age, very many for whom the development of individuality is an indispensable need. Thus I have formed the private and tentative opinion that it is just the mature man who, in our times, has the greatest need of some further education in individual culture after his youthful education, in school and perhaps in the university, has formed him on exclusively collective lines and soaked him through and through with the collective mentality.   [XIII, 101 (G, 68 f)

To be old is extremely unpopular. It is generally forgotten that not to be able to grow old is just as ridiculous as to be unable to outgrow childhood. A man of thirty who is still infantile is certainly to be pitied, but a youthful seventy-year-old, is that not delightful? But actually both are perverse, an offence to our sense of taste, psychological monstrosities. A young man who does not fight and conquer has missed the best of his youth, and an old man who does not understand how to listen to the secret of the stream which rushes from the summits to the valleys is as meaningless; he is a psychic mummy, nothing but a piece of petrified past. He stands outside his real life, repeating himself like a machine to the very height of deadening futility. What kind of a civilization, to require such ghostlike figures!   [XXVII, 217

To the psychotherapist an old man who cannot bid farewell to life appears as feeble and sickly as a young man who is unable to embrace it. And as a matter of fact, in many cases it is a question of the selfsame childish covetousness, of the same fear, the same obstinacy and wilfulness, in the one as in the other.
[XIX, 272 (J, 128 f)

A human being would certainly not grow to be seventy or eighty years old if this longevity had no meaning for the species to which he belongs. The afternoon of human life must also have a significance of its own and cannot be merely a pitiful appendage to life's morning. The significance of the morning undoubtedly lies in the development of the individual, our entrenchment in the outer world, the propagation of our kind and the care of our children. This is the obvious purpose of nature. But when this purpose has been attained—and even more than attained—shall the earning of money, the extension of conquests, and the expansion of life go steadily on beyond the bounds of all reason and sense? Whoever carries over into the afternoon the law of the morning—that is, the aims of nature—must pay for so doing with damage to his soul just as surely as a growing youth who tries to salvage his childish egoism must pay for this mistake with social failure. [xix, 268 (j, 125 f)

We must not forget that only a very few people are artists in life; that the art of life is the most distinguished and rarest of all the arts. Who ever succeeded in draining the whole cup with grace? So for many people all too much unlived life remains over—sometimes potentialities which they could never have lived with the best of wills. [xix, 270 (j, 127 f)

Our religions were always "schools for forty-year-olds" in the past, but how many people regard them as such today? How many of us older persons have really been brought up in such a school and prepared for the second half of life, for old age, death, and eternity? [xix, 268 (j, 125)

Just as a childish person shrinks back from the unknown in the world and in human existence, so the grown man shrinks back from the second half of life. It is as if unknown and dangerous tasks were expected of him; or as if he were threatened with sacrifices and losses which he does not wish to accept; or as if his life up to now seemed to him so fair and so precious that he could not do without it.—Is it perhaps at bottom the fear of death? That does not seem to me very probable, because as a rule death is still far in the distance, and is therefore regarded somewhat in the light of an abstraction. Experience shows us rather that the basis and cause of all the difficulties of this transition are to be found in a deep-seated and peculiar change within the psyche. [xix, 263 f (j, 122)

Personality develops itself in the course of life from germs that are hard or impossible to discern, and it is only our actions that reveal who we are. We are like the sun that nourishes the life of the earth and brings forth every kind of lovely, strange, and evil thing; we are like the mothers who bear in their wombs unknown happiness and suffering. At first we do not know what deeds or misdeeds, what destiny, what good or evil we contain, and only the autumn can show what the spring has engendered; only in the evening will it be seen what the morning began.

[XXVII, 187 f (F, 287)

Man has two aims: The first is the aim of nature, the begetting of children and all the business of protecting the brood; to this period belongs the gaining of money and social position. When this aim is satisfied, there begins another phase, namely, that of culture. For the attainment of the former goal we have the help of nature, and moreover of education; but little or nothing helps us towards the latter goal. Indeed, often a false ambition survives, in that an old man wants to be a youth again, or at least feels he must behave like one, although within himself he can no longer make believe. It is this that makes the transition from the natural to the cultural phase terribly difficult and bitter for many people. They cling to the illusions of youth, or at least to their children, in order to preserve in this way a fragment of illusion. One sees this in mothers, who find in their children their only justification, and who imagine they have to sink away into empty nothingness when they give them up. It is no wonder, then, that many bad neuroses develop at the beginning of the afternoon of life. It is a kind of second puberty period, a like repetition of storm and stress, not infrequently accompanied by all the tempests of passion. But the problems which appear in this age are no longer to be solved by the old rules; the hand of the clock cannot be turned back; what youth found and must find outside, the man of middle life must find within himself. [LI, 135 f (D, 77 f)

The psychic depths are nature, and nature is creative life. It is true that nature tears down what she has herself built up— yet she builds it once again. Whatever values in the visible world are destroyed by modern relativism, the psyche will produce their equivalents. [XIX, 427 (J, 248)

There is no human terror or abnormity that did not lie in the womb of a loving mother. As the sun shines upon the just and the unjust, and as women who bear and give suck protect the children of God and of the devil with equal love, unconcerned about the possible results, so we, too, are parts of this singular nature and, like it, carry within us the unpredictable.

[xxvii, 187 (f, 286)

It is the way of moralists to put little trust in God, as if they thought the fair tree of humanity flourished only by virtue of being propped up and trained on a trellis; whereas Father Sun and Mother Earth have allowed it to grow for their delight in accordance with laws of the deepest wisdom.   [v, 257 (d, 16 f)

It is evident that the rapid development of the towns, with the specialization of work brought about through the extraordinary division of labour, the increasing industrialization of the country, and the growing security of life deprive humanity of many opportunities of giving rein to its emotional energy. The farmer has a wealth of variety in his work and secures unconscious satisfaction through its symbolical content—a satisfaction which the workers in offices and factories do not know and can never enjoy. What do these know of the farmer's real life with nature; of those beautiful moments when, as lord and fructifier of the earth, he drives his plough through the ground, when with kingly gesture he scatters the seed for the future harvest; of his deep and justifiable fear of the destructive power of the elements, his joy in the fruitfulness of his wife who bears him the daughters and sons, who mean increased working power and prosperity? From all this, we city-dwellers, modern work-machines, are far, far removed. Is not the fairest and most natural of all satisfactions beginning to fail us, when we can no longer regard with unmixed joy the harvest of our own sowing, the "blessing" of children? Marriages in which all the modern devices are not practised are rare indeed. Is not this a first farewell to the joy which Mother Nature bestowed on her first-born son? From all this where is satisfaction to come from?

[v, 258 (d, 17)

If one wishes to see the undisturbed workings of Nature, one must not try to dictate to her.   [xi, 5

Nature has the primary claim on mankind, and only long after that comes the luxury of reason. The medieval ideal of a life lived for death should gradually be replaced by a more natural attitude to life, in which the natural claims of man are fully acknowledged, so that the desires of the animal sphere need no longer drag down the higher values of the spiritual sphere in order to be able to function at all.   [IV, 296 f

We should not rise above the earth with the aid of "spiritual" intuitions and run away from hard reality, as so often happens with people who have brilliant intuitions. We can never reach the level of our intuitions and should therefore not identify ourselves with them. Only the gods can pass over the rainbow bridge; mortal men must stick to the earth and are subject to its laws.   [LVIII, 165 (M, 148)

Reduction to the natural condition is for man neither an ideal nor a panacea. If the natural were really the ideal condition, then the primitive would be leading an enviable existence. But that is by no means so, for together with all the other sorrows and fatigues of human life, the primitive is tortured by superstitions, anxieties, and compulsions to such a degree that, if he lived in our civilization, he could not be described as other than profoundly neurotic, if not indeed mad.   [XIII, 84 (G, 56)

In the light of the possibilities revealed by intuition, man's earthliness is certainly a lamentable imperfection; but this very imperfection is part of his innate being, of his reality. He is compounded not only of his best intuitions, his highest ideals and aspirations, but also of the odious conditions of his existence, such as heredity and the indelible sequence of memories which shout after him: "You did it, and that's what you are!" Man may have lost his ancient saurian's tail, but in its stead he has a chain hanging on to his psyche which binds him to the earth—an anything-but-Homeric chain of conditions which weigh so heavy that it is better to remain bound to them, even at the risk of becoming neither a hero nor a saint. (History gives us some justification for not attaching any absolute value to these collective norms.) That we are bound to the earth does not mean that we cannot grow; on the contrary, it is the *sine qua non* of growth. No noble, well-grown tree ever disowned its dark roots, for it grows not only upwards but downwards as well. [LVIII, 165 f (M, 148)

The man in the first half of life, with its biological orientation, can usually, thanks to the youthfulness of his whole organism, afford to expand his life and make something of it that is generally serviceable. But the man in the second half of life is orientated towards culture, the diminishing powers of his organism permitting him to subordinate his instincts to the viewpoint of culture. [XIII, 102 (G, 69)

The development of culture is a process which consists, as we know, of a progressive taming of the animal side of man. It is a process of domestication which cannot be carried out without rebellion on the part of the animal nature which craves for freedom. From time to time a sort of delirium sweeps through mankind as it strives to fit itself into the mould imposed by culture. The ancient world experienced this frenzy in the wave of Dionysian orgies which came surging up from the East and which became an important and characteristic part of the culture of antiquity. This orgiastic spirit contributed in no small measure to the fact that, in many of the sects and schools of philosophy of the final pre-Christian century, the stoical ideal developed into asceticism, and that the chaos of polytheism of that epoch gave rise to the ascetic religions of Mithras and Christ. A second wave of Dionysian delirium swept through Western mankind during the Renaissance. It is difficult to judge our own age. Amongst the revolutionary questions which the last half-century has thrown up, the "sexual question" has produced a whole literature of its own. In this "movement" are rooted the beginnings of psychoanalysis, the theory of which was thereby considerably influenced in a one-sided direction. No one is ever quite free from the tendencies of his age. Since then, the "sexual question" has been pushed into the background to a great extent by problems of world politics. But this does not alter the fundamental fact that mankind's instinctive nature is forever straining against the bonds imposed by culture. The name changes, but the fact remains the same.

[LI, 36 f

Both these necessities exist in ourselves: Nature and culture. We cannot only be ourselves, we must also be related to others. Hence a way must be found that is not a mere rational compromise; it must also be a state or process that wholly corresponds with the living being, it must be a *semita et via sancta,* as the prophet says, a *via directa ita ut stulti non errent per eam.* ("A path and a holy way"; "a straight way so that fools shall not err therein."—Isaias 35:8.) [IX, 126 (I, 113)

No one can begin with the present; he must slowly grow into it, for without the past there is no present. The young man has not yet a past and, therefore, no present. Hence he does not create culture but merely existence. It is the privilege and task of riper age, that has passed the meridian of life, to produce culture. [X, 44 (G, 186 f)

When nature is left to herself energy is transformed along the lines of natural "gradients"; by this means, natural phenomena are produced, but not work. So also man when left to himself lives as a natural phenomenon and, in the proper meaning of the word, produces no work. It is culture that provides the machine through which the natural potentials are employed for the achievement of work. That man should ever have discovered this machine must be due to something rooted deep in his nature, in the very nature, indeed, of the living creature as such. For living matter is itself a transformer of energy, life participating, in some still unknown fashion, in the transformation process. Life takes place through the fact that it makes use of natural physical and chemical conditions as a means to its existence. [XIII, 70 (G, 45 f)

The opposites always balance on the scales—a sign of high culture. One-sidedness, though it lends momentum, is a mark of barbarism. [XV, 533 (H, 82)

129

Conscious capacity for one-sidedness is a sign of the highest culture. But involuntary one-sidedness, i.e., inability to be anything but one-sided, is a sign of barbarism. For the barbarian, this tendency to fall a victim to one-sidedness in one way or another, thereby losing sight of his whole personality, is a great and constant danger. [IX, 293 (I, 255 f)

The virgin earth demands that at least the unconscious of the conqueror sinks to the level of the autochthonic inhabitants. Thus in the American a distance separates the conscious from the unconscious that is not found in Europeans. It is a tension between a high level of culture in the conscious and an unmediated unconscious primitivity. But this tension provides a psychic potential that endows the American with an indomitable spirit of enterprise and an enviable enthusiasm which we in Europe do not know. The very fact that we are still in possession of our ancestor-spirits and that for us everything is historically mediated certainly gives us a contact with our unconscious, but we are also caught by this contact. In fact, so fast are we in an historical vice that great catastrophes are needed to loosen us from it, and to make us change our political behaviour from what it was five hundred years ago. The contact with the unconscious chains us to our earth and makes it hard for us to move, a fact that is to our disadvantage in respect to progressiveness and the many values of a plastic attitude.

[XIX, 209 (G, 140)

The greater the contrast, the greater is the potential. Great energy only comes from a correspondingly great tension between opposites. [XLVIII, 55

Hence no culture is ever really complete that swings towards a one-sided orientation, i.e., when at one time the cultural ideal is extroverted, the chief value being given to the *object* and the objective relation, while at another the ideal is introverted when the supreme importance lies with the individual or *subject* and his relation to the idea. In the former case, culture takes on a collective character, in the latter an individual.

[IX, 106 (I, 95)

No one makes history who does not dare to risk everything

for it, even his own skin. For he carries through the experiment, which is his own life, to the bitter end; and in so doing he interprets his life, not as a continuation but as a beginning. Continuation is a business already provided for in the animal, but to initiate is the prerogative of man, the one thing of which he can boast that transcends the animal.   [x, 41 (G, 184 f)

Money-making, social existence, family, and posterity are nothing but plain nature—not culture. Culture lies beyond the purpose of nature.   [xix, 269 (J, 126)

We Occidentals had learned to tame and subject the psyche, but we knew nothing about its methodical development and its functions. Our civilization is still young, and we therefore required all the devices of the animal-tamer to make the defiant barbarian and the savage in us in some measure tractable. But when we reach a higher cultural level, we must forego compulsion and turn to self-development.   [xix, 38 (J, 62)

And how is it now? If we were to express any opinion at all, we must confess that we manifestly need both civilization *and* culture, a shortening of the secondary function for the one and a prolongation for the other. For we cannot create the one without the other, and we are, unhappily, bound to admit that in humanity today there is a lack on either side. Or, to express ourselves more guardedly, where one is in excess, the other is deficient; for the continual harping upon progress has become untrustworthy and is under suspicion.
                    [ix, 399 (i, 352)

That which filled the Greeks with horror is still true today, but it is only true for us if we are able to give up a vain illusion of our times, i.e., that we are different and more moral than the ancient Greeks. We have merely succeeded in forgetting that there is an indissoluble bond between us and the man of antiquity. The realization of the existence of such a link would open a way to the real understanding of the spirit of antiquity such as never existed before, a way of inner sympathy on the one hand and of intellectual understanding on the other. By the indirect route of the buried foundations of our own souls we can realize the living spirit of the culture of antiquity, and this gives us a fixed point outside our own culture from which alone it is possible to get an objective understanding of its tendencies. That at least is what we hope from the rediscovery of the immortality of the Oedipus problem.   [IV, 5

Doubt concerning our culture and its values is the neurosis of this period. If our convictions were indisputable then they could not be doubted.   [XLV

Whoever is rooted in the soil endures. Remoteness from the unconscious, and therefore from the determining influence of history, means an uprooted state. That is the danger to the conqueror of foreign lands. It is also the danger confronting every individual who through one-sidedness in any kind of ism loses his relation with the dark, maternal, earthly origin of his being.   [XIX, 209 f (G, 140)

It is one of the most fundamental characteristics of every civilization that it has permanence and a man-made steadiness over against the senseless upheavals of nature. Every house, every bridge, every road, is a static and enduring achievement wrung from nature.   [XII, 10

The idea wants changelessness and eternity. Whoever lives under the supremacy of the idea strives for permanence; hence everything that pushes towards change must be against it.
                [IX, 138 (I, 124)

THE INDIVIDUAL AND THE COMMUNITY

To say anything fundamental about the civilized man of today is one of the most difficult and thankless of tasks. For we
can only speak as one of them, being caught in the same
presuppositions and blinded by the same prejudices as those
about whom we should be able to talk broadly and objectively.
[xix, 211

The modern man—or, let us say again, the man of the immediate present—is rarely met with. There are few who live up
to the name, for they must be conscious to a superlative degree.
Since to be wholly of the present means to be fully conscious
of one's existence as a man, it requires the most intensive and
extensive consciousness, with a minimum of unconsciousness.
It must be clearly understood that the mere fact of living in
the present does not make a man modern, for in that case everyone at present alive would be so. He alone is modern who is
fully conscious of the present.   [xix, 402 (j, 227)

We may define that man as normal who can somehow exist
under any circumstances that yield him in one way or another
the necessary minimum of the means of life. But countless is
the number of those for whom this is impossible; such normal
men are not to be found in any abundance.   [li, 101 (d, 54)

We always find in the patient a conflict which at a certain
point is connected with the great problems of society. Hence,
if analysis is pursued to this point, the apparently individual
conflict of the patient is revealed as a universal conflict of his
environment and epoch. Neurosis is thus, strictly speaking,
nothing less than an individual attempt, however unsuccessful,
at the solution of a universal problem. This must be so, for a
universal problem is not an *ens per se,* but exists only in the
hearts and minds of individuals.   [v, 268 f (d, 22 f)

A man can hope for satisfaction and fulfilment only in what

133

he does not yet possess; he cannot find pleasure in something of which he has already had too much. To be a socially adapted being has no charms for one to whom to be so is mere child's play. Always to do what is right becomes a bore for the man who knows how, whereas the eternal bungler cherishes the secret longing to be right for once in some distant future.—The needs and necessities of individuals vary. What sets one free is for another a prison—as for instance normality and adaptation. Although it is a biological dictum that man is a herd animal and is only healthy when he lives as a social being, yet the first case we observe may seem to upset this statement, and to prove that man is only healthy when leading an abnormal and unsocial life. [xix, 30 f (j, 55 f)

Man is not a machine in the sense that he can consistently maintain the same output of work. He can only meet the demands of outer necessity in an ideal way if he is also adapted to his own inner world, that is to say, if he is in harmony with himself. Conversely, he can only adapt to his inner world and achieve unity with himself when he is adapted to the environmental conditions. [xiii, 66 f (g, 43)

The old religions with their sublime and their ridiculous, their noble and horrible symbols, are not born out of the blue, but out of this very human soul that lives in us at this moment. All those things live in us in their primordial forms, and at any time they may break in upon us with destructive force, in the form of mass-suggestion, for example, against which the individual is defenceless. Our frightful gods have only changed their names—now they rhyme with "ism." Or is there any one bold enough to claim the World War or Bolshevism as an ingenious discovery? Just as our outer lives, therefore, are conditioned by a world in which at any time a continent may be submerged, or a pole be shifted, or a new pestilence break out, so our inner lives are determined by a world in which at any moment something similar may happen, albeit in the form of an idea, but no whit less dangerous and uncertain on that account. Failure to adapt to this inner world is an omission fraught with

just as serious results as is ignorance and incapacity in the outer
world.   [XI, 146 (D, 223 f)

There are many people whose conscious attitude is not deficient as regards adaptation to their surroundings but only as
regards the expression of their own character. These are people whose conscious attitude and achievements where adaptation is concerned overreach their individual possibilities; that
is, they appear better and of more value than they really are.
This outer "plus" on achievement is naturally never provided
by individual means alone, but mostly by the dynamic reserves
of collective suggestion. Such people climb up to a higher level
than befits their nature, for instance by means of the effect of
some collective ideal, or the attraction of a collective prejudice,
or by the support of the social mass. Such people are really not
equal inwardly to their outer stature.   [XIII, 146

Just as we naturally tend to assume that the world is such as
we see it, so we also naïvely assume that mankind is such as we
imagine it to be; although in this latter case no physics yet exist
to demonstrate the disparity between perception and reality.
Although the possibility of gross error is many times greater
than in the case of sensory perception, we yet continue, quite
unabashed and usually totally naïve, to project our own psychology on to our fellow beings. Everyone creates for himself
in this way a series of more or less imaginary relationships
which are based entirely on such projections.   [XIII, 158 f

The overwhelming majority of mankind are quite incapable
of putting themselves individually into the mind of another.
It is indeed quite a rare art, and at best cannot reach very far.
Even that man whom we think we know best and who assures
us himself that we know him through and through is at bottom
quite foreign to us. He is in fact different, and the most and
the best we can do is, at least, to divine this "otherness," to respect it, and to guard against the outrageous stupidity of wishing to interpret it.   [XI, 174 (D, 244)

It is well known that for the primitive that which is strange is hostile and evil. With us, in the later Middle Ages, the words which now mean what is foreign [*Fremde*] and what is miserable [*Elend*] were still identical. This qualification has a purpose, and therefore the normal man feels no necessity to make these projections conscious, although this state is dangerously illusory. The psychology of war has clearly brought this condition to light: everything which our own nation does is good, everything which the other nations do is wicked. The centre of all that is mean and vile is always to be found several miles behind the enemy's lines. This same primitive psychology appears in the individual, so that every attempt to make these eternally unconscious projections conscious is felt to be very uncongenial. Certainly we wish to have better relations with our fellow men, but naturally on condition that our fellow men fulfil our expectations, in other words, that they are willing to carry our projections. If we are to make these projections conscious, however, then a difficulty may easily arise in our relations to other people, for the bridge of illusion is missing over which love and hate can freely flow, and over which all those supposed virtues which hope to "raise" and "improve" others can also be so smoothly and satisfactorily carried over to the other man. [XIII, 158 f

It is so much easier to preach the universal panacea to everybody else than to take it oneself—and, as we all know, things are never so bad when everybody is in the same boat. No doubts can exist in the herd; the bigger the crowd the better the truth —and the greater the catastrophe. [LVII, 644 (M, 563)

Whatever mankind is fighting about in the outer world is also a battle within our own inner selves. For we must finally admit the fact that mankind is not a conglomeration of separate individualities, but contains such a high degree of psychological collectivity that in comparison the individual appears merely as a variation. How shall we judge a matter fairly if we cannot admit that it is also our own problem? Whoever can confess this to himself will first attempt to solve it in himself, and this in fact opens the way to the greater general solutions. [III, 313

What may be said of humanity in general is also valid for each individual, since humanity consists only of individuals, and as the psychology of humanity is so also is the psychology of the individual. In the World War we experienced a fearful reckoning with the rational purposiveness of civilized organization. What we call "will" in the individual is in the nation called "imperialism." For will is a demonstration of power over destiny, that is to say, an exclusion of the fortuitous. Civilized organization is rational, brought about through will and purpose—purposive sublimation of free and indifferent forms of energy. It is the same in the individual; and just as the idea of a universal cultural organization has received a fearful correction through this war, so must the individual during the course of his life often have to learn that so-called "disposable" forms of energy are not to be disposed of by him.

[LI, 91 f (D, 50)

We can best approximate to the truth if we picture to ourselves the conscious and personal psyche resting upon the wide foundation of an inherited and universal disposition of the mind, which as such is unconscious. Thus our personal psyche would be related to the collective psyche in much the same way as the individual is related to society. [XI, 45 (D, 150)

All human control comes to an end when the individual is caught in a mass movement and when the archetypes begin to function. We can observe the same phenomenon in the life of the individual when he is confronted with situations that cannot be dealt with in any way with which he is familiar.

[XXXVI, 667 (K, 13)

This war has thrown out the unanswerable accusation to civilized man that he is still a barbarian, and at the same time it has shown what inflexible retribution lies in store for him whenever he is tempted to make his neighbour responsible for his own bad qualities. Yet the psychology of the individual corresponds to the psychology of the nations. What the nations do each individual does, and as is the individual, so is the nation. Only in the change of attitude of the individual can begin the change in the psychology of the nation. [LI, 8 f (D, xii)

137

When fate, for four whole years, played out a war of monumental frightfulness on the stage of Europe—a war that nobody wanted—nobody dreamt of asking exactly who or what had caused the war and its continuation. Nobody realized that European man was possessed by something that robbed him of all free will. And this state of unconscious possession will continue undeterred until we Europeans become scared of our "god-almightiness." Such a change can begin only with individuals, for the masses are blind brutes, as we know to our cost.

[LVIII, 643 (M, 563)

When a problem that is at bottom personal, and therefore apparently subjective, impinges upon outer events which contain the same psychological elements as the personal conflict, it is suddenly transformed into a general question that embraces the whole of society. In this way the personal problem gains a dignity that was hitherto wanting, since a state of inner discord has an almost mortifying and degrading quality, so that one sinks into a humiliated condition both without and within, like a state dishonoured by civil war. It is this that makes one shrink from displaying before a larger public a purely personal conflict, provided, of course, that one does not suffer from an over-daring self-esteem. But when it happens that the connection between the personal problem and the larger contemporary events is discerned and understood, a relativity is established that promises release from the isolation of the purely personal; in other words, the subjective problem is amplified to the dimensions of a general question of our society.   [IX, 116 (I, 103 f)

Inasmuch as collectivities are mere accumulations of individuals, their problems are also accumulations of individual problems. One set of people identifies itself with the superior man and cannot descend, and the other set identifies itself with the inferior man and wants to reach the surface. Such problems are never solved by legislation or tricks. They are only solved by a general change of attitude. And the change does not begin with propaganda and mass meetings or with violence. It begins with a change in individuals. It will continue as a transformation of their personal likes and dislikes, of their outlook on life and of their values, and only the accumulation of such individual changes will produce a collective solution.

[XLVI, 142 f (B, 95)

When we consider the history of humanity, we see only the very outer surface of events and even these are warped by the dim mirror of tradition. What really happened escapes historical research, for the real historic happening is deeply hidden, lived by all and perceived by none. It is the most private, the most subjective, psychic life and experience. Wars, dynasties, social revolutions, conquests, and religions are all the most superficial symptoms of a secret psychic fundamental attitude in the individual, unknown to him and therefore not recorded by any chronicler. The great events of world history are in themselves of small importance. What is important in the final reckoning is only the subjective life of the individual. This alone makes history, and it is in it alone that all the great changes begin, and all future and all world history arise as an enormous summation from this hidden source of the individual. In our most private and subjective lives, we are not only these who suffer but also those who make the age. Our age—it is we ourselves!   [XXVII, 55 f

I hold the view that the greatest changes in human history are to be traced back to internal causal conditions, and that they are founded upon internal psychological necessity. For it often seems that external conditions serve merely as occasions on which a new attitude long in preparation becomes manifest. The development of the Christian era is an example of this. Political, social, and religious conditions influence the unconscious, since all the factors which are suppressed in the conscious religious or philosophical attitude of human society accumulate in the unconscious. This gradual accumulation means a gradual increase of the energy of the unconscious contents. Certain individuals gifted with particularly refined intuition become aware of the change going on in the collective unconscious, and sometimes even succeed in translating perceptions of it into communicable ideas. The new ideas spread more or less rapidly in accordance with the state of readiness in the unconscious of other people. In proportion to the more or less universal unconscious readiness, people are ready to accept

139

new ideas, or else to show particular resistance to them. New ideas are not only the enemies of old ones; they also appear often in an extremely unacceptable form. [xiii, 220 f (G, 265)

Like the ancients, who with a view to individual development catered to the claims of an upper class by an almost total suppression of the great majority of the common people (helots and slaves), the subsequent Christian world reached a condition of collective culture through an identical process, albeit translated as far as possible into the individual sphere (or raised to the subjective level, as we prefer to express it). While the value of the individual was proclaimed to be an imperishable soul by the Christian dogma, it became no longer possible for the inferior majority of the people to be suppressed for the freedom of a superior minority, but now the superior function was preferred over the inferior functions in the *individual*. In this way the chief importance was transferred to the one valued function, to the prejudice of all the rest. Psychologically this meant that the external form of society in antique civilization was translated into the subject, whereby in individual psychology an inner condition was produced which had been external in the older civilization, namely, a dominating, preferred function, which became developed and differentiated at the expense of an inferior majority. By means of this psychological process a collective culture gradually came into existence, in which *les droits de l'homme* certainly had an immeasurably greater guarantee than with the ancients. But it had this disadvantage, that it depended upon a subjective slave-culture, i.e., upon a transfer of the antique majority enslavement into the psychological sphere, whereby collective culture was undoubtedly enhanced while individual culture depreciated. Just as the enslavement of the mass was the open wound of the antique world, the enslavement of the inferior function is an ever-bleeding wound in the soul of man today.

[ix, 103 f (i, 93 f)

The ego lives in space and time and must adapt itself to their laws if it is to exist at all. If it is absorbed by the unconscious to such an extent that the latter alone has the power of decision, then the ego is stifled, and there is no longer any medium in which the unconscious could be integrated and in which the work of realization could take place. The separation of the empirical ego from the "eternal" and universal man is therefore of vital importance, particularly today, when mass-degeneration of the personality is making such threatening strides. Mass-degeneration does not come only from without: it also comes from within, from the collective unconscious. As regards the former, some protection was afforded by the *droits de l'homme* which at present are lost to the greater part of Europe, and even where they are not actually lost we see political parties, as naïve as they are powerful, doing their best to abolish them in favour of the slave state, with the bait of social security. Against the demonism from within, the Church offers some protection so long as it wields authority. But protection and security are only valuable if they do not cramp life excessively; and in the same way the superiority of consciousness is desirable only if it does not suppress and exclude too much of our existence. As always, life is a voyage between Scylla and Charybdis. [LX, 210 f (N, 477)

As the unconditional authority of the Christian *Weltanschauung* loses more and more ground, we shall become increasingly aware of the "blond beast" stirring in its subterranean prison, and threatening us with an outbreak that will have devastating consequences. [VIII, 471 (K, 73)

Dionysus is the abyss of passionate dissolution, where all human distinctions are merged in the animal divinity of the primordial psyche—a blissful and terrible experience. Humanity, sheltering behind the walls of its culture, believes it has escaped this experience, until it succeeds in letting loose another orgy of bloodshed. All well-meaning people are amazed when this happens and blame high finance, the armaments industry, the Jews, or the Freemasons. [LVIII, 134 (M, 118)

The catastrophe of the Great War and the subsequent extraordinary manifestations of a profound mental disturbance were needed to arouse a doubt that everything was well with the white man's mind. When the war broke out we had been

141

quite certain that the world could be righted by rational means. Now we behold the amazing spectacle of States taking over the age-old claim of theocracy, that is, of totality, inevitably accompanied by suppression of free opinion. We again see people cutting each other's throats to support childish theories of how to produce paradise on earth. It is not very difficult to see that the powers of the underworld—not to say of hell—which were formerly more or less successfully chained and made serviceable in a gigantic mental edifice, are now creating, or trying to create, a State slavery and a State prison devoid of any mental or spiritual charm. There are not a few people, nowadays, who are convinced that mere human reason is not entirely up to the enormous task of fettering the volcano.   [XLVI, 87 f (B, 58 f)

There is indeed reason enough why man should be afraid of those non-personal forces because they never, or almost never, appear in our personal dealings and under ordinary circumstances. But if, on the other hand, people crowd together and form a mob, then the dynamics of the collective man are set free—beasts or demons which lie dormant in every person till he is part of a mob. Man in the crowd is unconsciously lowered to an inferior moral and intellectual level, to that level which is always there, below the threshold of consciousness, ready to break forth as soon as it is stimulated through the formation of a crowd.   [XLVI, 26 f (B, 15 f)

The change of character that is brought about by the uprush of collective forces is amazing. A gentle and reasonable being can be transformed into a maniac or a savage. One is always inclined to lay the blame on external circumstances, but nothing could explode in us if it had not been there. As a matter of fact, we are always living upon a volcano and there is, as far as we know, no human means of protection against a possible outburst which will destroy everybody within its reach. It is certainly a good thing to preach reason and common sense, but what if your audience is a lunatic asylum or a crowd in a collective seizure? There is not much difference either, because the madman as well as the mob is moved by non-personal, overwhelming forces.   [XLVI, 27 f (B, 16 f)

As a reaction to the former exaggerated individualistic trend, a compensatory regression to the collective man has set in. Collective man has become paramount, and his authority simply consists of the weight of the masses. No wonder that we have a feeling of impending disaster, as if an avalanche had broken loose which no mortal power is capable of holding up. Collective man is threatening to suffocate the individual, the very individual who is absolutely indispensable, for it is on his sense of responsibility that every human achievement is ultimately founded. [xxvii, 64 (k, 76)

No one can flatter himself that he is immune from the spirit of his own epoch, or even that he possesses a full understanding of it. Irrespective of our conscious convictions, each one of us, without exception, being a particle of the general mass, is somewhere attached to, coloured by, or even undermined by the spirit which goes through the mass. Freedom stretches only as far as the limits of our consciousness. [xlviii, 54 f

Contemporaries are in the great majority only fitted to maintain and appraise the immediate present, thus helping to bring about that same fatal issue whose confusion the divining, creative mind had already sought to unravel. [ix, 382 (i, 319)

If I undergo what is called a communal experience within the group, this occurs at a deeper level of consciousness than when I experience something alone. Therefore the group-experience is much more frequent than an individual experience of transformation. It is also much easier to achieve, for the collective presence of many people has a great suggestive power. The individual within the mass is extremely suggestible. As soon as he becomes part of the mass, man is below his usual level. Of course he can retain the memory of the ethically superior being which he once was, but when he is in the mass this memory is no more than an illusion. It suffices for something to happen—for instance, a proposal is made which the whole mass adopts, and he is also for it even if the proposal is immoral. Within the mass man feels no sense of responsibility, but also no fear. [xlviii, 418

The fact that individual consciousness means separation and hostility has been experienced innumerable times by humanity, both individually and as a whole. And just as in the individual the period of division (inner conflict) is a period of illness, so it also is in the life of a people. We can hardly deny any longer that our present age is such a period of division and sickness. The political and social conditions, the religious and philosophic ruptures, modern art and modern psychology, all indicate the same verdict. And does anyone who has even a trace of a human sense of responsibility feel at all happy about it? If we are honest, we must admit that in this modern world no one is quite at ease; in fact we become increasingly uneasy. The word "crisis" is also a *medical* term to denote the dangerous height of an illness. [xxvii, 41 f

Whenever any contents of the collective unconscious become animated, the conscious feels disturbed, more often apparently in a disagreeable than in an agreeable way. This may be due to the fact that disagreeable experiences always make a greater impression than agreeable ones. In any case animation of the collective unconscious creates a certain confusion in the conscious. If this animation is due to a complete breakdown of all conscious hopes and expectations, the danger arises that the unconscious may take the place of conscious reality. Such a state is morbid. If, on the other hand, the animation of the collective unconscious is due to psychological processes in the unconscious of the whole people, the individual may well feel threatened or at least disoriented, but this state is not morbid— at any rate, not so far as the individual is concerned. The mental condition of the whole people, however, could then be compared to a psychosis. [xiii, 221 f (G, 265)

Great conglomerations of people are always the breeding grounds of psychic epidemics. [xlvii, 420

It is difficult to judge the present age in which we are living. But if we look back at the spiritual case history of humanity, then we see earlier onslaughts of the same illness which we can more easily judge. One of the worst cases was the Roman world-illness of the first Christian centuries. The phenomenon of dissociation appeared in an unexampled disruption of political and social conditions, of religious and philosophical convictions, and in a deplorable decline of the arts and sciences. If we reduce humanity of that epoch to one single human being, we have a personality highly differentiated in every way, which had first conquered its surroundings with a superior self-assurance, but then, after these successful achievements, had scattered its energy in so many individual occupations and interests, and had thereby forgotten its own origin and tradition and even its own memory to such an extent, that it now appeared to itself to be "this" or "that" and thus fell into a disastrous conflict with itself. The conflict eventually led to such a state of weakness that the formerly conquered world around broke up in a devastating way and completed the process of destruction.

[xxvii, 42 f

Individuals in society, and above all in the State, may control the stream of life to a certain extent and regulate it like a canal. But when it comes to the life of the nations, the water is like a great rushing river which lies far beyond the control of man, in the hands of one who has always been stronger than man. The League of Nations was given international authority, but some people now regard it as a child in need of care and protection, and others as a miscarriage. Therefore there is no bridle on the life of the nations and it rolls on unconsciously, with no idea of where it is going, like a rock crashing down the side of a hill, until it is stopped by an obstacle which is stronger than itself. Political events thus move from one impasse to the next, like the water in a stream that finds itself caught in gullies, whirlpools, and marshes.   [xxxvi, 666 f (к, 12 f)

We have to look for the sense, for at first we can only see nonsense, especially in our present-day world. It is really one of the most difficult things of all to discover any sense in it. And the search is enormously complicated by the fact that there are already so many "senses"; millions of short-lived, short-legged, short-breathed "purposes" which appear to all who are involved in them up to their necks to be extremely full of sense, the more so the more senseless they really are. This desperate scene becomes oppressive when, removed from the limited and less painful individual sphere, it unfolds itself as the so-called soul of a people. [XII, 3

But since every person is blindly convinced that he is nothing but his very modest and unimportant consciousness, which neatly fulfils duties and earns a moderate living, nobody is aware that this whole rationally organized crowd, called a state or a nation, is run by a seemingly impersonal, imperceptible, but terrific power, checked by nobody and by nothing. This ghastly power is mostly explained by fear of the neighbouring nation, which is supposed to be possessed by a malevolent devil. As nobody is capable of recognizing where and how much he himself is possessed and unconscious, one simply projects one's own condition upon the neighbour, and thus it becomes a sacred duty to have the biggest guns and the most poisonous gas. The worst of it is that one is quite right. All one's neighbours are ruled by an uncontrolled and uncontrollable fear just like oneself. In lunatic asylums it is a well-known fact that patients are far more dangerous when suffering from fear than when moved by wrath or hatred. [XLVI, 89 (B, 60)

Within the mass, an increasing degree of *participation mystique* prevails, which is nothing else than an unconscious identity. Take, for instance, a man at the theatre: everybody looks at everybody else, all eyes are looking to see what the other eyes are doing, and all hang upon the invisible threads of a mutual unconscious relationship. When this condition increases, the person is actually carried by the general wave of this state of identity. It can be a pleasant feeling: one sheep among ten thousand sheep. Or if I take the throng to be a great and glorious unity, then I am a hero, raised with the whole group. When I come to myself again, I discover that my name is so-and-so, and that I live in such-and-such a street on the third floor, and that this whole experience was really wonderful. I only hope that it will happen again tomorrow so that I may once again feel like a whole people, which is much better than merely to feel like citizen so-and-so. Since it is an easy, comfortable way of raising the personality up a step, man has

146

always formed groups which make possible the collective experience of transformation, often in a state of delirium. This re-identification with lower more primitive states of consciousness is always coupled with a feeling of increased zest for life.

[XLVII, 419

Man has one capacity, which is of the greatest possible service for collective aims, but which is quite the most harmful for individuation, namely, the power of imitation. Social psychology cannot dispense with imitation, for without it mass organizations, the State, and the ordering of society are simply impossible. Imitation embraces suggestibility, i.e., the influence of suggestion and mental contagion: it must be evident therefore that imitation, and not laws and statutes, is responsible for the ordering of society. But every day, on the other hand, we can see how the mechanism of imitation is used, or rather misused, for the purpose of personal differentiation. A distinguished personality, an unusual characteristic or activity, is simply imitated, whereby a certain superficial distinction from the immediate environment is achieved. As punishment for this—one is almost bound to express it in these terms—the essential resemblance to the spirit of the environment is intensified to the point of an unconscious compulsive union with it. Usually this falsified attempt at individual differentiation does not go beyond a pose, and the imitator stays on his former level, only several degrees more sterile than before.

[XI, 59 f (D, 161 f)

The element of differentiation is the individual. All the highest achievements as well as all the vilest deeds are individual. The greater a community is, and the more the summation of collective factors peculiar to every large community is supported by conservative prejudice to the detriment of everything individual, the more will the individual be morally and spiritually crushed. And thus the only source of moral and spiritual progress is choked up. Naturally, in such an atmosphere, the only things that can flourish are society and all the collective elements in the individual. All that is individual in a man has to go under, which means it is repressed. The individ-

147

ual elements are forced into the unconscious, where they become transformed regularly into the principle of evil. The destructive and anarchical tendencies thus produced have a bearing socially, it is true, through certain prophetically inclined individuals, or through conspicuous crimes like regicide and the like, but in the great mass of the community they remain in the background, and are seen only indirectly in the inevitable moral degeneration of society.   [xi, 55 (d, 158)

It is a well-known fact that the morality of a society as a whole is in inverse ratio to its size; for the more individuals congregate together, the more individual factors become blotted out. This means the decay of morality, which rests entirely upon the moral feeling of the individual, the indispensable condition of which is freedom. It follows that every man is unconsciously a worse man, in a certain sense, when he is in society than when acting alone; he is carried by the group and to that extent is relieved of his individual responsibility.

[xi, 55 f (d, 158 f)

A large company that is made up of entirely admirable people resembles, in respect to its morality and intelligence, an unwieldy, stupid, and violent animal. Hence the larger the organization, the more is its immorality and blind stupidity inevitable. (*Senatus bestia, senatores boni viri.*) By automatically stressing the collective qualities in its individual representatives, society will necessarily set a premium on everything that is average and that tends to vegetate in an easy, irresponsible way. It is unavoidable that individuality will be driven to the wall. This process begins in school, continues at the university, and rules everything in which the state has a hand. In a smaller social body, the individuality of its members is better safeguarded, their relative freedom is greater, and hence there is a wider possibility of conscious responsibility. Without freedom there can be no morality.   [xi, 56 f (d, 159)

The populace always stands at a low level however high it wishes to climb above its neighbours. A gathering of a hundred highly intelligent men, when summed up, forms one big idiot, because every talent, whether of intellectual or moral nature, is in the final count an individual differentiation. Differentiation is synonymous with difference. Differences do not accumulate; they mutually efface each other. What does accumulate is the general human factor, the "human-all-too-human," ultimately all that is primitive, stupid, indolent, and without will-power. Thus spirituality is never superfluous; it is a rare and inestimable treasure. [xii, 2

The stacking together of the paintings of the great masters in museums is a catastrophe, and a collection of a hundred good intellects produces collectively one idiot. [xxix, 79

Our admiration of our great organizations would soon dwindle were we to become aware of the other side of the wonder, namely, the tremendous heaping up and accentuation of all that is primitive in man and the unavoidable disintegration of his individuality in favour of that monstrosity which every great organization, on its nether side, is. A man of today who corresponds more or less to the collective moral ideal has made his heart into a den of murderers. [xi, 56 f (d, 159)

Nature cares nothing whatsoever about a higher level of consciousness; quite the contrary. And then society does not value these feats of the psyche very highly; its prizes are always given for achievement and not for personality—the latter being rewarded, for the most part, posthumously. [xix, 258 f (j, 118)

The levelling down of humanity into a herd, by suppressing the natural aristocratic or hierarchic structure, must inevitably lead sooner or later to a catastrophe. For if all that is distinguished is levelled down, then all orientation is lost and the yearning to be led becomes inevitable. [liii, 10 f

The attempts which are being made to achieve individual consciousness and to mature the personality are, regarded from the social point of view, still too weak to carry any weight at all in face of historical necessity. If the social order in Europe is not to be shaken to its foundations, then authority must at all costs be immediately re-established. This is probably what lies behind the tendency which has arisen in Europe to set up the collectivity of the State as a substitute for the collectivity of the Church. Just as the Church was once absolute in its endeavour to make theocracy a reality, so the State now makes an absolute claim to exclusive totality. The ruling principle of spirit has not been replaced by a ruling principle derived from nature or from the *lumen naturae*, as Paracelsus called it, but by the total incorporation of the individual into a political collectivity called "the State." [LIX, 12 (K, 28)

Society as a whole needs the magically effective person; accordingly it makes use of the will to power in the individual and of the will to submit in the many as vehicles to this end. Together these two components create personal prestige. This latter phenomenon possesses, as is shown in the history of political beginnings, the very greatest importance for the common life of the people. [XI, 51 (D, 155)

The crowd in itself is always anonymous and irresponsible. So-called Fuehrers are the inevitable symptoms of a massmovement. The true leaders of men are always those who carry themselves, and relieve the crowd at least of their own weight, in that they consciously do not allow themselves to be carried away by the blind laws of nature that move the masses.—But who can hope to withstand the overwhelming force that is drawing people like a maelstrom, in which they all cling together and drag each other down? Only he who is rooted in the inner as well as the outer world. [XXVII, 64 (K, 76)

One might think that a man of genius could browse in the greatness of his own thoughts and dispense with the cheap applause of the mob which he despises. But actually he falls a victim to the more mighty herd instinct; his searching, his findings, and his call are inexorably meant for the crowd and must be heard. [IV, 13

The importance of personal prestige can hardly be overstated, because it also involves the very real danger of a regressive loss of individuality in the collective psyche, not only for the distinguished individual, but also for his followers. This possibility is most likely to occur when the goal of the prestige, namely, general recognition, has been reached. The person then becomes a collective truth. When this point is reached it is always the beginning of the end. To gain prestige is not only a positive achievement for the distinguished individual; it is also an asset to his clan. The individual distinguishes himself by his deeds, the many by their renunciation of power. So long as this attitude needs to be defended and maintained against adverse environmental influences, the achievement remains positive; but as soon as there are no more obstacles, and general recognition is attained, the prestige loses its positive value and becomes, as a rule, a dead letter. A schismatic movement is now due, whereby the process repeats itself. [XI, 52 (D, 156)

My occupation, it is true, is my special activity; but it also has a collective factor, which has come about historically through the co-operation of many people, and its dignity rests upon the collective approval to which it owes its existence. When, therefore, I identify myself with my profession or my title, I behave as though I myself were also the whole complex of social factors of which a profession consists, or as though I were the bearer not only of the office but also and at the same time of the approval of society that supports it. In so doing, I have made an extraordinary extension of myself, and have usurped qualities which do not belong to me, but are outside of me. [XI, 38 (D, 145 f)

There exists a deep gulf between what a man is and what he represents, i.e., between the man as an individual and his function-capacity as a collective being. His function is developed at the expense of his individuality. Should he excel, he is merely identical with his collective function; but should he not, then, although certainly esteemed as a function in society, he is as an individuality wholly on the side of his inferior, undeveloped functions, and therefore simply barbarous, whereas the former has more fortunately deceived himself concerning his actually existing barbarism. [IX, 107 (I, 96)

Through his identification with the collective psyche, man

151

is invariably tempted to force the demands of his unconscious upon others, since the state of identity with the collective psyche is always accompanied by a feeling of general validity (godlikeness) which simply disregards the differences in the personal psychology of his fellow men. (The feeling of general validity comes from the universality of the collective psyche.) A collective attitude naturally presupposes the same collective attitude in others. But that means a ruthless disregard not only of individual distinctions but also of those of a more general kind within the collective psyche itself, such, for example, as differences of race. This disregard of individual distinctiveness naturally means the suffocation of the single individual, the consequence of which is a rapid obliteration of the element of differentiation in the community.   [xi, 54 f (d, 157 f)

If man cannot exist without society, neither can he exist without oxygen, water, albumen, fat, and so on. Like these, society is one of the necessary conditions for his existence. It would be ludicrous to maintain that man exists in order to breathe air. It is equally ludicrous to say that man exists for the sake of society. "Society" is nothing more than the concept of the symbiosis of a group of human beings. A concept is not a carrier of life. The sole and natural carrier of life is the individual, and this holds true throughout nature.

[lix, 14 (k, 31)

Although general biological instinct-forces make the moulding of personality possible, individuality is nevertheless essentially different from general instincts; indeed, it stands in the most direct opposition to them, just as the individual is as a personality always distinct from the collective. Its essence consists precisely in this distinction. What every ego-psychology must therefore exclude and ignore is just the collective element that is essential to instinct-psychology, for it is describing that very ego-process which is differentiated from collective instincts.

[ix, 86 (i, 78 f)

For the discovery of the truly individual elements in ourselves, a fundamental and unflinching reflection is required; and then, suddenly, we become aware of the immense difficulty of the task which individuality necessarily entails.

[xi, 60 (d, 162)

When we examine ourselves closely, we are astonished to see how much of our so-called individual psychology is really collective. So much is this the case that what is individual seems to be completely overshadowed and obliterated by it. But inasmuch as individuation is a quite indispensable psychological requirement, it is possible to infer from this estimation of the superior force of the collective what extremely careful attention is demanded by this tender plant, individuality, if it is not to be completely smothered by the collective.

[XI, 58 f (D, 161)

We tend to indulge in the ridiculous fear that man, as he really is, is an absolutely impossible being, and that if all men were as they really are, a terrible social catastrophe would result. Many modern individualists imagine, in a very one-sided way, that man as he really is is merely that eternally dissatisfied, anarchist, covetous element in human nature and quite forget that the very same human race has also created the strictly set forms of modern civilization, which have shown a greater permanence and strength than the undercurrent of anarchism. The fact of the superior strength of the social personality is an essential condition of life for humanity. If it were not so, then mankind would cease to exist. The craving and rebelliousness which we meet in the psychology of the neurotic subject is not mankind as it really is, but an infantile caricature. In reality the normal man is "an upholder of the state and a moral citizen"; he makes laws and keeps to them; and not because he is compelled to do so by outside forces—that would be a childish idea—but because he prefers law and order to moods, disorder, and lawlessness. [VI, 106 f

The difficulty of the psychological differences of men, this most necessary factor in providing the vital energy of a human society, no social legislation will surmount. It may well serve a useful purpose, therefore, to speak of the heterogeneity of men. These differences involve such different claims to happiness that even the most consummate legislation could never give them approximate satisfaction. No general external form could be devised, however equitable and just it might appear, that would not involve injustice for one or other human type. That in spite of this fact, every kind of enthusiast—political, social, philosophical, and religious—is at work endeavouring to find those general and uniform external conditions which shall signify a more general opportunity for happiness seems to me to be linked up with a general attitude to life too exclusively oriented by external facts. [ıx, 694 (ı, 618 f)

Although it is certainly a fine thing that every man should stand equal before the law, that every man should have his political vote, and that no man through inherited social position and privilege should unjustly overreach his brother, nevertheless it is distinctly less beautiful when the notion of equality is extended to other provinces of life. A man must needs have a very clouded vision or must regard human society from a very misty distance to cherish the view that a uniform distribution of happiness can be won through a uniform regulation of life. Such a man must already be somewhat deluded if he can really cling to the notion that, for instance, the same amount of income, or the same external opportunities of life, must possess approximately the same significance for all. But what would such a legislator do with all those for whom life's greatest possibility lies not without, but within? Were he just, he would have to give at least twice as much to one man as to another, since to the one it means much, to the other little.

[ıx, 693 f (ı, 618)

The misfortune lies in this: that never, under any circumstances, do *les lois des nations* possess that admirable accord with the laws of nature which could enable the civilized to be at the same time a natural state. If such a settlement could be regarded as at all possible, it could be conceived only as a compromise wherein neither of the two conditions would attain its own ideal but both would remain far below it. Whoever wishes to attain the ideal of either state will have to rest with the statement that Rousseau himself formulated: *"Il faut opter entre faire un homme ou un citoyen: car on ne peut faire à la fois l'un et l'autre"* ("One must choose whether to make a man or a citizen; for at the same time one cannot make both").

[ıx, 126 (ı, 112 f)

We can think of a human being as the leader of a small army in the struggle with his environment, a war not infrequently on two fronts, before him the battle for existence, in the rear the battle against his own rebellious instinctive nature. Even to those of us who are not pessimists our existence feels more like a battle than anything else. A state of peace is a desideratum, and when a man has found peace with himself and the world, it is indeed a noteworthy event.   [xix, 299 (G, 143)

The optimum of life is not to be found upon the line of crude egoism, since man, whose fundamental make-up discerns an absolutely indispensable meaning in the happiness he brings to his neighbour, can never win his life's optimum upon the line of egoism. An unbridled craving for individual pre-eminence is equally unfitted to achieve this optimum, since the collective element is so strongly rooted in man that his yearning for fellowship destroys all pleasure in naked egoism. The optimum of life can be gained only by obedience to the tidal laws of the libido, by which systole alternates with diastole—laws which provide happiness and the necessary limitations, even setting the life-tasks of the individual nature, without whose accomplishment life's optimum can never be achieved.

[ix, 301 f (i, 263)

The reality of man is no fair semblance, but a true likeness of that eternal human nature which links together all humanity, an image of human life in its heights and depths which is common to all of us. In this reality we are no longer differentiated persons (*persona* = mask), but are conscious of the common human bonds. In this reality we leave aside the social and superficial distinctions of our personalities, and reach down to the real problems of the present day, problems which do not arise out of myself—or at least so I imagine. But in this reality I can no longer deny the fact that I feel and know myself to be one of many, and what moves the many moves me.

[x, 35 (G, 181)

We cannot be ashamed of ourselves as a nation, nor can we change ourselves as such. Only those individuals can change or improve themselves who are able to develop spiritually beyond the national prejudices. The national character is an involuntary fate which is imposed upon the individual like a beautiful or an ugly body. It is not the will of the individual which conditions the rise and fall of a nation, but super-personal factors, the spirit and the earth, which mould the people by incomprehensible ways out of a dark background. It is therefore illusory to praise or blame nations, for no one can change them. Furthermore the idea of "nation" (as also that of "state") is a personification which really only corresponds with a certain nuance of the individual psyche. The living being is a separate being, and the nation has no such separate life of its own and is therefore not an end in itself. The nation is nothing but a character, either a disadvantage or an advantage, and is therefore at the best only a means to an end.   [xii, 9

The secret of the earth is not a joke and not a paradox. We need only see how in America the skull- and hip-measurements of all European races become Indianized in the second generation. That is the secret of the American soil. And every soil has its secret, of which we carry an unconscious image in our souls: a relationship of spirit to body and of body to earth.   [xviii, 471

The Swiss national character, built up during hundreds of years, is no coincidence but a meaningful reaction to the contradictory, disintegrating, and therefore dangerous influences of the surroundings. Just as Switzerland must understand why a mentality like Keyserling's criticized it so sharply, so also it must understand that just its characteristics which are most open to attack are part of its indispensable possession.   [xii, 11

Our most lovely mountain, which dominates Switzerland far and wide, is called the Jungfrau. The Virgin Mary is the patron saint of Switzerland, and Tertullian says of this Virgin: "*Illa terra virgo nondum pluviis rigata . . .*" ("This virgin land has not been watered by rain . . ."), and St. Augustine says: "*Veritas de terra orta est, quia Christus de Virgine natus est*" ("Truth is born of the earth, because Christ was born of the Virgin")—which is a living reminder that the Virgin Mother is the earth. Since ancient times, the astrological sign of the zodiac for Switzerland has been either the Virgin or the Bull; both are so-called earth-symbols, and this is an infallible sign that the ancient astrologers had already recognized the chthonic character of the Swiss. From this close tie with the earth come all the good and the bad characteristics of the Swiss, their deep-rootedness, their limitations, their lack of spirituality, their parsimony, their love of solid values, their obstinacy, their rejection of everything foreign, their suspiciousness, their terrible Swiss-German dialect, and their indifference or neutrality, politically expressed. Switzerland consists of many valleys, deep furrows in the earth's crust, in which the settlements of man are embedded. There are no great plains where the choice of a spot to live in is immaterial, where there are no sunny parts and shady parts, and there are no wide coastlines bordering the oceans of the world with their suggestion of far-off lands. In the very backbone of the continent, burrowing into the earth, the troglodytic Alpine people live, surrounded by mighty nations to whom the wide world belongs, with their colonies and their natural resources to enrich them. The soul of the Swiss clings to that which he has, for the rest belongs to the others, the mighty. Under no circumstances will he allow his possessions to be taken from him. His people is a small people and his possessions are few. If he should lose them, how should he ever replace them? [xii, 7

We are in reality unable to borrow or absorb anything from outside, from the world, or from history. What is essential to us can only grow out of ourselves. When the white man is true to his instincts, he reacts defensively against any advice that one might give him. What he has already swallowed he is forced to reject again as if it were a foreign body, for his blood refuses to assimilate anything sprung from foreign soil.
[xxviii, 203 (f, 31)

It is true that an earlier and deeper level of psychic development can be tapped, where it is still impossible to distinguish between an Aryan, Semitic, Hamitic, or Mongolian mentality, since all human races have a common collective psyche. But with the beginning of racial differentiation, essential differences are developed in the collective psyche. For this reason, we cannot transplant the spirit of a foreign race *in globo* into our mentality without sensible injury. [xi, 54 (d, 157 f)

From the standpoint of maintaining the species, a more or less purely instinctive choice might be considered the best, but from the psychological standpoint it is not always fortunate, since there often exists great disparity between the purely instinctive and the individually differentiated personality. In such a case the race might indeed be invigorated by a purely instinctive choice, but individual happiness may be destroyed.

[XIX, 279 (G, 191 f)

It is sometimes said that the Swiss has a particular resistance to the problem of himself. I must protest against this accusation. The Swiss *is* introspective but he would not admit it for anything in the world, even when he notices the wind in his own land. We thus pay our silent tribute to the Germanic time of storm and stress, but we never mention it, which enables us to feel vastly superior. Yet it is the German who has the best chance to learn; in fact, he has an opportunity which is perhaps unique in history. He is experiencing the perils of the soul from which Christianity tried to rescue mankind, and he can learn to realize the nature of these perils in his own innermost heart.

[XXXVI, 663 f (K, 9)

Does a neutral Switzerland, with its backward, earthy nature, fulfil a significant function in the European system? I believe that this question should be answered in the affirmative. For the political or cultural question has not only one aspect—spirit, progress, change—but also the other side of it—remaining steady and standing firm. The eternal progress is known to go downhill at times; and in contrast to a perilously rapid tempo, a halt may mean real salvation. The nations also become weary and long for a stabilization of political and social factors. What did the Pax Romana mean to Imperial Rome?   [XII, 10

There are two kinds of interference against which the Swiss raises his hackles: the political and the spiritual. It is quite obvious why he must defend himself to the utmost against political interference (this extreme resistance is the art of neutrality born of necessity). But that he should also defend himself against spiritual interference is more mysterious, yet undoubtedly true. I can confirm this from my own practical experience: the British, the Americans, and the Germans, as patients, are far more receptive to new ideas than the Swiss. An idea usually means for them no particular risk, whereas it does for a Swiss. For him a new idea is something like an unknown, dangerous animal which is to be avoided if possible or at least only approached with caution.   [XII, 9

If it is true that we are the most backward, conservative, obstinate, self-satisfied, and bristly of all nations, then this means for the European that he is sound at his centre, deep-rooted, unconcerned, self-confident, conservative, and backward, i.e., still deeply bound to the past and neutral between the fluctuating and contradictory aims and opinions of the other nations or functions. It would be no unworthy role for Switzerland to represent the earth-heaviness of Europe and to fulfil the function of a centre of gravity.   [XII, 9

It is the tragedy of all innovations that the good is always thrown out with the bad. Thank heavens that the craze for innovations is not a Swiss national weakness par excellence, but we live in a bigger world which is shaken by the unknown fever of innovation. In face of this fearful and grandiose display, we demand from our young people more urgently than ever before the quality of constancy, not only as a guarantee for the permanence of our own country but also for the sake of European culture which will gain nothing if the achievements of our Christian past are to be replaced by their very opposite.—The talented man is he who carries the torch and he is chosen for this high duty by nature herself.   [LIII, 8

Self-divestiture in favour of the collective corresponds to a social ideal; it even passes for social duty and virtue, although it can also be misused for egoistical purposes. Egoists are often called "self-centred." This, naturally, has nothing to do with the concept of "self," as I am using it here. On the other hand, self-realization seems to stand in opposition to self-divestiture. This misunderstanding is quite general, and it arises from the fact that not enough distinction is made between individualism and individuation. Individualism is a purposeful attempt to stress and make conspicuous some ostensible peculiarity, in opposition to collective considerations and obligations. But individuation means precisely a better and more complete fulfilment of the collective dispositions of mankind, since an adequate consideration of the peculiarity of the individual is more conducive to a better social achievement than when the peculiarity is neglected or repressed. [xi, 91 f (d, 183 f)

The revolution in our conscious outlook, brought about by the catastrophic results of the World War, shows itself in our inner life by the shattering of our faith in ourselves and our own worth. We used to regard foreigners—the other side—as political and moral reprobates; but the modern man is forced to recognize that he is politically and morally just like anyone else. Whereas I formerly believed it to be my bounden duty to call other persons to order, I now admit that I need calling to order myself. [xix, 411 (j, 234)

THE WORLD OF VALUES

Man, and man only
Can do the impossible;
He 'tis distinguisheth
Chooseth and judgeth;
He to the moment
Endurance can lend.

He and he only
The good can reward,
The bad can punish,
Can heal and can save;
All that wanders and strays
Can usefully blend.

—GOETHE, "The Godlike"

AWARENESS AND CREATIVE LIVING

Knowledge rests not upon truth alone, but upon error also.
⌊xix, 79 (j, 136)

I do not call the man who admits his ignorance an obscurantist; I think it is much rather the man whose consciousness is not sufficiently developed to be aware of its ignorance.
[lviii, 644 (m, 564)

I cannot accept that point of view which suppresses certain possible working hypotheses because they may not be valid forever or because they may be erroneous. [iv, 413

The ideal and the purpose of science do not consist in giving the most exact possible description of facts—science cannot yet compete with cinematographic and phonographic records; it can fulfil its aim and purpose only in the establishment of law, which is merely an abbreviated expression for manifold and yet correlated processes. This purpose transcends the purely experimental by means of the concept, which, in spite of general and proved validity, will always be a product of the subjective psychological constellation of the investigator. In the making of scientific theory and concept much that is personal and incidental is involved. There is also a psychological personal equation, not merely a psychophysical. [ix, 18 (i, 16)

We can see colours but not wave-lengths. This well-known fact must nowhere be more seriously held in view than in psychology. The operation of the personal equation has already begun in the act of observation. One sees what one can best see from oneself. Thus, first and foremost, one sees the mote in one's brother's eye. No doubt the mote is there, but the beam sits in one's own—and may somewhat hinder the act of seeing. I misdoubt the principle of "pure observation" in so-called objective psychology, unless one confines oneself to the eyepieces of the chronoscope, or to the ergograph and such "psychological" apparatus. With such methods one also insures oneself against too great a yield of experimental psychological facts.

But the personal psychological equation becomes even more important in the presentation or the communication of observations, to say nothing of the interpretation and abstraction of the experimental material. Nowhere, as in psychology, is the basic requirement so indispensable that the observer and investigator should be adequate to his object, in the sense that he should be able to see not the subject only but also the object. The demand that he should see *only* objectively is quite out of the question, for it is impossible. We may well be satisfied if we do not see *too* subjectively.   [ɪx, 18 f (ɪ, 16 f)

Every psychologist should first and foremost be convinced that his point of view is primarily his own subjective prejudice. This prejudice is however as good as another, and can very probably serve as a basic assumption for many other people. It is therefore usually worth while applying such a point of view as widely as possible. It will doubtless bear fruit of a certain usefulness. But under no circumstances should we indulge in the unscientific illusion that a subjective prejudice can represent a universal basic psychic truth. No true science can result from such an illusion, only a belief whose shadow-side is impatience and fanaticism. Contradictory views are necessary to the birth of a science; only they should not be set up in opposition to each other, but should be synthesized as soon as possible.   [xxv, 639

In the century and a half which has elapsed since the *Critique of Pure Reason,* the realization has gradually gained ground that thought, reasoning, understanding, etc., are not processes with an independent existence of their own, free from all subjective conditionality and obeying only the eternal laws of logic; they are rather psychic functions which are co-ordinated and subordinated to a personality. The question is no longer: has a thing been seen, heard, handled, weighed, counted, thought about, and deemed to be logical? The question now runs: *who* has seen, *who* has heard, *who* has thought about it? Beginning with the "personal equation" in the observation and measurement of minimal processes, this criticism extends to the creation of an empirical psychology such as no previous age had known. Nowadays we are convinced that

164

there are psychological premises in all fields of knowledge which definitely influence the choice of material, the method of working, the type of conclusion reached, and the construction of hypotheses and theories. We even believe that the personality of Kant was the determining factor underlying his *Critique of Pure Reason*. Not only our philosophers but also our own philosophical tendencies and indeed our so-called "best" truths become somewhat disturbed, if not dangerously undermined, at the thought of a personal premise. All creative freedom—we cry in protest—is thus taken from us: What! should a man be able to think, say, and do only that which he is?

[XLIII, 40 f

What to the causal view is fact to the final view is symbol; and conversely, what to the one standpoint is essential is to the other inessential. We are therefore forced to resort to the antinomic postulate and to consider the world also as a psychical phenomenon. Certainly it is indispensable for science to know how things are in themselves, but even science cannot escape the psychological conditions of knowledge; and psychology must be peculiarly alive to these conditions. [XIII, 41 f (G, 25)

It is, for instance, an immediately intelligible fact to an ordinary human intelligence that every philosophy that is not just a mere history of philosophy depends upon a personal psychological precondition. This precondition may be of a purely individual nature, and moreover would ordinarily be so regarded, if a true psychological criticism existed at all. Because it has always been taken for granted, we have thereby overlooked the fact that what we regarded as individual prejudice was certainly not so under all circumstances, since the standpoint of the philosopher in question often boasted a very imposing following. His standpoint was acceptable to these men not because they echoed him without thinking but because it was something they could fully understand and appreciate. Such an understanding would be quite impossible if the standpoint of the philosopher were merely individually determined, for it is quite certain in that case that he would neither be fully understood nor even tolerated. The peculiar character of the standpoint which is understood and appreciated by his following must, therefore, correspond to a typical personal attitude, which in the same or similar form finds many representatives in human society. As a rule, the partisans of either side attack each other merely externally, always seeking out the joints in their opponent's individual armour. Such a dispute, as a rule, bears little fruit. It would be of considerably greater value if the contest were transferred to the psychological realm, whence it actually originates. Such a transposition would soon reveal the fact that many different kinds of psychological attitudes exist, each of which has a right to existence, although necessarily leading to the setting up of incompatible theories. As long as one tries to settle the dispute by forms of external compromise, one merely satisfies the modest claims of shallow minds that have never yet glowed with the passion of a principle.   [ix, 694 f (i, 619)

Since I am not a philosopher but an empiricist, I cannot allow myself to assume that my own particular temperament, i.e., my individual attitude towards problems of thought, is of general validity. Apparently philosophers may do so, for they constantly assume that their disposition and attitude are general and refuse to recognize their individual problems as an important condition of their philosophy.   [xliii, 404

The newest developments in psychology show with an ever greater clarity that not only are there no simple formulae from which the world of the soul might be derived, but also that we have never yet succeeded in defining the psychic field of experience with adequate certainty. Indeed, scientific psychology, despite its immense extension on the surface, has not even begun to free itself from a mountain-high mass of prejudices which persistently bars its entrance to the real soul. Psychology as the youngest of the sciences has only just developed and therefore is suffering from all those children's diseases which afflicted the adolescence of the other sciences in the late Middle Ages. There still exist psychologies which limit the psychic field of experience to consciousness and its contents or which understand the psychic to be only a phenomenon of reaction without any trace of autonomy. The existence of an unconscious psyche has not yet attained undisputed validity, despite the presence of an overwhelming amount of empirical material

which could prove beyond all peradventure that there can be
no psychology of consciousness without the recognition of the
unconscious. Without this foundation, no datum of psychology,
if it be in any way complex in nature, can be dealt with. Moreover, the actual soul with which we have to deal in life and in
reality is complexity itself.   [xxxiii, 10 (a, ix f)

It is really time that academic psychology became converted
to reality and sought to know something about the real human
soul and not merely about laboratory experiments. It should
no longer be possible for professors to forbid their students to
study psychoanalysis or to use the analytical ideas, and our
psychology should no longer be reproached for "taking everyday experiences into account" in an unscientific way. I know
that general psychology would reap the greatest benefit from
a serious study of the problem of dreams, for instance, if it
could only at last free itself from the totally unjustifiable assumption that dreams have their origin in somatic stimuli. The
overrating of the somatic factor in psychiatry also is one of the
chief reasons why pathological psychology does not progress
when it is not directly fertilized by analysis. The dogma that
"mental diseases are diseases of the brain" is a survival of the
materialism of the eighteen-seventies. It has become a prejudice which has not the least justification and which inhibits all
progress.   [xiii, 182 f

People are indignant at the thought of "metaphysical phan-
toms," if anyone explains cellular processes according to the
vitalistic point of view, but at the same time a physical hypothesis is taken to be very "scientific" although it is no less fantastic.
Nevertheless it fits into the materialistic prejudice, and therefore every kind of nonsense which promises to change psychological phenomena into physical has the sanction of science. It
is to be hoped that the time is no longer far distant when this
relic of a rusty materialism which has become devoid of thought
can finally be dropped by our scientists.   [xiii, 184

Only he who regards world events as a chain of more or less
erroneous coincidences, and therefore believes in the constant
need of the educating hand of man endowed with reason, can

come to the conclusion that the psychoanalyst's method of research was a "wrong road" which should be marked "dangerous." Apart from the deeper insight into psychological determination, we have to thank this "wrong road" for the raising of questions of incalculable consequence. We should rejoice and be thankful that Freud had the courage to follow this path. It is not such things that hinder the progress of science but rather the conservative clinging forever to views once held, that typical conservatism of authority, the childish pride of the scholar in his infallibility and his fear of being wrong. This unwillingness to make any sacrifice does more harm to the reputation and greatness of scientific knowledge than an honest mistake. When will the unnecessary squabbling about who is right cease? If we look back on the history of science, how many have been right and how many have remained right?

[VI, 44

To a certain intellectual mediocrity, characterized by enlightened rationalism, a scientific theory that simplifies matters is a very good means of defence, because of the tremendous faith of modern man in anything which bears the label "scientific." Such a label sets your mind at rest immediately, almost as well as *Roma locuta causa finita*.   [XLVI, 83 f (B, 55 f)

In the field of psychology, theories are among the most devastating things. Of course we need certain theoretical standpoints for the sake of their orientation and heuristic value. But they should always be taken as merely helpful concepts, which can be laid aside at any moment. We know so little about the psyche that it is positively ridiculous to believe that we are so far advanced as to be able to make general theories about it. We have not even established the empirical extent of the phenomenology of the psyche. How then can we even dream of making general theories? A theory, however, is the best shield behind which to conceal lack of experience and sheer ignorance. But the consequences are grievous: narrow-mindedness, superficiality, and scientific sectarianism.   [II, 7

168

It is natural that the latest nominalism should claim a general validity, although it is based on a definite and therefore limited presupposition depending on temperament. Its claim runs: valid is that which comes from outside and can therefore be verified. The ideal case would be experimental confirmation. The antithesis to this says: valid is that which comes from inside and cannot be verified. The hopelessness of this standpoint strikes us at once. The natural philosophy of ancient Greece, which tends to materialism, combined with the reasoning of Aristotle won a late but definite victory over Plato. But in every victory lies the germ of future defeat.   [XLII, 405

Psychology, as one of the psyche's many expressions of life, works with ideas and conceptions which are themselves drawn from archetypal structures and therefore produce merely a somewhat more abstract form of myth. Psychology thus translates the archaic language of myths into a modern mythological theme, which is not yet recognized as such, and this mythological theme forms an element of the myth termed "science." This useless activity is myth, living and lived, and therefore satisfying and even healing to people of suitable temperament.
                    [XLIX, 132

Medieval alchemy prepared the greatest attack on the divine order of the universe which mankind has ever dared. Alchemy is the dawn of the age of natural sciences which, through the *daemonium* of the scientific spirit, drove nature and her forces into the service of mankind to a hitherto unheard of degree. Here are the real roots, the secular psychic processes of preparation for those factors which are at work in the world today. Technics and science have indeed conquered the world, but whether the soul has gained thereby is another matter.
                    [XLVIII, 72 f

It is not possible to derive any philosophical system from the elementary thoughts of primitive man. They furnish us only with antinomies. And yet it is just these which are the inexhaustible source of all mental effort and provide the problems of thought in all times and in all civilizations.   [XIX, 245 (J, 172)

Science comes to a stop at the frontiers of logic, but nature does not—she thrives on ground as yet untrodden by theory. *Venerabilis natura* does not halt at the opposites; she uses them to create, out of opposition, a new birth.   [LX, 230 (N, 499)

But a man is only a true philosopher when he succeeds in transmuting a primitive and purely natural vision into an abstract idea belonging to the universality of consciousness. It is this achievement, and this alone, which is his personal value, and which he must appraise as such. The personal value (in other words) lies in the philosophical achievement and not in the primary vision. The genesis of the vision is the same with the philosopher, the idea just accruing to him as a part of general human property, in which, theoretically, every one shares. The golden apples come from the same tree, whether culled by a locksmith's imbecile apprentice or by a Schopenhauer.

[XI, 40 f (D, 147 f)

I do not regard the work of science as a competition to be right at all costs but as a labour for the increase and deepening of knowledge.   [IV, 413

Our psychology is a science which can be reproached at worst with having discovered the dynamite with which terrorists also work. What the moralist, the practical man in general, does with it is not our business and we have no intention of interfering. Plenty of officious and unsuitable people are sure to push their way in and do the most foolish things with it, but even this cannot affect us. Our aim is simply and solely scientific knowledge, which cannot afford to be concerned with the turmoil that it has caused. Should religion and morals be blown to pieces by it, so much the worse for him if they have not more stability. Knowledge is also a force of nature which goes its way with an inner and irresistible necessity. Here likewise there can be no "hushing up" and bargaining, only an unconditional acceptance.   [III, 314

Until recently psychology was a special branch of philosophy, but now we are coming to something which Nietzsche foresaw—the ascendancy of psychology in its own right. It is even

170

threatening to swallow philosophy. The inner resemblance of the two disciplines consists in this, that both are systems of opinion about subject-matter which cannot be fully experienced and therefore cannot be comprehended by a purely empirical approach. Both fields of study thus encourage speculation, with the result that opinions are formed in such variety and profusion that heavy volumes are needed to contain them all, whether they belong to the one field or to the other. Neither discipline can do without the other, and the one always furnishes the implicit—and frequently even unconscious—primary assumptions of the other. [xxvii, 9 (j, 207)

The assumption that there exists only one psychology or only one fundamental psychological principle is an intolerable tyranny, belonging to the pseudo-scientific prejudice of the normal man. People are always speaking of *the* man and of his "psychology," which is invariably traced back to the "nothing else but." In the same way one always talks of *the* reality, as though there were only one. Reality is that which works in a human soul and not that which certain people assume to be operative and about which prejudiced generalizations are wont to be made. Moreover, however scientifically such generalizations may be advanced, it must not be forgotten that science is not the *summa* of life, that it is indeed only one of the psychological attitudes, only one of the forms of human thought.
[ix, 60 (i, 56)

Yet there is not *one* modern psychology—there are several. This is curious enough when we remember that there is only one science of mathematics, of geology, zoology, botany, and so forth. But there are so many psychologies that an American university was able to publish a thick volume under the title *Psychologies of 1930*. I believe there are as many psychologies as philosophies, for there is also no one single philosophy, but many. I mention this for the reason that philosophy and psychology are linked by indissoluble bonds which are kept in being by the interrelation of their subject-matters. Psychology takes the psyche for its subject-matter, and philosophy—to put it briefly—takes the world. [xxvii, 8 f (j, 206)

Has it ever been known—except in the very dark ages of history—that a scientific truth needed to be raised to the dignity of a dogma? Truth can always stand on its own; only opinions that have shaky foundations require the prop of dogmatizing. Fanaticism is the ever-present brother of doubt.   [xxvi, 2

Dogma and science, in my opinion, are incommensurable, and when melted together they damage each other. Dogma is of inestimable value as a religious factor, just because of its absolute standpoint. But science which presumes to ignore criticism and scepticism itself degenerates into a diseased cave-plant. Science needs the most extreme uncertainty as a life element. Wherever science shows a tendency towards dogma and consequently to intolerance and fanaticism, it is highly probable that a justifiable doubt is being hidden and an all-too-well-founded uncertainty is being explained away.   [xvii, 6

It is not every man's lot to be blessed with a faith which anticipates all solutions, and it is not given to all men to rest content and without further desire in the sunshine of revealed truth. That light, which is lit in the heart *per gratiam spiritus sancti,* just that *lumen naturae,* however small it may be, is more important to these, the seekers, or at least as important as the big light which "shineth in the darkness and the darkness comprehended it not." They found that in the very darkness of nature a light was hidden, a scintilla, without which the darkness itself would not be black.   [xlviii, 131

One-sidedness occurs again and again in the history of science. But this is not a reproach; on the contrary, we must be glad that there are men who have the courage to be extreme and one-sided. It is to them that we owe discoveries. It is only to be regretted when everyone passionately defends his own one-sidedness. Scientific theories are only suggestions as to how we could regard things.   [vi, 19

Science as such has no boundaries, and there is no such thing as a specialism which can boast of complete self-sufficiency. When it approaches the limits of its sphere it is bound to spill over into the adjoining territory if it is to make serious claim to the status of a science.   [lix, 3 f (k, 18)

Wherever we are unconsciously working against ourselves there is always impatience, irritability, and a powerless urge once and for all to subdue the opponent by every contrivable means. This state of things usually produces certain symptoms, among which is the use of a peculiar language: people then wish to impress the opponent by speaking forcefully, and therefore they use a special forceful style with new words, so-called neologisms, which can be described as "power-words." We meet this symptom not only in the psychiatric clinics but also in certain of our latest philosophers, and especially where-ever it is a matter of pushing through something incredible against an inner resistance. Then language swells and over-reaches itself and coins strange words, characterized by an un-necessary complexity. The words are expected to accomplish that which cannot be achieved by fair means. It is the ancient "magic of words," which can sometimes develop into a positive mania. [xlviii, 60

After all everyone carries the torch of knowledge only a short stretch, and no one is proof against error. Doubt alone is the father of scientific truth. He who combats dogma in a higher sense falls, tragically enough, all too easily under the tyranny of a half-truth. [xlv

Science as an end in itself is assuredly a high ideal, but its accomplishment brings about as many "ends in themselves" as there are sciences and arts. Naturally this leads to a high differ-entiation and specialization of the particular functions con-cerned, but it also leads to their aloofness from the world and from life, and an inevitable multiplication of specialized ter-rains, which gradually lose all connection with each other. The result of this is an impoverishment and stagnation that is not merely confined to the specialized terrains, but also invades the psyche of the man, who is thus divided up or reduced down to the specialist level. By this token must science prove her value to life; it is not enough that she be mistress—she must also be maid. By so doing she in no way dishonours herself.
[ix, 83 (i, 76)

Science is not, indeed, a perfect instrument, but none the less it is an invaluable, superior one which only works harm when taken as an end in itself. Scientific method must serve; it errs when it usurps a throne. It must be ready to serve all branches of science, because each, by reason of its insufficiency, has need of support from the others. Science is the best tool of the Western mind and with it more doors can be opened than with bare hands. Thus it is part and parcel of our understanding and only clouds our insight when it lays claim to being the one and only way of comprehending. [xiv, 10 (h, 78)

Whoever seeks to minimize the merits of Western science is undermining the main support of the European mind.
[xiv, 15 (h, 77 f)

When we are speaking of the relation of psychology to the work of art we are standing outside the realm of art, and here it is impossible for us not to speculate. We must interpret; we must find meaning in things, otherwise we should be quite unable to think about them. We must resolve life and happenings, all that fulfils itself in itself, into images, meanings, concepts; and thereby we deliberately detach ourselves from the living mystery. As long as we are caught up in the creative element itself we neither see nor understand; indeed we must not begin to understand, for nothing is more damaging and dangerous to immediate experience than cognition. But for the purpose of cognition we must detach ourselves from the creative process and regard it from without; only then does it become a picture that expresses meanings. Then we not only may but indeed must speak of "meaning." [xix, 63 f (g, 242)

Perhaps art itself does not intend to "signify," contains no sort of "meaning," at least not in the sense in which we are now speaking of "meaning." Perhaps it is like nature, which simply is, without any intention to "signify." Is "meaning" necessarily more than mere interpretation "secreted" into it by the need of an intellect hungry for meaning? Art, one might say, is beauty, and therein it finds its true aim and fulfilment. It needs no meaning. The question of meaning holds nothing productive for art. [xix, 63 (g, 242)

The great work is like a dream which, all obvious qualities notwithstanding, does not interpret itself, and is therefore unequivocal. No dream says "Thou shalt" or "This is the truth"; it presents a picture, the way nature lets a plant grow, and it is up to us to draw conclusions from it. If a man has an anxiety dream, he either has too much fear or too little, and if he dreams of the old wise man, he is either too much of a doctrinaire or he needs a teacher. And both are subtly the same, a point of which we are aware only when we let the work of art react approximately upon us the way it reacted on the poet. In order to understand its meaning, we must allow ourselves to be formed just as it formed the poet. And then we will also understand what his primal experience was: he has touched that salubrious and redeeming psychic depth where as yet no individual has secluded himself in the solitude of his consciousness in order to start forth on a painful road of errors, where all still feel the same vibration, and where, therefore, the sentiment and action of the individual reach out to all humanity.

[xvi, 330 (e, 44 f)

The plant is not a mere product of the soil, but a living process centred in itself, the essence of which has nothing to do with the character of the soil. In the same way the art-work must be regarded as a creative formation, freely making use of every precondition. Its meaning and its own individual particularity rests in itself, and not in its preconditions. In fact one might almost describe it as a being that uses man and his personal dispositions merely as a cultural medium or soil, disposing his powers according to its own laws, while shaping itself to the fulfilment of its own creative purpose.   [xix, 52 f (g, 234)

The unborn work in the soul of the artist is a force of nature that effects its purpose either with tyrannical might or with that subtle cunning which nature brings to the achievement of her end, quite regardless of the personal weal or woe of the man who is the vehicle of the creative force. The creative energy lives and waxes in the man as a tree in the earth from which it takes its nourishment. It might be well, therefore, to regard the creative process as a living thing, implanted, as it were, in the souls of men.   [xix, 58 (g, 238)

The irrational-creative, which stands out most distinctly in art, would ultimately mock at all rationalizing efforts. All ordinary expression may be explained causally, but creative expression, which is the absolute contrary of ordinary expression, will be forever hidden from human knowledge. We may continue to describe it and sense it, but in appearance only, and we will never understand it. The science of art and psychology will be dependent one upon the other, and the principle of the one will not negate that of the other.   [XVI, 316 (E, 29 f)

Only that aspect of art which consists in the process of artistic form can be an object of psychology; whereas that which constitutes the essential nature of art must always lie outside its province. This other aspect, namely, the problem of what is art in itself, can never be the object of a psychological but only of an aesthetic-artistic method of approach.   [XIX, 41 (G, 225)

The fact that in the child, the "war of faculties" not yet having declared itself, we find artistic, scientific, and religious possibilities still slumbering tranquilly together; or that with the primitive, dispositions towards art, science, and religion still maintain an undifferentiated co-existence in the chaos of a magical mentality; or that, finally, with animals, no trace of "mind" can as yet be discerned, but merely "natural instinct"— all these facts hold no shadow of evidence for that essential unity in the nature of art and science which alone could justify a reciprocal subsumption or, in other words, a reduction of the one into the other. For if we go back far enough in the state of mental development for the essential differences of the individual provinces of the mind to have become altogether invisible, we have not thereby reached a deeper principle of their unity but merely an earlier evolutionary state of undifferentiation in which neither province has as yet any existence at all. But this elementary state is not a principle from which any conclusion regarding the nature of later and more highly developed states might be inferred, notwithstanding, as is of course always the case, that a direct descent can be demonstrated.   [XIX, 42 f (G, 226 f)

Personal causality has as much and as little to do with the

work of art as the soil with the plant that springs from it. Doubtless we may learn to understand some peculiarities of the plant by becoming familiar with the character of its habitat. And for the botanist this is, of course, an important component of his knowledge. But nobody will maintain that he has thereby recognized all the essentials relating to the plant itself. The personal orientation that is demanded by the problem of personal causality is out of place in the presence of the work of art, just because the work of art is not a human being, but essentially supra-personal. It is a thing and not a personality; hence the personal is no criterion for it. Indeed the especial significance of the genuine art-work lies in the fact that it has successfully rid itself of the restraints and blind alleys of the personal and breathes an air infinitely remote from the transitoriness and short-winded excursions of the merely personal.

[xix, 51 f (G, 233 f)

For the essence of the work of art does not consist in the fact that it is charged with personal peculiarities—in fact, the more this is the case the less the question of art enters in—but that it rises far above the personal and speaks out of the heart and mind and for the heart and mind of humanity. The personal is a limitation, yes, even a vice of art. [xvi, 329 (E, 40 f)

The psychology of the creative is really feminine psychology, a fact which proves that creative work grows out of unconscious depths, indeed, out of the region of the mothers. If the creative element preponderates, the unconscious preponderates consequently as a force that shapes life and destiny as opposed to the conscious will, and consciousness is carried off by the force of a subterranean stream, a mere helpless spectator of events. The growing work is the poet's destiny and determines his psychology. It is not Goethe who makes Faust, but Faust that makes Goethe. And what is Faust? Faust is a symbol, not a mere semeiotic reference to something known long ago, but the expression of something primitively alive and effective in the soul of the German, which Goethe has helped to be born.

[xvi, 329 (E, 43)

Nothing would be more erroneous than to assume that the poet creates from the material of tradition. He works rather from the primal experience, the dark nature of which requires

177

mythological figures and thus draws avidly to itself everything
that is akin, to be used for self-expression. The primal experience is word- and imageless, for it is a vision in "the dark mirror." It is only a most powerful intuition that would like to
become expression. It is like a whirlwind carrying everything
before it, whirling it upward and thus gaining visible form.
And since this expression never attains the plentitude of the
vision and never exhausts its boundlessness, the poet requires
an almost gigantic material in order to even approximately express that of which he has had an intuition. And he also needs
a refractory and contradictory form of expression to conjure
the terrific paradoxicalness of this vision with approximate validity. Dante spreads out his experience between all the images
of Hell, Purgatory, and Heaven; Goethe needs the Blocksberg
and the Hellenic nether-world; Wagner the entire Nordic
mythology; Nietzsche returns to the hymnal style and to the
legendary seer of prehistoric times; Blake invents indescribable
figures; and Spitteler borrows old names for new characters.
And nothing is missing in the entire scale, from the incompre-
hensibly sublime down to the perversely grotesque.

[XVI, 324 (E, 36 f)

Just as the love experience is the real experience of a real
fact, so is the vision. Whether its object be of a physical, a psychic, or a metaphysical nature does not concern us. It is psychic
reality, having the same dignity as the physical. The experience
of human passion stands within the frontiers of consciousness;
the object of the vision, however, lies beyond. In the emotion
we experience known things, but intuition leads us to unknown
and hidden things, to things that are secret by nature, and
which, if they are ever conscious, are intentionally hidden and
secreted away; for this reason there clings to them, from time
immemorial, mystery, strangeness, and illusion. They are hidden from man, and he hides from them with Deisidaimonia,
seeking shelter behind the shield of science and the armour of
reason. The cosmos is his day-faith which shall protect him
from the night-fear of chaos.   [XVI, 332 (E, 34)

The intellect is sovereign of the scientific realm. But it is another matter when science steps across into the realm of practical application. The intellect, which was formerly king, is

now merely a resource, a scientifically perfected instrument, it is true, but still only an implement—no more the aim itself, but merely a condition. The intellect, and with it science, is now placed at the service of creative power and purpose. Yet this is still "psychology" although no longer science: it is a psychology in a wider meaning of the word, a psychological activity of a creative nature, in which creative phantasy is given priority. Instead of using the term "creative phantasy," it would be just as true to say that in a practical psychology of this kind the leading role is given to *life;* for on the one hand it is undoubtedly phantasy, procreating and productive, which uses science as a resource, but on the other it is the manifold demands of external reality which prompt the activity of creative phantasy. [IX, 82 f (I, 75 f)

If psychology remains only a science, we do not reach life— we merely serve the absolute aim of science. It leads us, certainly, to a knowledge of the actual state of affairs, but it always resists every other aim but its own. The intellect remains imprisoned in itself just so long as it does not willingly sacrifice its supremacy through its recognition of the value of other aims. It recoils from the step which takes it out of itself and which denies its universal validity, since from the standpoint of intellect everything else is nothing but phantasy. But what great thing ever came into existence that was not first phantasy?
[IX, 84 f (I, 77)

Why do we always forget that there is nothing powerful and beautiful in the whole field of human culture which did not originally spring from a sudden happy thought? What would become of humanity if no one had any more sudden intuitions? It would be much nearer the truth to look upon the conscious mind as a sack which contains nothing more than the ideas which have happened to fall into* it. We are never more painfully aware of the extent to which we depend on sudden ideas than when they refuse to "fall into" us. [XXVII, 49 f

If the play expires in itself without creating anything durable and living, it is only play; but in the alternative event it is

* [The original German word, *einfallen,* means both "to fall into" and "to occur."—TRANSLATOR.]

called creative work. Out of a playful movement of elements, whose associations are not immediately established, there arise groupings which an observant and critical intellect can only subsequently appraise. The creation of something new is not accomplished by the intellect, but by the play-instinct, from inner necessity. The creative mind plays with the objects it loves. Hence one can easily regard every creative activity whose potentialities remain hidden from the many as play. There are, indeed, very few creative men at whom the reproach of playing has not been cast.   [IX, 171 f (I, 155)

We know that every good idea and all creative work is the offspring of the imagination, and has its source in what one is pleased to term infantile phantasy. It is not the artist alone, but every creative individual whatsoever who owes all that is greatest in his life to phantasy. The dynamic principle of phantasy is play, which belongs also to the child, and as such it appears to be inconsistent with the principle of serious work. But without this playing with phantasy no creative work has ever yet come to birth. The debt we owe to the play of imagination is incalculable. It is therefore short-sighted to treat phantasy, on account of its daring or inacceptable character, as of small account.   [IX, 90 (I, 82)

To me, phantasy is actually the maternally creative side of the masculine spirit. When all is said and done, we are never proof against phantasy. It is true that there are worthless, inadequate, morbid, and unsatisfying fantasies whose sterile nature will be quickly recognized by every person endowed with common sense; but this of course proves nothing against the value of creative imagination. All the works of man have their origin in creative fantasy. What right have we then to depreciate imagination? In the ordinary course of things, fantasy does not easily go astray; it is too deep for that, and too closely bound up with the tap-root of human and animal instinct. In surprising ways it always rights itself again. The creative activity of the imagination frees man from his bondage to the "nothing but" and liberates in him the spirit of play. As Schiller says, man is completely human only when he is playing.
                    [XIX, 103 (J, 75 f)

The man who speaks with primordial images speaks with a thousand tongues; he entrances and overpowers, while at the same time he raises the idea he is trying to express above the occasional and the transitory into the sphere of the ever-existing. He transmutes personal destiny into the destiny of mankind, thus evoking all those beneficent forces that have enabled mankind to find a rescue from every hazard and to outlive the longest night. That is the secret of effective art.

[XIX, 70 f (G, 248)

The great poetry that creates from out the soul of mankind is inaccurately explained if we reduce it to the personal. For wherever the collective unconscious forces its way into experience and weds itself to the collective consciousness, there occurs a creative act which concerns the entire contemporaneous epoch. The work emerging from this is, in the deepest sense of the word, a message to the contemporaries. For this reason, *Faust* touches something in the soul of every German, for this reason also Dante's fame is immortal, and *The Shepherd of Hermas* has almost become a canonical book. Each period has its one-sidedness, its prejudices and psychic suffering. An epoch is like the soul of an individual; it has its particular, specifically limited state of consciousness and requires, therefore, a compensation which is accomplished by the collective unconscious in such a way that the poet or seer or leader lends himself to the unspoken things of the time and brings forth, through image or act, that which is awaited by the incomprehended common need, whether this be for good or evil, for the healing of an epoch or for its destruction.   [XVI, 325 (E, 38)

Delving once more into the primal state of the soul is the secret of artistic creation and the effect of art, for at this stage of experience it is no longer the individual but the people who experience something; nor is any longer the welfare of the individual at stake, but the life of the people itself. For this reason the great work of art is objective and impersonal, albeit touching the deepest things in us. For this reason the personal side of the poet is simply an advantage or an inhibition and never essential for his art. His personal biography may be that of a Philistine, of a worthy citizen, of a neurotic, of a fool, or of a criminal, all interesting and necessary but unessential as far as the poet is concerned. [XVI, 330 (E, 45)

Is it thinkable that a non-German would have written a *Faust* or a *Thus Spake Zarathustra?* Both allude probably to the same thing, to something vibrating in the German soul, a primal image, as Jakob Burckhardt put it once, the figure of a doctor and teacher of mankind, the archetype of the wise man, the helpful and redeeming man. This image has been engraved in the unconscious from time immemorial; there it sleeps until the unpropitiousness of the age awakens it, that is, till the time when a great error leads the people away from the right road. For wherever there open shifting paths we need the leader and the master and even the doctor. There are many primal images, but they do not appear in the dreams of the individual and not in the works of art until they have been excited by the deviation of the consciousness. But if consciousness is lost in a one-sided and therefore erroneous condition, these "instincts" are vivified and send their images into the dreams of the individual as well as into the visions of the artists and seers, in order to re-establish in this way the psychic balance. The psychic need of the people is fulfilled in the work of the poet, and therefore the work means more to the poet in action and truth than his personal destiny. [XVI, 329 f (E, 43 f)

The artist is the mouthpiece of the secrets of the psyche of his time—involuntarily, like every true prophet, and often unconsciously, like a sleep-walker. He believes himself to be speaking out of himself; but the spirit of the age speaks through him, and what it says is so, for it works. [XXVII, 156

The shaping of the primordial image is, as it were, a translation into the language of the present which makes it possible for every man to find again the deepest springs of life which would otherwise be closed to him. Therein lies the social importance of art; it is constantly at work educating the spirit of the age, since it brings to birth those forms in which the age is most lacking. Recoiling from the unsatisfying present the yearning of the artist reaches out to that primordial image in the unconscious which is best fitted to compensate the insufficiency and one-sidedness of the spirit of the age. The artist seizes this image, and in the work of raising it from deepest unconsciousness he brings it into relation with conscious values, thereby transforming its shape, until it can be accepted by his contemporaries according to their powers.   [XIX, 71 (G, 248)

The artist is essentially the instrument, and he stands below his work, for which reason we should never expect from him an interpretation of his own work. He achieved his highest with his composition. He must leave the interpretation to others and to the future.   [XVI, 330 (E, 44)

For art is innate in the artist, like an instinct that seizes and makes a tool out of the human being. The thing that in the final analysis wills something in him is not he, the personal man, but the aim of art. As a person he may have caprices and a will and his own aims, but as an artist he is in a higher sense "man," he is the *collective man*, the carrier and shaper of the unconsciously active soul of mankind. This is his office, the burden of which often preponderates in such a way that human happiness and everything that to the ordinary mortal spells life worth living falls hopelessly its victim.   [XVI, 328 (E, 41 f)

Creative genius is never one but many, and therefore it speaks in the stillness of the soul to the many to whom it represents meaning and fate as much as it does to the individual artist.   [XXVII, 164

Whether the poet knows that his work is generated in him and grows and ripens there, or whether he imagines that he creates out of his own will and from nothingness, it changes in no way the curious fact that his work grows beyond him. It is, in relation to him, like a child to its mother.   [XVI, 329 (E, 43)

Usually the development of a talent is not in proportion to the ripeness of the rest of the personality; and we often have the impression that the creative personality grows at the expense of the human personality. Sometimes there is such a discrepancy between the genius and his humanity that we cannot help wondering whether a little less genius would not have been better. What is great intelligence worth together with moral inferiority? There are not a few talented individuals whose value is paralysed or even perverted by their human inadequacy. Talent is not necessarily a blessing; it is so only if the rest of the personality keeps pace with it.   [LIII, 6

The artist's relative lack of adaptation becomes his real advantage; for it enables him to keep aloof from the highways, the better to follow his own yearning and to find those things of which the others are deprived without noticing it. Thus, as in the case of the single individual whose one-sided conscious attitude is corrected by unconscious reactions towards self-regulation, art also represents a process of mental self-regulation in the life of nations and epochs.   [XIX, 72 f (G, 249)

Genius forces its way against all odds, for it is part of its very nature to be unconditional and untamable. But so-called "misunderstood genius" is a doubtful phenomenon. Usually it turns out to be inadequacy searching for a soothing self-justification.
                                                                 [LIII, 7
Talent can be impeded, crippled, perverted, or it can be encouraged, developed, and improved. But genius is a *rarissima avis* like the phoenix with whose appearance we cannot reckon. It is simply there by God's good grace, in its whole strength, conscious or unconscious. Talent, on the other hand, occurs with a certain regularity which can be statistically registered, and does not by any means always possess a corresponding dynamic character.   [LIII, 7

To be "normal" is a splendid ideal for the unsuccessful, for all those who have not yet found an adaptation. But for people who have far more ability than the average, for whom it was never hard to gain successes and to accomplish their share of the world's work—for them, restriction to the normal signifies the bed of Procrustes, unbearable boredom, infernal sterility, and hopelessness.   [XIX, 30 (J, 55)

To be in advance of others is always to invite a flogging, and if the gifted child does not get it from the teacher, he gets it from fate, but mostly from both. The talented individual does well to get used in good time to the fact that a greater ability leads to being an exception with all the risks this implies, particularly that of an exaggerated self-conceit. Only humility and obedience can protect a person against this, and even these not always. [LIII, 7

The greatness of historical personalities has never consisted in their unconditional subjection *to* convention, but, on the contrary, in their liberating freedom *from* convention. They thrust themselves up like mountain peaks out of the mass that clung to its collective fears, convictions, laws, and methods, and chose their own way. And to the ordinary human being it always seemed wonderful that someone should prefer to the beaten path, with its known destination, a small and steep path that leads into the unknown. This is why it was always believed that such a man, if not out of his mind, was yet inhabited by a demon or god; the miracle of a man acting otherwise than in the way humanity had always acted could be explained only as due to his being gifted with demonic power or divine spirit.
[XXVII, 192 f (F, 290 f)

Creative life is always on the yonder side of convention. This is how it comes about that, when the mere routine of life in the form of traditional conventions predominates, a destructive outbreak of the creative forces *must* follow. But such an outbreak is only catastrophic as a mass phenomenon, and never in the individual who consciously subordinates himself to these higher powers and places his abilities at their service.
[XXVII, 198 f (F, 295)

Every creative man is a duality or a synthesis of paradoxical qualities. On the one hand he is human-personal, on the other hand an impersonal-creative process. As a human being he may be healthy or morbid; his personal psychology can and should be explained, therefore, in a personal way. But as an artist he can only be understood through his creative act.
[XVI, 327 (E, 41)

It is thus obvious that the artist must be explained through his art and not through the inadequacies and personal conflicts of his nature, which are mere consequential phenomena of the

185

fact that he is an artist, that is, a man who from birth is charged with a greater task than the common mortal. The fact that he has greater capacity requires also a greater expenditure of energy, for which reason the "more" on the one side is accompanied necessarily by a "less" on the other. [xvi, 329 (e, 43)

There is rarely a creative man who does not have to pay a high price for the divine spark of his great gifts. It is as if everyone were born with a certain capital of life energy. The strongest force in him will wrest for itself most of the available energy, while for the rest there remains too little for any value to develop out of it. On the contrary, the human element is frequently bled for the benefit of the creative element and to such an extent that it even brings out the bad qualities, as for instance, ruthless naïve egoism (so-called "autoeroticism"), vanity, all kinds of vices—and all this in order to bring to the human "I" at least some life-strength, since otherwise it would perish from sheer inanition. [xvi, 328 (e, 42)

Great talents are the most lovely and often the most dangerous fruits on the tree of humanity. They hang upon the most slender twigs that are easily snapped off. [lim, 6

PROBLEMS OF SELF-REALIZATION

Nothing is so jealous as a truth.   [LVIII, 210 (M, 190)

The investigation of truth begins with each case anew, because any living truth is individual and not to be derived from any previously established formula. Each individual is an experiment of ever-changing life, and an attempt at a new solution or new adaptation.   [XL, 40 (G, 349)

No doubt it is a great nuisance that mankind is not uniform but compounded of individuals whose psychic structure spreads them over a span of at least ten thousand years. Hence there is absolutely no truth that does not spell salvation to one person and damnation to another. All universalisms get stuck in this terrible dilemma.   [LVIII, 52 (M, 36)

At no time did barbarism consist in a state where reason or truth have an insufficient effect; it appears only when man expects such an effect from them, or, we might even say, it is because man provides reason with too much efficacy from a superstitious over-valuation of "truth." Barbarism is one-sidedness, lack of moderation—bad proportion generally.
      [IX, 115 f (I, 103)

Our world is so exceedingly rich in delusions that a truth is priceless, and no one will let it slip because of a few exceptions with which it cannot be brought into accord. Whoever doubts this truth is of course looked upon as a faithless reprobate, while a note of fanaticism and intolerance creeps into the discussion on all sides.—And yet each of us can carry the torch of knowledge but a part of the way, until another takes it from him. Could we but accept this in an impersonal way—could we but grasp the fact that we are not the personal creators of our truths, but only their exponents, who thus make articulate the psychic needs of our day—then much of the poison and bitterness might be spared and we should be able to perceive the profound and super-personal continuity of the human mind.
      [XIX, 27 f (J, 53 f)

Convictions are an assurance and a reliable track for certain stretches of the way. Then comes a painful change which is experienced as something disintegrating and immoral, until a new conviction takes the place of the old one. In so far as the essence of human nature always remains the same, certain moral values possess an eternal validity. But the most exact observance of the decalogue does not prevent subtle infamies, and the infinitely more exalted principle of Christian brotherly love can lead to confusion and the clash of conflicting duties, the tangled skein of which can often only be cut by a very unchristian sword.   [XLVIII, 172

Convictions easily turn into self-protective devices; if this happens they tend to become rigid; but this is contrary to the sense of life. The test of a firm conviction is its elasticity and flexibility; like every other exalted truth, it thrives best by the admission of its errors.   [LV, 160 (K, 39)

Convictions and moral values would have no sense if they were not believed and given an exclusive worth. And yet they are merely human time-conditioned explanations and statements, of which we know very well that they are capable of all sorts and kinds of modifications, as the past has shown and the future may again reveal.   [XLVIII, 171

There appears to be a conscience in mankind which severely punishes the man who does not somehow and at some time, at whatever cost to his pride, cease to defend and assert himself, and instead confess himself fallible and human. Until he can do this, an impenetrable wall shuts him out from the living experience of feeling himself a man among men.   [XIX, 10 (J, 39 f)

Error is just as important a condition of life as truth. [VI, 110

Admittedly, a fact never exists only as it is in itself, but also as we view it.   [IX, 429 (I, 375)

I respect the honest man who lives in his modest house and by his "motto" shows the world that he has his own consciousness of worth and can ignore the opinion of others. He is an "aristocrat" in his own way, not *au-dessus de la mêlée,* as a feudal baron might be, but—though this may sound a bit misleading—*au-dessous de la mêlée.* This is not merely a play upon words: the tumult and outcry occur where opposites clash, and that is always the middle level between the higher and the lower. The distinguished are above it, the undistinguished below it. So long as the distinguished man remains above it, he is outside the entanglement, and the undistinguished man is also outside it so long as he remains below the level. Above and below were ever brothers, as the wise saying in the *Tabula smaragdina* puts it: "Heaven above, Heaven below. . . ."

[xii, 6

In our all-absorbing everyday life, there is unfortunately little that is unusual which is at the same time healthy. There is little room for obvious heroism. Not that the call to heroism does not reach us! On the contrary, that is just the damnable and burdensome part of it, our banal everyday life makes banal demands on our patience, our devotedness, endurance, self-sacrifice, and so on, which we must fulfil modestly and without any heroic gestures to court applause, and which actually need a heroism that is not seen from without. It does not shine and is not praised, and it seeks ever again the disguise of everyday apparel. [li, 87 f

It is not good and wise speech which counts, but actions alone: neither is it any use to live according to accepted moral principles, for obedience to moral customs and laws can just as well be a cloak for a subtle lie which is just too artful to be noticed by our fellow men. We may perhaps, through belief in our own most patent rectitude, succeed in escaping all adverse criticism and in deceiving ourselves. But deep down below the surface of the average conscience, a still small voice says to us: "Something is out of tune," however much our rightness may be confirmed by public opinion or the moral code. [xviii, 13

Be the man through whom you wish to influence others. Mere talk has always been considered hollow, and there is no trick, however cunning, by which one can evade this simple rule for long. The fact of being convinced, and not the subject-matter of conviction—it is this which has always carried weight.

[XIX, 34 (J, 59)

Everything that exists acts, for otherwise it would not be actual. It is actual thanks only to its inherent energy. Being is a field of force. [XIX, 241 (J, 169)

The ethical problem is a matter of passionate importance to a moral man, and it is rooted in the deepest instinctive processes of his nature, as well as in his most ideal aspirations. It is for him a devastatingly real problem. Can we wonder, then, that the deeps of his nature should give their answer to it?

[XI, 108 (D, 196)

It is a matter of everyday experience that our affects are never on a level with our judgment. [LX

In actual truth, we do not by any means enjoy complete freedom, for we are constantly threatened by certain psychic factors which, being "facts of nature," can take possession of us. This happens when we reabsorb certain metaphysical projections to any extent, and we are almost defenceless, as we at once identify with every impulse instead of seeing it as something outside ourselves, whereby it would at least be kept at arm's length and could not immediately storm the citadel of the ego.

[XLVI, 157

Lack of freedom and possession are synonyms, and therefore there is always something in the psyche which takes possession and limits or suppresses moral freedom. In order on the one hand to keep this true but very unpleasant fact secret, and on the other to find the courage for freedom, we have become accustomed to use what is really an apotropaic language when we say, "I have the tendency, or the habit, or a feeling, or a resentment . . . ," instead of stating the truth: "the tendency, or the habit, or the feeling of resentment has me." The latter mode of expression would, however, cost us our last illusion of freedom. But I wonder whether that would not be better in a higher sense than to allow ourselves to be still further deceived by our own speech. [XLVI, 156 f

As a being who is merely created, or developing out of an unconscious precondition, man has no freedom, and consciousness no *raison d'être*. Psychological judgment must take account of the fact that, in spite of all causal dependence, man possesses a feeling of freedom which is identical with the autonomy of the conscious mind. In spite of the fact that everything proves the dependence and preconditioned state of the ego, it still cannot be convinced of its own lack of freedom.   [L, 138

The existence of ego-consciousness only makes sense if it is free and autonomous. This statement is admittedly an antinomy but it also gives a complete picture of the actual state of things. Of course the emphasis laid on dependence and freedom differs according to time, place, and the individual. In reality, both dependence and freedom are always present: the supremacy of the Self and the hubris of the conscious mind. Ego-consciousness, if it obeys only itself, is always on the way to the illusion of feeling itself Godlike and superhuman. But on the other hand, total acceptance of dependence leads to a fatalistic childishness and to a spiritual arrogance which estranges a man from the world and humanity.   [L, 139

Everyone has a certain psychic disposition which limits his freedom to an enormous extent, indeed, makes it almost illusory. Not only philosophically is "freedom of will" an imponderable problem, but also practically, for there is hardly anyone who is not to a great extent, or even mainly, governed by tendencies, habits, instincts, prejudices, resentments, and all sorts of complexes. All these facts of nature function exactly like a whole Olympus of gods who must be propitiated, served, feared, and honoured not only by the individual possessor of this company of gods but also by his personal surroundings.
                    [XLVI, 156

Although it may reasonably be doubted whether man has made any marked or even perceptible progress in morality during the known five thousand years of his civilization, yet it cannot be denied that there has been a notable development in consciousness and its functions. Above all, there has been a tremendous extension of consciousness in the form of *knowledge*. Not only have the individual functions become differentiated, but to a large extent they have been brought under the control of the ego—in other words, man's will has developed. This is particularly striking when we compare our mentality with that of primitives. The security of our ego has, in comparison with earlier times, greatly increased and has even taken such a dangerous leap forward that, although we sometimes speak of "God's will," we no longer know what we are saying, for in the same breath we assert, "Where there's a will there's a way." And who would ever think of appealing to God's help rather than to the goodwill, the sense of responsibility and duty, the reason or intelligence, of his fellow men?

[LX, 51 f (N, 368)

The will is a great magician, and furthermore it is strangely paradoxical. It feels itself to be free and declares that it is free. We have the feeling of freedom, in spite of the fact that one can prove beyond all doubt that quite definite causes were there to produce with the greatest compulsion such and such an effect. On the other hand, we know that there is nothing which has not its cause; and so the will must also be determined by a cause. But the will feels itself to be free, because it has a piece of that dark, creative force in us which somehow makes us and makes our lives; which works upon the body, maintaining or destroying our structure, and making new men. In the will this energy comes to some extent within the domain of our human consciousness and brings with it that absolute, sovereign feeling of eternal freedom which no philosophy can undermine. We can set up against it as many philosophical systems as we like, but the feeling of freedom is still there. It is impossible to destroy it with philosophy, for it is a curious primordial fact of nature. [XXXIV, 10

We are still so barbarous that faith in the laws of human nature and the human path appears as a dangerous and non-ethical naturalism. Why is this? Because under the barbarian's thin skin of culture the wild beast lurks in readiness, amply justifying his fear. But the beast that is caged is not thereby conquered. There is no morality without freedom. When a barbarian loosens the animal within him, he is not free but bound. Barbarism must first be vanquished before freedom can be won.

Theoretically this takes place when an individual perceives and feels the basic root and motive power of his own morality as an inherent element of his own nature, and not as external prohibition.　　　　　　　　　　　　　　　　　　　　[IX, 302 (I, 264)

The moral laws are not merely an evil against which we should revolt, but a necessity produced by the innermost needs of man. The moral law is nothing else than an outer manifestation of the inborn urge of man to repress and tame himself. This urge to domestication or civilization is lost in the unfathomable, misty depths of the history of human development, and can never be thought of as the result of a certain code of laws imposed upon mankind from outside. Man himself, obeying his own instincts, has created his own laws.　　　　　　[VI, 122

Morality is no misconception, conceived by an ambitious Moses upon Sinai, but something inherent in the laws of life and fashioned like a house or a ship or any other cultural instrument in the normal process of life. The natural flow of libido, this very middle path, involves a complete obedience to the fundamental laws of human nature, and there can positively be no higher moral principle than that harmony with natural laws whose accord gives the libido the direction in which life's optimum lies.　　　　　　　　　　　　　　　　[IX, 301 (I, 263)

It should never be forgotten—and this must be said to the Freudian school—that morality was not brought down from Sinai in the form of tables and imposed upon the people. Morality is a function of the human soul which is as old as mankind. Morality is not imposed upon us from outside; we carry it *a priori* within ourselves, not the laws but the moral essence, without which life in a community would be impossible. Therefore morality exists in every grade of society. It is our instinctive regulation of behaviour which also rules the herd life among animals. But the moral law is valid only within a group of human beings living together. Beyond this group, it ceases to apply, and in its place the old truth prevails: *Homo homini lupus* ("Man is to man as a wolf"). With the growth of civilization, an ever greater number of men can be brought under the sway of the same moral laws: but as yet it has never been possible to make the moral law rule beyond the frontiers of the society, that is, in the free space between independent societies. There, as in ancient times, lawlessness and disorder prevail and the worst immorality, as however only the enemy of the moment will say aloud.   [LI, 49 f

We must never forget that what today is deemed a moral law will tomorrow be cast into the melting-pot and transformed, so that in the near or distant future it may serve as the basis of a new ethical structure. This much we ought to have learned from the history of civilization, that the forms of morality belong to the category of transitory things.   [VII, 50 (C, 276)

"Morality is the only thing that cannot be improved, since every modification of habitual morality is, in its application, an immorality." In this *bon mot* there is something more serious, since it also carries an undeniable fact of feeling, against which many a pioneer has stumbled.   [x, 12 (G, 167)

Psychoanalysis has been reproached for liberating man's (happily) repressed animal instincts and thus bringing about incalculable evil. This apprehension shows how little confidence is felt in the efficacy of the moral principles of today. The illusion is cherished that *only* the morality of precept and principle holds men back from unbridled licence. A much more efficacious regulative principle, however, is necessity, which sets bounds far more real and convincing than any moral principles.
[v, 270 (D, 24)

Every one of us gladly turns away from his problems; if possible, they must not be mentioned, or, better still, their existence is denied. We wish to make our lives simple, certain, and smooth—and for that reason problems are taboo. We choose to have certainties and no doubts, results and no experiments, without even seeing that certainties can arise only through doubt and results through experiment. The artful denial of a problem will not produce conviction; on the contrary, a wider and higher consciousness is called for to give us the certainty and clarity we need.   [XIX, 250 (J, 111)

Nowadays the individual still feels himself inhibited by the hypocrisies of public opinion, and therefore prefers to lead a secret separate life while publicly adhering to morality. But things might change considerably if everyone suddenly found the moral mask too foolish, and people began to be conscious of how dangerously their inner beasts were lying in wait for each other. Then an orgy of depravity might sweep over humanity—this is the dream, the wishful dream, of the morally deficient today. They forget the breath-taking struggle for life which would quickly put down such an orgy with a firm hand.

[IV, 222

The sense of moral inferiority always indicates that the missing element is something which, if one listens to feeling, should not be missing; in other words, it is something that could be conscious if one took enough trouble. The feeling of moral inferiority does not arise from the collision with the generally accepted and, in a sense, arbitrary moral law, but from an inner conflict with the Self, which, for the sake of psychic equilibrium, demands that the deficit be redressed. Whenever a sense of inferiority appears, it is an indication of two things. In the first place, it means that there is an unconscious component that needs to be assimilated; and secondly, the possibility of assimilation actually exists. In the last resort it is a man's moral qualities which force him, either by direct recognition of the necessity, or indirectly, by means of a painful neurosis, to assimilate his unconscious personality and to hold it in consciousness.

[XI, 27 f (D, 136 f)

Wherever an inferiority complex exists, there is a good reason for it. There is always something inferior there, although not just where we persuade ourselves that it is. Modesty and humility do not by any means signify an inferiority complex. These are virtues, to be highly prized and deeply admired; they are not complexes. They prove that their fortunate possessor is not a presumptuous fool, but knows his own limitations, and will therefore never stumble beyond his human domain, dazzled, boasting, and intoxicated by his own imagined greatness.

[LVI, 18

Those people who imagine themselves to be so secure are in reality insecure. Our life is insecure and therefore a certain feeling of insecurity is much nearer to the truth than the illusion and bluff of security. In the long run it is the better adapted man who wins and not the man illegitimately sure of himself and at the mercy of dangers from without and within. Money and power are not the only criteria! The ultimate criterion is peace of mind. [LVI, 18

We must always take into account that there are, on the one hand, innumerable people who cannot distinguish between a really witty joke and mere nonsense, and on the other, a good number who are so convinced of their own cleverness that in their whole life they have never come across anything but idiots. [XLII, 31

People all too often have a pathetic assurance, thanks to which they commit nothing but foolish mistakes. It is better to be uncertain of ourselves, because then we are more modest and humble. It is true, however, that an inferiority complex always contains in it the danger of over-reaching itself and compensating for the supposed deficiency by a flight into the opposite extreme. [LVI, 18

The question of where we are going is of course extremely important; but equally important, it seems to me, is the question of *who* is going where. The "who" always implies a "whence." It takes a certain greatness to gain lasting possession of the heights, but anybody can overreach himself.

[LVIII, 166 (M, 148)

People who have an exaggerated ethical ideal, who always think, feel, and act altruistically and idealistically, avenge themselves for their intolerable ideals by subtly planned maliciousness, which of course does not become conscious as such, but which leads to misunderstandings and unhappy situations. All these difficulties appear to them as "especially unfortunate circumstances," or the fault and the malice of other people, or tragic complications. Consciously they imagine they are rid of the conflict, but it is still there, unseen, to be stumbled over at every step. [IV, 62

But besides the possibility of becoming a prophet, a subtler and apparently more legitimate joy beckons, namely, one can become the disciple of a prophet. For the great majority this is an altogether ideal technique. Its advantages are these: the *odium dignitatis,* namely the superhuman responsibility of the prophet, becomes the so much sweeter *otium indignitatis.* The disciple is unworthy; modestly he sits at the feet of the "master," guarding himself from having ideas of his own. Spiritual laziness becomes a virtue; it is permissible to bask in the sun of at least a semi-divine being. The archaism and infantilism of the unconscious fantasies are not debited to his own account, since all responsibility is laid at the "master" 's door. Through his deification of the "master," the disciple, without apparently noticing it, waxes in stature; moreover, does he not possess the great truth—not his own discovery, of course—but at least received from the "master" 's own hands? Naturally, the disciples always cleave together, not indeed out of love, but with the very understandable intention of receiving an effortless confirmation of their own convictions by creating a collective harmony.   [xi, 86 f (D, 181)

Christ the ideal took upon himself the sins of the world. But if the ideal is wholly outside, then the sins of the individual are also outside, and consequently he is more of a fragment than ever, since superficial misunderstanding conveniently enables him, quite literally, to "cast his sins upon Christ" and thus to evade his deepest responsibilities—which is contrary to the spirit of Christianity.   [LVIII, 20 (M, 9)

I cannot love anyone if I hate myself. That is the reason why we feel so extremely uncomfortable in the presence of people who are noted for their special virtuousness, for they radiate an atmosphere of the torture to which they subject themselves. In reality it is not a virtue but a vice. And thus, from so-called goodness, which was once really good, something which is no longer good has arisen; it has become an evasion. Nowadays any coward can make himself respectable by going to church and loving his neighbour. But it is simply an untrue state, an artificial world.   [xxxiv, 88

To live in perpetual flight from ourselves is a bitter thing, and to live with ourselves demands a number of Christian virtues which we must apply to our own case, such as patience, love, faith, hope, and humility. It is all very fine to make our neighbour happy by applying them to him, but the demon of self-reflection so easily claps us on the back and says, "Well done!" And because this is a great psychological truth it must be stood on its head for an equal number of people so as to give the devil something to carp at. But—does it make us happy when we have to apply these virtues to ourselves? when I am the recipient of my own gifts, the least among my brothers whom I must take to my bosom? when I must admit that I need all my patience, my love, my faith, and even my humility, and that I myself am my own devil, the antagonist who always wants the opposite in everything? Can we ever really endure ourselves? "Do unto others . . ."—this is as true of evil as of good.   [LX, 228 (N, 497)

It is always better to learn to bear with ourselves rather than to wage war against ourselves; and not to work our own inner difficulties into useless fantasies but to translate them into actual experience. Then at least we live and do not merely consume ourselves in fruitless conflicts. If men can be trained to look dispassionately at the lower side of their natures, it may be hoped that in this way they may also learn to understand and to love their fellow men better. To forswear hypocrisy and to adopt an attitude of tolerance towards oneself can only have good results for the just estimation of one's neighbour, since men are all too prone to transfer to their fellow men the injustice and violence that they do to their own natures.   [v, 271

We always understand others in the same way in which we understand, or try to understand, ourselves. That which we do not understand in ourselves we do not understand in others either, and vice versa. Thus the way is thoroughly paved to insure that the image we make of another is usually mainly a subjective one. Even an intimate friendship does not in any way guarantee an objective judgment of the other.   [XIII, 161 f

Strife and misunderstanding are, assuredly, constant requi-

sites for the tragicomedy of human life, but it is none the less
undeniable that the advance of civilization has led from the
right of the strongest to the establishment of laws, and therewith to the creation of a court of justice and a standard of rights
which are superordinated above the contending parties. It is
my conviction that a basis for the adjustment of conflicting
views could be found in the recognition of types of attitude,
not however of the mere existence of such types but also of the
fact that every man is so imprisoned in his type that he is
simply incapable of a complete understanding of another standpoint. Without a recognition of this far-reaching demand a violation of the other's standpoint is practically inevitable.

[ix, 696 (i, 620)

In daily life it happens all the time that we presume that the
psychic processes of other people are the same as ours. We suppose that what is pleasing or desirable to us is the same to
others, and that what seems bad to us must also seem bad to
them. It is only of late that our courts of law have adopted a
psychological standpoint and admitted the relativity of guilt in
pronouncing sentence. Unsophisticated people are still moved
to rancour by the tenet *quod licet Jovi non licet bovi*. Equality
before the law still represents a great human achievement; it has
not yet been superseded. And we still attribute to "the other
fellow" all the evil and inferior qualities that we do not like to
recognize in ourselves. That is why we have to criticize and
attack him. What happens in such a case, however, is that an inferior "soul" emigrates from one person to another. The world
is still full of *bêtes noires* and of scapegoats, just as it formerly
teemed with witches and werewolves.   [xix, 234 (j, 163)

That the subjective observation and interpretation agrees
with the objective facts of the psychological object is evidence
for the interpretation only in so far as the latter makes no pre-
tence to be universal, but intends to be valid only for that field
of the object that is under consideration. To this extent it is just
the beam in one's own eye that enables one to detect the mote
in the brother's eye. The beam in one's own eye, in this case,
does not prove (as said) that the brother has no mote in his. But
the impairment of vision might easily give rise to a general
theory that all motes are beams. The recognition and taking to

199

heart of the subjective limitation of knowledge in general, and of psychological knowledge in particular, is a basic condition for the scientific and accurate estimation of a psyche differing from that of the observing subject. This condition is fulfilled only when the observer is adequately informed concerning the compass and nature of his own personality. He can, however, be sufficiently informed only when he has in great measure freed himself from the compromising influence of collective opinion and feeling, and has thereby reached a clear conception of his own individuality. [IX, 19 (I, 17)

We always proceed on the naïve assumption that we are masters in our own house. The first thing we have to do is to accustom ourselves to the idea that, even in our most intimate psychic life, we live in a kind of house through the doors and windows of which we look out upon a world, and that the objects or contents of this world, although profoundly affecting us, do not belong to us. For many, this hypothesis is by no means easy to conceive, just as they cannot readily recognize and accept the fact that their neighbour's psychology is not necessarily identical with their own. [XI, 148 f (D, 225)

We have an abysmal horror of the horribleness of our personal unconscious. Therefore Europeans prefer to tell others what they should do. The fact that the improvement of the whole of humanity must begin with the individual, in fact with myself, is a thing which we cannot drive into our heads. Many even think that it is pathological to look into one's own inner self: as a theologian once assured me, it leads to melancholia.
[XLIV, 50

The actual existence of an enemy on whom we can pile all our malice means an unmistakable lightening of our conscience. We can then say without the least hesitation who the real culprit is, i.e., it is perfectly clear to us that the cause of misfortune is to be found outside and not in our own attitude. [XIII, 172

We can understand why the inner friend so often appears as an enemy, and why he is so far away and his voice so low. "Who is near to Him is near to the fire." [XLVII, 427

Our unwillingness to see our own faults and the projection of them is the beginning of most quarrels, and is the strongest guarantee that injustice, animosity, and persecution are not ready to die out. [LVI, 15

A man's hatred is always concentrated upon that which makes him conscious of his bad qualities. [IX, 374 (I, 331)

Everything that works from the unconscious appears projected on others. These others are not wholly guiltless, to be sure, for even the worst projection is at least hung on a hook, perhaps a very small one, but still a hook offered by the other person. [XIII, 90 (G, 61)

He who does not possess an unusual amount of self-realization cannot stand above his projections but is always below them, for the natural mental condition presupposes the presence of these projections. It is the natural state of things that the contents of the unconscious should be projected. [XIII, 159

The most important thing seems to us that we should be able to stand the test of our own judgment. Looked at from without, this attitude appears as self-righteousness, but it is only so if we are incapable of self-criticism. If we have self-criticism, then criticism from outside will only affect us externally and cannot reach our hearts, for we feel that a stricter judge sits within us than any who could judge us from without. And furthermore, what innumerable opinions people have! As many heads, as many different judgments! We find that our own judgment has after all as much worth as the judgments of others. We can never do right by all of them, and therefore it is better to be at peace with oneself. [XII, 5

In every human being, there sits a merciless judge who apportions guilt to us even when we are not conscious of any wrong. Although we do not know of it, it is as if it were known somewhere. [XLVIII, 73 f

How can anyone see straight when he does not even see him-

201

self and that darkness which he himself carries unconsciously into all his dealings? [XLVI, 151 (B, 102)

The "other" within us always seems to us strange and unacceptable. But if we allow ourselves to be affected and hurt by it, then it goes into us, and we are the richer for a piece of self-knowledge. [XII, 8

Only a fool is interested in other people's guilt, since he cannot alter it. The wise man learns only from his own guilt. He will ask himself: Who am I that all this should happen to me? To find the answer to this fateful question he will look into his own heart. [LVIII, 169 (M, 152)

A true man knows that his most bitter foe, or indeed a whole host of enemies, does not equal that one worst adversary, that "other self" who "bides within his breast." Nietzsche had Wagner in himself; and that is why he envied him *Parsifal*. But, what was worse, he, Saul, had also Paul within himself. That is why Nietzsche became stigmatized by the spirit. Like Saul, he had to experience Christification when the "other" presented him with the challenge, *Ecce homo*. Which was it who "broke before the cross," Wagner or Nietzsche? [LI, 63 (D, 31)

We are the Dioscuri, of whom one was mortal and the other immortal, and who are always together and yet can never quite become one. The process of transformation aims at bringing us near to this inner relationship, but consciousness feels resistances against it because the other seems strange and sinister, and because we cannot get used to the idea of not being the sole master in our own house. We should prefer to be always only an ego and nothing else. But we are faced with that inner friend or foe, and it depends on us whether he is our friend or our foe. [XLVII, 425

The "other" within is just as one-sided in his way as the ego in another way. But from the conflict of the two truth and meaning can arise, only, however, if the ego is willing to concede the "other" a personality in a just manner. [XLVII, 427

Nowhere are we nearer to the most exalted mystery of all origins than in the knowledge of our own self, which we fondly imagine we already know. But the depths of the universe are better known to us than the depths of the Self, where we can listen almost directly to the creative essence and its growth without however understanding it. [xix, 332

We can get lost in something which has strongly moved us, if we do not realize in time why we have become so affected by it. We should really once for all ask ourselves the question: Why has this idea laid hold of me and affected me so much? What does it mean in relation to myself? This modest doubt can save us from becoming so entirely the victim of an idea of our own that we are swallowed by it for good and all. [xlv

Conscience, and particularly bad conscience, can be a gift from heaven; a genuine grace, if used as a superior self-criticism. Self-criticism, as an introspective, discriminating activity, is indispensable to any attempt to understand one's own psychology. If you have done something which puzzles you and you ask yourself what has prompted you to such an action, you need the motive of a bad conscience and its corresponding discriminating faculty in order to discover the real motive of your behavior. It is only then that you are able to see what motives are ruling your deeds. The sting of bad conscience even spurs you on to discover things which were unconscious before and in this way you might cross the threshold of the unconscious mind and become aware of those impersonal forces that make you the unconscious instrument of the wholesale murderer in man.
[xlvi, 90 f (b, 61)

It is considered egoistic or unhealthy to be occupied with oneself. "One's own society is the worst"; "it makes one quite melancholy"—such are the splendid testimonials that are subscribed to our human make-up. But they are deeply ingrained in the Western attitude. Does he who thinks in this way ever clearly present to himself what sort of delight others must take in the company of such dirty-souled cowards? [xi, 142 (d, 221)

Brooding is a sterile activity, which runs round in a circle, never reaching a sensible goal. It is not work, but a weakness, even a vice. On the other hand, if we do not feel at one with ourself it is legitimate to make ourself the object of a serious inquiry, just as we can seriously investigate our own conscience without lapsing into moral weakness. He who feels in a bad way with himself and wishes to improve, briefly he who wishes to "become something," must take counsel with himself. For unless a man changes inwardly as well, external changes in the situation are either unimportant or even harmful.   [LVI, 16 f

Every progress of humanity, every achievement in the field of perception, has been bound up with progress in self-realization. Man has distinguished himself from the object, and has then confronted nature in an active way. Therefore a new orientation of the psychological attitude will also have to follow the same path.   [XIII, 176

The greatest of all illusions is to think that anything could ever satisfy us. It is this illusion that makes things seem intolerable and bars the way to all progress, and it is one of the most difficult things to overcome.   [XLII, 35

It is not enough to jump up, puff oneself out, and shout, "I take the responsibility!" Not only humanity, but fate also, would like to know in such a case who has promised to take this great step and whether he is capable of assuming the responsibility. Of course anyone can say so. It is not the post which makes the man, but the man who does his work. Therefore self-investigation, with the help of a second person or even several, is (or rather should be!) the essential precondition for the taking on of higher duties, even if it is only a question of realizing the meaning of individual life in the best possible form and to the greatest possible extent. Nature always does this, although without responsibility, for this latter is the fated and divine lot of man.   [LVI, 17

The method is only the way and direction laid down by a man in order that his action may be the true expression of his nature. If it fails to be this, then the method is nothing more than an affectation, something artificially pieced on, rootless and sapless, serving only the illegitimate goal of self-deception. It becomes a means of fooling oneself and of evading what is perhaps the implacable law of one's being.　　[xiv, 11 f (h, 79)

The judgment of others is not *eo ipso* a standard of values; in some cases it is only useful information. The individual is capable, nay, he is even called upon to set up and use his own standard of values. Ethics are in the final count an individual affair.　　[xii, 5 f

Since great innovations always begin in the most improbable places, the fact, for example, that a man is not nearly as ashamed of his nakedness as he used to be might be the beginning of a recognition of himself as he is. Hard upon this will follow the recognition of many other things that are now strictly taboo, because the reality of the earth will not for ever remain veiled, like the *virgines velandae* of Tertullian. Moral unmasking is only one step further in the same direction, and behold, there stands a man as he is, and confesses himself to be as he is. If he does this in a meaningless way, he is a chaotic fool, but if he knows the significance of what he does, he can belong to a higher order of man who, regardless of suffering, makes real the Christ-symbol.　　[xiv, 72 (h, 134 f)

We can obviously make a wrong use of self-knowledge, just as of any other knowledge.　　[lvi, 18

If there ever was a time when individual consciousness was the absolutely indispensable and only right thing, it is now, in our present catastrophic epoch. Yet whoever attains to individual consciousness must necessarily break through the frontiers of the unconscious, for this contains what, above all else, he needs to know.　　[li, 9 (d, xii)

Because each individual needs upheaval, inner discord, the break-up of the existing order, and renewal, this does not mean that he should force these things upon his fellow men under the hypocritical cloak of Christian love, or sense of social responsibility, or any other beautiful synonym for the unconscious urge to personal power. Individual consciousness, the return of the individual to fundamental human nature, to his own being with its individual and social destiny—it is here that the process of healing can begin for that blindness which reigns at the present time. [LI, 11 (D, xiv)

BETWEEN GOOD AND EVIL

There are times in the history of the world (our own may be one of them) when something that is good must make way; what is destined to be better thus appears at first to be evil. This last sentence shows how dangerous it is even to touch upon these problems, for how easy it would be, according to this, for evil to smuggle itself in by simply explaining that it is the potentially better!   [xxvii, 210 (f, 304)

The inner voice brings to consciousness whatever the whole —whether the nation to which we belong or humanity of which we are a part—suffers from. But it presents this evil in individual form, so that at first we would suppose all this evil to be only a trait of individual character.   [xxvii, 208 f (f, 303)

We are so accustomed to hear that everybody has his "difficulties and problems" that we simply accept it as a banal fact, without considering what these difficulties and problems really mean. Why is one never satisfied with oneself? Why is one unreasonable? Why is one not always good and why must one ever leave a cranny for evil? Why does one sometimes say too much and sometimes too little? Why does one do foolish things which could easily be avoided with a little consideration? What is it that is always frustrating us and thwarting our best intentions? Why are there people who never notice these things or cannot even admit their existence? And finally, why do people in the mass beget the historical lunacy of the last thirty years? Why couldn't Pythagoras, twenty-four hundred years ago, have established the rule of wisdom once and for all, or Christianity have set up the Kingdom of Heaven upon earth?
[lx, 45 f (n, 362)

Look at the devilish means of destruction! They are invented by perfectly harmless gentlemen, reasonable, respectable citizens, being all we hope to be. And when the whole thing blows up and causes an indescribable inferno of devastation, nobody seems to be responsible. It simply occurs, yet it is all man-made.
[xlvi, 88 f (b, 60)

The dammed-up instinct-forces in civilized man are immensely more destructive, and hence more dangerous, than the instincts of the primitive, who in a modest degree is constantly living his negative instincts. Consequently no war of the historical past can rival a war between civilized nations in its colossal scale of horror. [IX, 199 (I, 175)

Let man but accumulate his materials of destruction, and the devil within him will soon be unable to resist putting them to their fated use. It is well known that fire-arms go off of themselves if only enough of them are together. [XIX, 413 (J, 236)

The incompleteness of humanity is always a dissonance in the harmony of our ideal. Unfortunately no one lives in the world as it is desired to be, but in the world of actuality, where good and evil wage their war of mutual destruction, and where the hands which are meant for creating and building cannot avoid getting dirty. Whenever there is something really critical or doubtful in question, there is always someone who assures us, amid much applause, that nothing has happened and everything is in order. [X, 36 (G, 182)

The Church has the doctrine of the devil, of an evil principle, whom we like to imagine complete with cloven hoofs, horns, and tail, half man, half beast, a chthonic deity apparently escaped from the rout of Dionysus, the sole surviving champion of the sinful joys of paganism. An excellent picture, and one which exactly describes the grotesque and sinister side of the unconscious, for we have never really come to grips with it and consequently it has remained in its original savage state. Probably no one today would still be rash enough to assert that the European is a lamblike creature and not possessed of the devil. The frightful records of our age are plain for all to see, and they surpass in hideousness everything that any previous age, with its feeble instruments, could have hoped to accomplish. [LX, 46 (N, 363)

Thanks to the development of the feeling-values, the splendour of the shining Godhead has increased to an immeasurable degree, but man himself has swallowed the darkness and out of it has produced sin, original sin, and the main wickedness of heart. Indeed the devil has been largely disposed of, i.e., intro-jected, so that even the medieval European was able to confess: *omne bonum a Deo, omne malum a homine*. In recent times this development has taken a diabolical turn in the opposite direc-tion and the wolf in sheep's clothing goes about whispering in our ears that evil is really nothing but a misunderstanding of good. People imagine that darkness has thus been done away with for good and all and never stop to think what an insidious poisoning of the human soul has in consequence set in. Man thereby makes himself into the devil, for the latter is the half of an archetype whose irresistible power causes even the non-believing European to cry out "Oh, God!" on all appropriate and inappropriate occasions. [XLIII, 439

Western man has already whittled down his own soul to such an extent that he is now compelled to deny the very essence of that psychic power which is and always will be beyond man's control, namely the Godhead itself, in order to be master of good as well as of evil, which he has already swallowed.

[XLIII, 440

Evil needs to be pondered just as much as good, for good and evil are ultimately nothing but ideal extensions and abstrac-tions of doing, and both belong to the chiaroscuro of life. In the last resort there is no good that cannot produce evil and no evil that cannot produce good. [LVIII, 53 (M, 36)

Only that which acts is actual. If something which seems to me an error shows itself to be more effective than a truth, then I must first follow up the error, for in it lie power and life, which I lose if I hold to what seems to me true. Light has need of darkness—otherwise how could it appear as light?

[XXI, 24 f (J, 277)

We know of course that without sin there is no repentance and without repentance no redeeming grace, also that without original sin the redemption of the world could never have come about—but we assiduously avoid investigating whether in this very power of evil God may not have placed some special purpose which it is most important for us to know. One often feels driven to some such view when, like the psychotherapist, one has to deal with people who are confronted with their blackest shadow. [LVIII, 51 (M, 36)

The word "human," which resounds so beautifully, means fundamentally nothing beautiful, virtuous, or intelligent, but just a low average. This is the step which Zarathustra could not take, the step to the "ugliest man," to the real human creature. The struggle and the fear that always mark the recoil from this step show how great is the attraction and seductive power of the underworld. Its power is undeniable, and to deny it is no deliverance; it is merely a sham, an essential misconstruction of its value and meaning. For where is a height without an equal depth, and how can there be light that throws no shadow? No good ever appears that an evil does not oppose. "Thou canst be delivered from no sin thou hast not committed," said Carpokrates, a deep saying for all who wish to understand, and a brilliant opportunity for all who prefer to draw false conclusions. But all that is below, and that longs to take its share in the lives of more conscious and, therefore, more complete men, is not a persuasive prompting to mere pleasure, but something that man fears. [x, 43 (G, 186)

Mankind is constantly inclined to forget that what was once good does not remain good eternally. He goes along the old ways that once were good, long after they have become injurious to him; only through the greatest sacrifices and with what untold suffering can he rid himself of this delusion and discern that what was good once is now perhaps grown old and is good no longer. This is so in the little things as in the big.
[IX, 264 (I, 229)
Whatever the metaphysical position of the devil may be, in psychological reality evil signifies an effective and even threatening limitation of good, so that it is not too much to say that in this world not only day and night but also good and evil hold the balance, and that this is the reason why the victory of the good is always a special act of grace. [L, 54

We have certain ideas as to how a civilized, educated, moral human being should live, and from time to time we do our best to fulfil these ambitious expectations ourselves. But since nature has not blessed all her children with the same favours, some are more gifted and others less. Thus there are people who are able to live "correctly" and respectably, and there is no fly to be found in the ointment. Either their sins are small sins, if they commit any at all, or else they are unaware of them. But nature is by no means merciful to unconscious sinners. She punishes them just as severely as if they were guilty of a conscious transgression. As Drummond once said, we find that it is just the most pious people who are unconscious of their other side and who develop especially hellish moods which make them unbearable to their nearest and dearest. The fame of holiness may reach far and wide, but to have to live with a saint can cause either an inferiority complex or even a wild outbreak of immorality in individuals who are morally less gifted. Morality appears to be a gift like intelligence. It cannot be pumped into a system in which it is not inborn without doing harm.

[XLVI, 136 f

We quite forget that we can be as deplorably overcome by a virtue as by a vice. There is a sort of frenzied, orgiastic virtuousness which is just as infamous as a vice and leads to just as much injustice and violence.   [IV, 221 f

The world insists on a certain code of behaviour, and the professional people strive to live up to what is expected of them. The man who succeeds in doing this is, to say the least of it, a bluffer. The danger is that of becoming identical with the "persona," the professor, for instance, with his text-book or the tenor with his voice. When this happens the harm has already been done. Such a man lives only in his own biography. He can no longer do the simplest thing in a natural, human way. For now it is as if everything were already written ". . . and then he went to such and such a place and said so and so. . . ." The garment of Deianira has grown on to his skin, and it needs the desperate resolve of a Hercules to tear this Nessus shirt from his body and enter the consuming flames of immortality in order to be transformed into what he really is. With a little exaggeration, we might also say that the persona is that which in

211

reality we are not but which in our own and other people's opinions we are. In any case the temptation to be what we appear to be is great, for the persona is usually paid in ready money. [XLVII, 414 f

A consciousness that is purely personal emphasizes its peculiar and exclusive right to its contents with a certain anxiety, seeking therewith to construct a totality. But all the contents that do not readily fit into this totality are either overlooked and forgotten or repressed and denied. This is also a kind of self-education, but it is too arbitrary and does too great violence to the facts. In favour of an ideal image, into which one would prefer to mould oneself, too much that is generally human has to be sacrificed. These "personal" people are accordingly always very sensitive, for something is only too liable to happen that will bring to consciousness some unwelcome part of their real (individual) character. [XI, 62 f (D, 164)

The identification with one's profession or office is certainly a seductive possibility. Otherwise why should so many men be content to be nothing more than this general worth which society accords them? To look for a personality behind this shell would be fruitless. The opening up would be a massive undertaking, but inside it we should find only a pitiable little man. This is why the profession, or whatever this outer shell may be, is so seductive; it offers an easy compensation for personal insufficiency. [XI, 41 f (D, 148)

A man cannot get rid of himself in favour of an artificial personality without punishment. The mere attempt to do so releases, in all ordinary cases, unconscious reactions in the form of moods, affects, fears, compulsive ideas, feelings, vices, etc. In his private life, the "strong man" socially is often a mere child in relation to his own feeling, and his public discipline (which he often demands unquestioningly from others) goes to pieces entirely in private. His "joy in his work" assumes a melancholy or hypochondriac face at home. Behind the mask, his "spotless" public morality begins to look rather remarkable—we will not mention deeds, only fantasies; but women, too,

could say something about such men. And his children may
have definite views about his "selfless altruism."

[XI, 127 f (D, 210)

Obviously whoever builds up too good a persona has to pay
for it in irritability. Bismarck had hysterical weeping fits, Wagner a correspondence about the belt of a silk dressing-gown,
Nietzsche wrote letters to a "dear Lama," Goethe indulged in
conversations with Eckermann, etc. But there are also much
subtler things than the banal "lapses" of heroes. I once made
the acquaintance of a very fine and honourable man, in fact
one might almost have called him a saint. I studied him for
three whole days, and never a mortal shortcoming did I find
in him. My feeling of inferiority grew ominous, and I began
seriously to think of how I might better myself. But on the
fourth day his wife consulted me. . . . Well—nothing of the
sort has ever happened to me since. But I learned this from it:
that every man who becomes one with his persona can allow
every disturbing element to be manifested by his wife, without
her noticing the fact. But she pays for her self-sacrifice with a
bad neurosis.   [XI, 126 f (D, 209)

The meeting with ourselves belongs to the more unpleasant
things that may be avoided as long as we possess living symbol-
figures in which all that is inner and unknown is projected. The
figure of the devil, in particular, is a most valuable and acceptable psychic possession, for as long as he goes about outside in the form of a roaring lion, we know where evil lurks;
namely, in that incarnate Old Harry where it has been in this or
that form since primeval times. With the rise of consciousness
since the Middle Ages, to be sure, he has been considerably reduced in stature. But to take his place there are human beings
to whom we gratefully resign our shadows. With what pleasure, for instance, we read newspaper reports of crime! A true
criminal becomes a popular figure because he unburdens in no
small degree the consciences of his fellow men, for now they
know once more where evil is to be found.   [XXXI, 200 (F, 69)

The man who looks into the mirror of the waters does, indeed,
see his own face first of all. Whoever goes to himself risks a con-

frontation with himself. The mirror does not flatter, it faithfully shows whatever looks into it; namely, the face we never show to the world because we cover it with the persona, the mask of the actor. But the mirror lies behind the mask and shows the true face. This confrontation is the first test of courage on the inner way, a test sufficient to frighten off most people.

[xxxi, 199 f (f, 69)

Simple things are always the most difficult. In actual life it requires the greatest discipline to be simple, and the acceptance of oneself is the essence of the moral problem and the epitome of a whole outlook upon life. That I feed the hungry, that I forgive an insult, that I love my enemy in the name of Christ —all these are undoubtedly great virtues. What I do unto the least of my brethren, that I do unto Christ. But what if I should discover that the least among them all, the poorest of all the beggars, the most impudent of all the offenders, the very enemy himself—that these are within me, and that I myself stand in need of the alms of my own kindness, that I myself am the enemy who must be loved—what then? As a rule, the Christian's attitude is then reversed; there is no longer any question of love or long suffering; we say to the brother within us "Revenge!" and condemn and rage against ourselves. We hide it from the world; we refuse to admit ever having met this least among the lowly in ourselves. Had it been God himself who drew near to us in this despicable form, we should have denied him a thousand times before a single cock had crowed.

[xxi, 19 (j, 271 f)

Unfortunately there is no doubt about the fact that man is, as a whole, less good than he imagines himself or wants to be. Everyone carries a shadow, and the less it is embodied in the individual's conscious life, the blacker and denser it is. If an inferiority is conscious, one always has a chance to correct it. It is constantly in contact with other interests, so that it is steadily subjected to modifications. But if it is repressed and isolated from consciousness, it never gets corrected.   [xlvi, 137 f (b, 93)

There is really something terrifying about the fact that man has also a shadow-side to his nature which is not just made up of small weaknesses and blemishes, but possesses a positively demoniacal impetus. The individual human being seldom knows anything about it; for, as an individual, it seems to him incredible that he could somewhere or somehow outreach himself. But let these harmless beings form a mob, and the result can be a delirious monster, and every individual is only the smallest cell in the body of the monster, where, for good or ill, he can do nothing else but join in the blood-lust of the beast, even upholding it with all his might. Out of a dim presentiment of the possibilities lurking in the dark side of human nature, we refuse to recognize it. We struggle blindly against the healing dogma of original sin, which is nevertheless so utterly true. We even hesitate to admit the conflict of which we are so painfully aware. [LI, 54 f

The educated man tries to repress the inferior one in himself, without realizing that by this he forces the latter to become revolutionary. [XLVI, 143 (B, 95)

We carry our past with us, to wit, the primitive and inferior man with his desires and emotions, and it is only by a considerable effort that we can detach ourselves from this burden. If it comes to a neurosis, we have invariably to deal with a considerably intensified shadow. And if such a case wants to be cured it is necessary to find a way in which man's conscious personality and his shadow can live together. [XLVI, 138 (B, 93)

As a rule those tendencies that represent the amount of anti-social elements in man's psychical structure—what I call the "statistical criminal" in everybody—are suppressed, that is, consciously and deliberately disposed of. But tendencies that are merely repressed are usually only doubtful in character. They are not indubitably antisocial, but are rather unconventional and socially awkward. The reason one represses them is equally doubtful. Some people repress them from sheer cowardice, others from a merely conventional morality, and others again from the motive of respectability. Repression is a sort of half-conscious and half-hearted letting go of things, a dropping of hot cakes or a reviling of grapes which hang too high, or a

looking the other way in order not to become conscious of one's
desires.   [XLVI, 135 f (B, 91)

The maddest and most moving dramas are not played, as we
know, on the stage, but in the hearts of respectable citizens
whom we pass by without a thought, and who at best show the
world what battles are raging within them only if they have a
nervous breakdown. What the layman finds most difficult to
understand is that the patient himself has frequently no idea
that civil war has broken out in his unconscious. But if we think
how many people there are who understand nothing at all
about themselves, we need not wonder overmuch that there are
some who have no idea of their actual conflicts.   [V, 255 f

To cherish secrets and to restrain emotions are psychic mis-
demeanours for which nature finally visits us with sickness—
that is, when we do these things in private. But when they are
done in communion with others they satisfy nature and may
even count as useful virtues. It is only restraint practised in
and for oneself that is unwholesome. It is as if man had an in-
alienable right to behold all that is dark, imperfect, stupid, and
guilty in his fellow beings—for such, of course, are the things
that we keep private to protect ourselves. It seems to be a sin
in the eyes of nature to hide our insufficiency—just as much as
to live entirely on our inferior side.   [XIX, 10 (J, 39)

If the repressed tendencies—the shadow, as I call them—were
decidedly evil, there would be no problem whatever. But the
shadow is merely somewhat inferior, primitive, unadapted, and
awkward; not wholly bad. It even contains inferior, childish, or
primitive qualities which would in a way vitalize and embellish
human existence, but "it is not done."   [XLVI, 141 f (B, 94 f)

In reality, however, the acceptance of the shadow-side of human nature verges on the impossible. Consider for a moment
what it means to grant the right of existence to what is unreasonable, senseless and evil! Yet it is just this that the modern
man insists upon. He wants to live with every side of himself—
to know what he is. That is why he casts history aside. He wants
to break with tradition so that he can experiment with his life

216

and determine what value and meaning things have in themselves, apart from traditional presuppositions.

[XXI, 23 (J, 275 f)

A mere suppression of the shadow is just as little of a remedy as is beheading for headache. To destroy a man's morality does not help either, because it would kill his better self, without which even the shadow makes no sense. The reconciliation of these opposites is a major problem, and even in antiquity it bothered certain minds. [XLVI, 138 f (B, 93 f)

Taking it in its deepest sense, the shadow is the invisible saurian tail that man still drags behind him. Carefully amputated, it becomes the serpent of healing of the mystery. Only monkeys parade with it. [XXXI, 227 (F, 93)

If you imagine someone who is brave enough to withdraw these projections, all and sundry, then you get an individual conscious of a pretty thick shadow. Such a man has saddled himself with new problems and conflicts. He has become a serious problem to himself, as he is now unable to say that *they* do this or that, *they* are wrong, *they* must be fought against. He lives in the "house of self-collection." Such a man knows that whatever is wrong in the world is in himself, and if he learns only to deal with his own shadow then he has done something real for the world. He has succeeded in removing an infinitesimal part, at least, of the unsolved gigantic social problems of our day. [XLVI, 150 f (B, 101 f)

The shadow is a tight pass, a narrow door, whose painful constriction is spared to no one who climbs down into the deep well-spring. But one must learn to know oneself in order to know who one is. For what comes after the door is, surprisingly enough, a boundless expanse full of unprecedented uncertainty, with apparently no inside and no outside, no above and no below, no here and no there, no mine and no thine, no good and no bad. It is the world of water, where everything living floats in suspension; where the kingdom of the sympathetic system, of the soul of everything living, begins: where *I* am inseparably

217

this and that, and this and that are I; where I experience the other person in myself, and the other, as myself, experiences me. The unconscious is anything but a capsulated, personal system; it is the wide world, and objectivity as open as the world. [xxxi, 200 f (f, 70)

It is naturally a fundamental error to believe that if we see an anti-value in a value, or an untruth in a truth, the value or the truth is then invalid. They have only become relative. Everything human is relative, because everything depends upon an inner polarity, for everything is a phenomenon of energy. And energy itself necessarily depends on a previous polarity without which there can be no energy. There must always be high and low, hot and cold, etc., so that the process of adjustment, which is energy, can occur. The tendency to deny all previous values in favour of their opposites is therefore just as exaggerated as the former one-sidedness. Where generally accepted and undoubted values are suddenly thrown away, there is a fatal loss. Whoever acts in this way ends by throwing himself overboard with the discarded values. [li, 137

The difficulty lies in striking the dead centre. For this an awareness of the two sides of man's personality is essential, of their respective aims and origins. These two aspects must never be separated through arrogance or cowardice.
[lviii, 166 (m, 148)

Our mistake would lie in supposing that what is radiant no longer exists because it has been explained from the shadow-side. Yet the shadow belongs to the light as the evil belongs to the good, and vice versa. Therefore I cannot regret the shock that was felt at the exposure of our occidental illusions and pettiness; on the contrary, I welcome this exposure and attach to it an almost incalculable significance. It is one of those swings of the pendulum which, as history has so often shown, set matters right again. It forces us to accept a present-day philosophical relativism such as has been formulated by Einstein for mathematical physics, and which is fundamentally a truth of the Far East whose ultimate effects upon us we cannot foresee. [xix, 20 f (j, 47 f)

Our knowledge of good and evil has decreased with our increasing knowledge and experience, and in the future it will diminish still further, although we cannot ignore the ethical values. In this extreme uncertainty we need the enlightenment of a holy and "whole-making" spirit; and whatever this may be it is certainly not our reason. [L, 64

Even on the highest summits we are never beyond good and evil, and the more we learn of the inextricable interweaving of good and evil the more uncertain and confused will our moral judgment become. Moreover it is of no use whatsoever to throw out the moral criterion like old scrap-iron and to "set up new tables" (after a well-known example). For as it always was and till the end of time shall be: an injustice purposely thought out and committed against our soul will avenge itself, whether the world has taken on another aspect or not. [L, 64

On paper the moral code looks clear and neat enough; but the same document written on the "living tables of the heart" is often a sorry tatter, particularly in the mouths of those who talk the loudest. We are told on every side that evil is evil and that there can be no hesitation in condemning it, but that does not prevent evil from being the most problematical thing in the individual's life and the one which demands the deepest reflection. What above all deserves our keenest attention is the question: "Exactly *who* is the doer?" For the answer to this question ultimately decides the value of the deed. It is true that society attaches greater importance at first to what is done, because it is immediately obvious; but in the long run the right deed in the hands of the wrong man will also have a disastrous effect. No one who is far-sighted will allow himself to be hoodwinked by the right action of the wrong man, any more than by the wrong action of the right man. [LVIII, 52 f (M, 36)

If, as many are fain to believe, the unconscious were only nefarious, only evil, then the situation would be simple and the path clear: to do good and to eschew evil. But what is "good" and what is "evil"? The unconscious is not just evil by nature, it is also the source of the highest good: not only dark

219

but also light, not only bestial, semihuman, and demonic but superhuman, spiritual, and, in the classical sense of the word, "divine." [LX, 46 f (N, 364)

Christianity has made the antinomy of good and evil into a world problem and, by formulating the conflict dogmatically, raised it to an absolute principle. Into this as yet unresolved conflict Christian man is cast as a protagonist of good and a fellow player in the world drama. To be a follower of Christ means, in its deepest sense, a suffering that is unendurable to the great majority of mankind. Consequently the example of Christ is in reality followed either with reservations or not at all, and the pastoral practice of the Church even finds itself obliged to "lighten the yoke of Christ." This means a pretty considerable reduction in the harshness and severity of the conflict and hence, in practice, a relativism of good and evil. Good is equivalent to the unconditional imitation of Christ and evil is its hindrance. Man's moral weakness and sloth are what chiefly hinder the imitation, and it is to these that probabilism extends a practical understanding which may sometimes, perhaps, come nearer to Christian tolerance, mildness, and love of one's neighbour than the attitude of those who see in probabilism a mere laxity. [LVIII, 39 f (M, 25)

"Love thy neighbour" is wonderful, since we then have nothing to do about ourselves; but when it is a question of "love thy neighbour as thyself" then we are no longer so sure, for we think that it would be egoism to love ourselves. To love oneself, there was no need to preach this to people in olden times, because they did so as a matter of course. But how does this stand nowadays? It would do us good to take the thing somewhat to heart, especially the phrase "as thyself." How can I love my neighbour, if I do not love myself? How can we be altruistic, if we do not treat ourselves decently? But if we treat ourselves decently, and if we love ourselves, then we discover what we are and what we should love. There is nothing for it but to put our foot into the serpent's mouth. He who cannot love, can never transform the serpent, and then nothing is changed. [XXXIV, 87

Christ espoused the sinner and did not condemn him. The true follower of Christ will do the same; and, since one should do unto others as one would do unto oneself, one will also take the part of the sinner who is oneself. And as little as we would accuse Christ of fraternizing with evil, so little should we reproach ourselves that to love the sinner who is oneself is to make a pact with the devil. Love makes a man better, hate makes him worse—even when that man is oneself.

[LVIII, 54 (M, 37)

The reality of evil and its incompatibility with good cleave the opposites asunder and lead inexorably to the crucifixion and suspension of everything that lives. Since "the soul is by nature Christian" this result is bound to come as infallibly as it did in the life of Jesus: we all have to be "crucified with Christ," i.e., suspended in a moral suffering equivalent to veritable crucifixion. In practice this is only possible up to a point, and apart from that is so unbearable and inimical to life that the ordinary human being can afford to get into such a state only occasionally, in fact as seldom as possible. For how could he remain ordinary in face of such suffering!   [LVIII, 38 f (M, 24)

It is no easy matter to live a life that is modelled on Christ's, but it is unspeakably harder to live one's own life as truly as Christ lived his. Anyone who did this would run counter to the forces of the past, and though he might thus be fulfilling his destiny, would none the less be misjudged, derided, tortured, and crucified.   [XXI, 20 (J, 273)

Life demands for its consummation and fulfilment a balance between joy and suffering; but since suffering is in itself unpleasant, people naturally prefer not to think about how much care and sorrow belong to the natural lot of man. So they use comforting words such as "progress" and "the greatest possible happiness," forgetting that happiness itself is poisoned when the measure of suffering has not been fulfilled.   [LV, 162 (K, 42)

Opposites can be reconciled practically only in the form of compromise, i.e., irrationally, wherein a *novum* arises between them which, though different from both, has the power to

221

take up their energies in equal measure as an expression of both and of neither. Such an expression cannot be contrived; it can only be created through living. [IX, 149 (I, 133)

Nature is ambiguous, and we cannot say that either Paracelsus or the alchemists were wrong if, with caution and a scrupulous sense of their responsibility, they spoke in parables. This method is really more suited to the subject. What lies between light and dark and what unites these opposites has a part in both sides and can just as well be studied from the left side as from the right, without our being any the wiser; we can only tear the opposites apart once again. Only the symbol can help, which by its paradoxical character represents that third factor which logic does not admit, but which in actual reality is a living truth. [XLVIII, 134 f

The symbol is the middle way, upon which the opposites unite towards a new movement, a watercourse that pours forth fertility after long drought. [IX, 367 (I, 324)

Most intense conflicts, if overcome, leave behind a sense of security and rest, or a brokenness, that it is scarcely possible to disturb again or to cure, as the case may be. But on the other hand, it needs just these widely split opposites and their conflagrations for the production of valuable and permanent results. [XIII, 45 (G, 28)

The possession of complexes, on the other hand, does not in itself signify a neurosis, for complexes are the normal focal points of psychic happenings, and the fact that they are painful does not show that there is a pathological disturbance. Suffering is not an illness, but the normal counterpole to happiness. A complex only becomes pathological when we delude ourselves that we have not got it. [LV, 159 (K, 39)

Suppression amounts to a conscious moral choice, but repression is a rather immoral penchant for getting rid of disagreeable decisions. Suppression may cause worry, conflict, and suffering, but it never causes a neurosis of one of the usual patterns. Neurosis is a substitute for legitimate suffering.

[XLVI, 136 (B, 91 f)

Not everyone is capable of self-surrender. There is no "ought" or "must" about it, for the very act of exerting the will inevitably places such an emphasis on "I will" that the opposite of self-surrender results. The Titans could not take Olympus by storm, still less a Christian heaven. The most healing of all experiences, and those which are most necessary for the soul, are a "precious thing hard to obtain," and their achievement demands something out of the ordinary from the ordinary man.

[LV, 162 (K, 43)

The most wounding, painful arrows do not come from outside through rumours which always attack from without; they come from the ambush, from our own unconscious. They it is that cause that helpless suffering, and not that which assails us from outside. [IV, 278

To depart from the truths of the blood produces neurotic restlessness, of which we might have had more than enough nowadays. Restlessness breeds senselessness, and the emptiness of a life which has no sense is a psychic suffering of which our age has not yet grasped the full extent and implications.

[XXVII, 230

Suppose I feel well and content with life, nobody can prove to me that I am not. Logical arguments simply glance off the experienced fact of feeling. Original sin, the meaning of life, and immortality are such facts of feeling. But to experience them is a charisma which no human art can bring to pass. Only unreserved self-surrender can hope to achieve such an aim.

[LV, 162 (K, 43)

The Christian doctrine of original sin on the one hand, and of the meaning and value of suffering on the other, has therefore a deep therapeutic value, and is undoubtedly much better suited to Western man than is Islamic fatalism. In the same way the belief in immortality contributes to that smooth flow of life into the future which is needed if arrest and regression are to be avoided. [LV, 162 (K, 42)

Everyday reasonableness, sound human judgment, and science as a compendium of common sense certainly help us over a good part of the road; yet they do not go beyond that frontier of human life which surrounds the commonplace and matter-of-fact, the merely average and normal. They afford, after all, no answer to the question of spiritual suffering and its innermost meaning. A psychoneurosis must be understood as the suffering of a human being who has not discovered what life means for him. But all creativeness in the realm of the spirit as well as every psychic advance of man arises from a state of mental suffering, and it is spiritual stagnation, psychic sterility, which causes this state. [xxi, 7 (j, 259 f)

To be adapted is certainly an ideal. Yet adaptation is not always possible; there are situations in which the only correct adaptation is patient endurance. [ix, 353 (i, 312)

But it is the same with every single human being and his reasonably ordered world. His reason has done violence to natural forces which seek their revenge and only await the moment when the partition falls to overwhelm the conscious life with destruction. Man has been aware of this danger since the earliest times, even in the most primitive stages of culture. It was to arm himself against this threat and to heal the damage done that he developed religious and magical practices. This is why the medicine-man is also the priest; he is the saviour of the body as well as of the soul, and religions are systems of healing for psychic illness. This is especially true of the two greatest religions of man, Christianity and Buddhism. Man is never helped in his suffering by what he thinks for himself, but only by revelations of a wisdom greater than his own. It is this which lifts him out of his distress. [xxi, 25 f (j, 278)

THE LIFE OF THE SPIRIT

For a long time spirit and the passion of the spirit were the greatest values, the things most worth striving for, in our peculiar Christian culture of the mind. Only after the decline of the Middle Ages, that is, in the course of the nineteenth century, when spirit began to degenerate into intellect, a reaction set in against the unbearable domination of intellectualism which led to the pardonable mistake of confusing intellect with spirit, and blaming the latter for the misdeeds of the former. Intellect does, in fact, violate the soul when it tries to possess itself of the heritage of the spirit. It is in no way fitted to do this, because spirit is something higher than intellect in that it includes not only the latter, but the feelings as well. It is a line or principle of life that strives after superhuman, shining heights. [xv, 533 (h, 81)

While our intellect has been achieving colossal things, our spiritual dwelling has fallen to pieces. We are thoroughly convinced that even with the latest and largest reflecting telescope, now being built in America, men will discover behind the farthest nebulae no empyrean where fire and water intermingle; and we know that our sight will wander despairingly through the emptiness of immeasurable extension. Nor are matters improved when mathematical physics reveals to us the world of the infinitesimally small—swarms of electrons into all eternity! In the end we dig up the wisdom of all times and peoples and find that everything most dear and precious has already been said in the most winning and lovely words. Like yearning children we stretch out our hands to it and suppose that, if we could grasp it, we would possess it too. But what we do possess is no longer valid, and our hands grow weary from reaching out, for riches lie everywhere as far as sight extends. All these possessions turn to water, and more than one magician's apprentice has finally been drowned in these waters called up by himself—unless he first succumbed to the saving delusion that *this* wisdom was good and *that* was bad. From these adepts come those disturbing invalids who believe they have a prophetic mission: that through the artificial sundering of true and false wisdom arises a cleft in the psyche, and from it a loneliness and craving like that of the alcoholic, who always hopes to find companions in his vice. When our natural inheritance has been dissipated, then—to use the language of Heraclitus—all spirit has descended from its fiery heights; to be sure, a different *descensus spiritus sancti*—every symbol is also prophetic. But when spirit becomes heavy it turns to water, and baptism in fire is replaced by baptism in water. In the night of the *Sabbathus sanctus* the magic formula of the priest still repeats this process—*"Descendat in hanc plenitudinum fontis virtus spiritus sancti"*—and the inevitable has happened: the soul has turned to water, as Heraclitus says, and with Luciferian presumption the intellect has usurped the seat whereon the spirit once throned. The spirit, indeed, may claim the *patris potestas* over the soul, but not so the earth-born intellect, which is man's sword or hammer, and not a creator of spiritual worlds, a father of the soul.   [xxxi, 194 f (F, 64)

Who knows how much Faust's imperturbable curiosity as he gazed on the spooks and the bogies of the classical Walpurgisnacht owed to the helpful presence of Mephisto and his matter-of-fact point of view! Would that more people could remember the scientific or philosophical reflections of the much-abused intellect at the right moment! Those who abuse it lay themselves open to the suspicion of never having experienced anything that would have taught them its value and shown them why mankind has forged this weapon with such unprecedented effort. One has to be singularly out of touch with life not to notice such things. The intellect may be the devil, but the devil is the "strange son of chaos" who can most readily be trusted to deal effectively with his mother. The Dionysian experience will give this devil plenty to do should he be looking for work, since the resultant settlement with the unconscious far outweighs the labours of Hercules. In my opinion it presents a whole world of problems which the intellect could not settle even in a hundred years—the very reason why it has so often gone off on a holiday to recuperate on lighter tasks. And this is also the reason why the psyche is forgotten so often and so long, and why the intellect makes such frequent use of magical, apotropaic words like "occult" and "mystic," in the hope that even intelligent people will think that these mutterings really mean something. [LVIII, 134 ff (M, 119)

In the case of civilized man the rationalism of the conscious, otherwise so useful to him, becomes a most formidable obstacle to a frictionless transformation of energy. The reason, always seeking to avoid what is to it an unbearable antinomy, places itself exclusively on the one side or the other, and seeks to hold with a grip of death to the values it has once established. This attempt continues so long as the fact of human reason passes for an "immutable substance" from which any symbolical idea is excluded. But reason is only relative, and eventually checks itself in its own antinomy. Also, it is only a means to an end, a symbolical expression for the point of intersection in a path of development. [XIII, 43 (G, 26)

Although the religious phenomenon of being seized and moved, almost possessed [*Ergriffenheit*], in common with all other emotional phenomena, throws all critical knowledge overboard as incommensurable, the human urge to know yet persists again and again with "ungodly" or Luciferian obstinacy and determination, even with positive necessity, regardless of whether it means gain or harm to the thinking man. Sooner or later, therefore, man will oppose his urge to know to his experience of being deeply moved, and will try to escape from the grasp of the experience in order to be able to form some judgment of the happening. If he can do this with reflection and conscientiousness, he will always discover that at least a part of his experience is of limited human significance. [LVII, 16 f

Most objective values—and reason itself among them—are firmly established complexes handed down to us through the ages, to the organization of which countless generations have laboured with the same necessity with which the nature of the living organism, in general, reacts to the average and constantly recurring conditions of the environment, confronting them with corresponding function-complexes—as, for instance, the eye, which so perfectly corresponds with the nature of light. We might, therefore, speak of a pre-existing, metaphysical world-reason, if, as Schopenhauer has already pointed out, the reaction of the living organism that corresponds with average external influence were not the indispensable condition of its existence. Human reason, therefore, is merely the expression of human adaptability to the average occurrence which has gradually become deposited in solidly organized complexes, constituting our objective values. [IX, 659 (I, 583 f)

The objective occurrence is both law-determined and accidental. In so far as it is law-determined, it is accessible to reason; in so far as it is accidental, it is not. One might reverse it and say that we apply the term law-determined to the occurrence appearing so to our reason, and where its regularity escapes us we call it accidental. The postulate of a universal lawfulness remains a postulate of reason only; in no sense is it a postulate of our functions of perception. Since these are in no way grounded upon the principle of reason and its postulates, they are, of their very nature, irrational. [IX, 532 (I, 468)

In practice, chance is everywhere, and so obtrusive that we might just as well put our causal philosophy back in our pocket. The whole richness of life is both law-abiding and lawless, rational and irrational. Therefore rationalism and the will which is based on it take us only a short stretch of the way. The further we extend the path chosen by rationalism, the more certain we may be that we are excluding the irrational potentialities of life, which have just as much right to be lived. It is true that man showed a certain purposefulness by being capable of directing his life at all. The development of reasonableness can be justly claimed to be the greatest achievement of humanity. But this does not mean that it must or will continue to be so under all circumstances. [LI, 89 f

Rational truths are not the last word, there are also irrational truths. In human affairs, what appears impossible upon the way of the intellect has very often become true upon the way of the irrational. Indeed, all the greatest changes that have ever af-

fected mankind have come not by the way of intellectual calcu-
lation, but by ways which contemporary minds either ignored
or rejected as absurd, and which only long afterwards became
fully recognized through their intrinsic necessity. More often
than not they are never perceived at all, for the all-important
laws of mental development are still to us a seven-sealed book.

[IX, 126 f (I, 113)

Old Heraclitus, who was indeed a very wise man, discovered
the most extraordinary of all psychological laws, namely, the
regulating function of the opposites. He called it *enantiodromia*
(a running contrariwise), by which he meant that everything
tends sooner or later to go over into its opposite. Thus the rational attitude of culture necessarily goes over into its opposite,
the irrational devastation of culture. One must not identify
oneself with reason, because man is not and cannot be wholly
rational, nor will he ever become so. This is a fact which should
be noted by all pedants of culture. The irrational cannot and
must not be wiped out. The gods cannot and must not die.

[LI, 130 f (D, 74)

I have no intention of depreciating the value of divine gift of
reason, the highest of human possessions. But as the sole ruling
power it has no meaning, just as light would have no meaning
in a world without darkness. The wise counsel of the mother
and her relentless law of natural limitation should indeed be
respected by man. He should never forget that the world exists
because its opposites counterbalance each other. The rational
side is balanced by the irrational, and the purposeful effort by
the given fact.   [XLIII, 427 f

Reason can provide this desired equilibrium only to the man
whose reason is already an organ of balance. But for how many
individuals and at what period of history has this actually been
the case? As a general rule, a man must also acquire the opposite of his own condition before he finds himself, willy-nilly,
in the middle way. For the sake of mere reason he can never
forego the appealing sensuousness of the immediate situation.
Against the power and temptation of the temporal, therefore,
he must set the joy of the eternal, and against the passion of
the sensual the ecstasy of the spiritual. As real as the one is for
him, the other must be compellingly effective.   [IX, 320 (I, 280)

Just the most unexpected, just the alarmingly chaotic, reveals the deepest meaning. And the more this meaning is recognized the more does the anima lose its impetuous, impulsive, and compulsive character. Dams against the flood of chaos slowly arise, for the meaningful divides itself from the meaningless. When sense and nonsense are no longer identical, the force of chaos is weakened by the subtraction of sense and nonsense; sense is endowed with the force of meaning, and nonsense with the force of meaninglessness. Thereby a new cosmos arises. [xxxi, 213 (F, 80)

Mental processes or consciousness in general involve such an effort for mankind that simplicity is given the preference under all circumstances, even when it does not at all correspond to the truth. But when it represents at least a half-truth, one is, so to speak, delivered up to it. The simpler nature affects the complicated one like a room that is too small, not allowing him enough space. The complicated nature, on the other hand, gives to the simpler one too many rooms with too much space, so that she never knows where she really belongs.

[xix, 285 f (g, 196 f)

Noble and ignoble are appraisals of worth and therefore subjective, arbitrary, and not to be included in an objective discussion. The word "aristocrat" is also an appraisal of worth. Let us therefore rather speak of the man of the spirit and the man of the earth. Spirit, as we know, is always thought of as "above," as a bright, fiery being of the air, a stirring "pneuma," while the earth lies solid, dark, and cool below. In the principles of ancient Chinese philosophy, this eternal image is expressed as Yang and Yin. The man of the spirit is Yang; his characteristic is an attitude conditioned by ideas (which is also described as "spirit"). The man of the earth is Yin, and his characteristic is an attitude conditioned by the earth. Yang and Yin are deadly enemies and yet need each other. The man who is permeated by his earth stands rooted in an ancient principle which lacks nothing as regards nobility and greatness; it is the eternal opponent and partner of the moving spirit. [xii, 6

The classical world contains a piece of nature and certain problems which Christianity was bound to overlook if it did not wish to hopelessly compromise the establishment of a spiritual point of view on a firm basis. No code of criminal law, no code of morals, nor even the most sublime casuistry will ever finally tabulate or pass a just sentence upon the confusions, the clash of duties, and the unseen tragedies of the natural man in his conflict with the urgencies of civilization. The "spirit" is the one aspect, nature the other. *Naturam expellas furca, tamen usque recurret!* Nature must not be allowed to win the game, and yet she cannot lose it. Wherever consciousness clings to too rigidly defined concepts and becomes caught up in rules and regulations of its own choosing—which is inevitable and belongs to the very nature of a civilized consciousness— then nature steps in with her inescapable demands. Nature is not only matter, she is also spirit. If it were not so, then the only source of the spirit would be human reason.   [xlviii, 169 f

We should not pretend to understand the world only by the intellect; we apprehend it just as much by feeling. Therefore the judgment of the intellect is, at best, only the half of truth, and must, if it be honest, also come to an understanding of its inadequacy.   [ix, 703 f (i, 628)

Besides the gifts of the head there are also gifts of the heart, which are no less important but can easily be overlooked, because in such cases the head is frequently weaker than the heart. And yet such people are often more useful and valuable for the welfare of society than those who are gifted in other ways.   [liii, 6

One can, it is true, understand a great deal with the heart, but then the mind often finds it difficult to follow up with an intellectual formulation which gives a suitable expression to what has been understood. There is also a form of understanding with the head, in particular that of the scientific mind, in which there is often too little room for the heart.   [liv, 46 (l, 175)

The utterances of the heart—in contrast to those of a dis-

criminating intellect—always apply to the whole. The strings
of the heart sing, like those of the Aeolian harp, only to the soft
breath of portending mood which does not drown the sound
but listens to it. What the heart hears are the great, all-embracing things of life, the experiences which we do not arrange but
which we ourselves suffer.   [xx, 9

I am convinced of what I *know*. Everything else is hypothesis
and beyond that I can leave a lot of things to the Unknown.
They do not bother me. But they would begin to bother me, I
am sure, if I felt that I *ought* to know something about them.
                                            [xlvi, 82 (b, 54)
A conclusive appeal to reason would be all very fine if man
were by nature an *animal rationale;* but he is not; he is quite
as much unreasonable as he is reasonable. Therefore reason is
often not sufficient to modify the instinctual drive and make it
conform to a rational order.   [lv, 158 (k, 38)

There are, it is true, arbitrary answers and solutions, but in
principle and in the long run they are neither desirable nor
satisfying. No Gordian knot can be permanently cut, for it has
the awkward property of always tying itself again.
                                            [lv, 159 (k, 38)

But the wheel of history cannot be turned backward, and we
can only strive towards that attitude which permits us to live
the unhampered destiny that our primitive nature instinctively
directs. Only in this condition can we be sure that we are not
perverting spirit into sensuality, and the latter into spirit; for
both must live, the one drawing its life from the other.
                                            [xix, 288 (g, 199)
Nothing is more disgusting than a secretly sexualized spirituality; it is just as unclean as an over-prized sensuality.
                                            [xix, 288 (g, 198)
When certain South American Indians actually and literally
define themselves as red parrots, and expressly reject any figur-
ative explanation, this has nothing in the least to do with
"moral" sexual repression, but is due to an unalterable law inherent in the thinking function, the law of independence and

emancipation from the concretism of sensual perceptions. It should be recognized that the thinking function possesses a separate principle, which only merges with the beginnings of sexuality in the polyvalent infantile germinal stage. A bending back of thought under a one-sided sexuality is an undertaking which runs counter to the basic facts of human psychology.

[II, 36

I am convinced that a true scientific spirit in psychology must also come to the conclusion that the dynamic processes of the psyche are not to be traced back to this or that particular instinct—which would bring psychology down to the level of the theory of heat. The scientific approach will rather include the instincts in the realm of the psyche and will draw the principle of the explanation from their mutual relationship. I have therefore emphasized that it would be well to assume a hypothetical factor, an "energy," as the psychological basis of explanation, and to define it as "libido" in the classical sense of the word, as an "impetuous craving," without stating anything about its material side. By means of such a factor, the dynamic processes can be explained unhesitatingly and without violating them in any way, which would be inevitable in the case of a concrete basis of explanation. [VIII, 467

Instinct is not a thing apart, and it cannot be isolated in practice. It is always bound up with archetypal contents which have a spiritual aspect, by which it both justifies and limits itself. In other words, the instinctual drive is always and inevitably linked up with something in the nature of a philosophy of life, however archaic, dim, and lacking in clarity this may be. Instinct forces man to think, and if he does not think of his own free will, there arises a compulsive thinking, for the two poles of the psyche, the physiological and the spiritual, are indissolubly bound up with one another. That is why the instincts cannot be freed without touching on the spirit, just as the spirit is condemned to meaningless activity if it is divorced from the instinctive sphere. [LV, 161 (K, 41 f)

What after all would spirit be, if it had no peer among the instincts to oppose it? It would be an empty form.

[XIII, 97 (G, 66)

We might call sexuality the spokesman of the instincts; therefore the spiritual standpoint sees it as its chief antagonist, not at all because sexual indulgence in and for itself is more immoral than excessive eating and drinking, avarice, tyranny, and other extravagances, but because the spirit senses in sexuality a peer, a counterpart related to itself. For just as the spirit would subordinate sexuality, like every other instinct to its form, so sexuality in its turn has an ancient claim upon the spirit, which once—in begetting, in pregnancy, in birth and childhood—it contained within itself; moreover the spirit can never dispense with the passion of sexuality in its creations.

[XIII, 96 f (G, 65 f)

I must also emphasize the fact that the spiritual principle does not, strictly speaking, collide with instinct, but only with blind instinctiveness, which really amounts to an unjustifiable preponderance of the instinctive nature over the spiritual. Spirituality appears in the psyche as an instinct also, as a real passion—indeed, "a consuming fire," as Nietzsche has expressed it, an analogy with the miracle of Pentecost. It is not derived from another instinct, as an "instinct-psychology" would have it; it is definitely a principle *sui generis,* an indispensable form of instinctual power. [XIII, 98 (G, 66)

It is recognized that man living in the state of nature is in no sense merely "natural" like an animal, but sees, believes, fears, worships things the meaning of which is not at all discoverable from the conditions of his natural environment. The underlying meaning of these things leads us in fact far away from all that is natural, obvious, or easily intelligible, and not infrequently contrasting most vividly with the instincts of every living creature. We need only remind ourselves of all those gruesome rites and customs of primitives against which every natural feeling rises in revolt, or of all those convictions and ideas which are in indisputable contradiction to the evidence of the facts. These things force us to the assumption that the spiritual principle, whatever that may be, enforces itself against the merely natural conditions with an incredible strength. One might say that this is also "natural," and that both forces have their origin in one and the same "nature." I do not in the least doubt this origin, but I must point out that this "natural" something presents a conflict between two principles to which, according to taste, one can give this or that name, and that this opposition is the expression, and perhaps also the foundation, of the tension which we term psychic energy.   [XIII, 88 f (G, 59 f)

The pre-existing paths are hard facts, as indisputable as the historical fact of man's having built a city out of his original dwelling-cave. This development was possible only through community culture, and the latter was possible only through the restriction of instinct. The curbing of instinct is maintained through mental processes with the same force and with the same results in the individual as in the history of peoples. The controlling of instinct is a normative or, more accurately, a law-giving process; and its power comes from the unconscious fact of inherited disposition, the deposits of the mental processes of the ancestors.   [XIII, 91 (G, 61)

The fact that all immediate experience is psychic and that immediate reality can only be psychic explains why it is that primitive man puts the appearance of ghosts and the effects of magic on a plane with physical events. He has not yet torn his naïve experiences into their antithetical parts. In his world, mind and matter still interpenetrate each other, and his gods still wander through forest and field. He is like a child, only half-born, still enclosed in a dream-state within his own psyche and the world as it actually is, a world not yet distorted by the difficulties in understanding that beset a dawning intelligence. When the primitive world disintegrated into spirit and nature, the West rescued nature for itself. It was prone to a belief in nature, and only became the more entangled in it with every painful effort to make itself spiritual. The East, on the contrary, took mind for its own, and by explaining away matter as mere illusion (Maya), continued to dream in Asiatic filth and misery. But since there is only *one* earth and *one* mankind, East and West cannot rend humanity into two different halves. Psychic reality exists in its original oneness, and awaits man's advance to a level of consciousness where he no longer believes in the one part and denies the other, but recognizes both as constituent elements of one psyche.   [XXVII, 26 f (J, 221)

The conflict of nature and mind is itself a reflection of the paradox contained in the psychic being of man. This reveals a material aspect and a spiritual aspect, which appear a contradiction as long as we fail to understand the nature of psychic life. Whenever, with our human understanding, we must pronounce upon something that we have not grasped or cannot grasp, then—if we are honest—we must be willing to contradict ourselves, and we must pull this something into its antithetical parts in order to deal with it at all. The conflict of the material and spiritual aspects of life only shows that the psychic is in the last resort an incomprehensible something. [xxvii, 23 f (j, 219)

It is sufficient to know that there is not a single important idea or view that does not possess historical antecedents. They are all founded upon archetypal, primordial forms, whose sensuous nature dates from a time when consciousness did not yet think but merely perceived. Thought was an object of inner perception, not intellection only, but sensed as a manifestation —seen or heard, so to speak. Thought was essentially revelation, not something invented, but something forced upon us or bringing conviction through its immediate actuality. Thoughts antedate the primitive ego-consciousness, and the latter is the object of thought, rather than its subject, according to the Pauline phrase *sicut et cognitus sum* or to the Cartesian *cogito ergo sum*. [xxxi, 215 f (f, 83)

Throughout our whole lives, we have, besides our newly won, directed, adapted thinking, a form of fantasy-thinking which is like the thinking of antiquity and of the barbaric age. In the same way as our bodies still retain the relics of older functions and conditions in a number of organs, our mind, which has apparently outgrown the archaic instinctive tendencies, nevertheless still bears the marks of the development which mankind has passed through and, in dreaming, repeats the ancient times, at last in its fantasies. [iv, 30

But an authority whose statesmanship is wise enough to leave sufficient free play to nature—of which spirit is a part—need not fear a premature decline. It is perhaps a humiliating sign of the spiritual immaturity of European man that he both needs and desires rather a large measure of authority. We are nevertheless faced with the fact that countless millions in Europe—with the unworthy complicity of so-called reformers whose childishness is equalled by their lack of tradition—have escaped from the *patris potestas* of kings and emperors only to fall helpless and senseless victims to any sort of power which cares to assume authority. The immaturity of man is a fact with which we have to reckon.   [LIX, 17 (K, 34)

Progress and development are ideals not lightly to be denied, but they lose all meaning if man only arrives at his new state as a fragment of himself, having left his essential hinterland behind him in the shadow of the unconscious, in a state of primitivity or, indeed, barbarism. The conscious mind, split off from its origins, incapable of realizing the meaning of the new state, then relapses all too easily into a situation far worse than the one from which the innovation was intended to free it—*exempla sunt odiosa!*   [XLIX, 136 (O, 129)

For whoever is psychologically so adapted as to perceive mainly the similarity of things, the collective or constellating concept is, so to speak, taken for granted, i.e., it frankly obtrudes itself with the undeniable actuality of the sense-perception. But, for the man who is psychologically so adjusted as to perceive mainly the diversity of things, the similarity of things is not exclusively assumed; what he sees is their difference, which indeed forces itself upon him with just as much actuality as similarity does to the other. It seems as though "feeling into" [*Einfühlung*] the object were the psychological process which brought the distinctiveness of the object into an especially bright light, and as though *abstraction* from the object were the process most calculated to blind one's eyes to the actual distinctiveness of individual things in favour of their general similarity, which is the very foundation of the idea.   [IX, 69 (I, 63 f)

Ideas represent forces that are beyond logical justification and moral sanction; they are always stronger than man and his brain. Man believes indeed that he moulds these ideas, but in reality they mould him and make him their unwitting mouthpiece. [XIX, 21 (J, 48)

As an empiricist, I must affirm that there is a sort of temperament for which ideas are realities and not mere nomina. By chance—I might almost say—we are now living, and have been for two hundred years, in an age in which it has become unpopular and even incomprehensible to suppose that ideas could be anything else than nomina. Anyone who still thought anachronistically and, following his own temperament, along Platonic lines had to realize with pain that the "heavenly," i.e., metaphysical, reality of the idea had been banished to the unverifiable realm of belief and superstition or left pityingly to the poet. The nominalistic point of view had once again overcome the realistic in the secular duel of universalities and the "primordial image" had vanished into *flatus vocis*. This swing-over was accompanied—even to a considerable extent caused—by the marked advance of empiricism, the advantages of which forced themselves all too clearly upon the mind. Since then the "idea" is no longer an *a priori*, but a secondary thing and a derivative. [XLIII, 404 f

It is true that widely accepted ideas are never the personal property of their so-called author; on the contrary, he is the bondservant of his ideas. Impressive ideas which are hailed as truths have something peculiar to themselves. Although they come into being at a definite time, they are and have always been timeless; they arise from that realm of procreative, psychic life out of which the ephemeral mind of the single human being grows like a plant that blossoms, bears fruit and seed, and then withers and dies. Ideas spring from a source that is not contained within one man's personal life. We do not create them; they create us. To be sure, when we deal in ideas we inevitably make a confession, for they bring to the light of day not only the best that in us lies, but our worst insufficiencies and personal shortcomings as well. [XIX, 74 f (J, 132)

Platonic freedom of the mind does not enable a judgment of

the whole, but tears apart the light side of the divine picture from its darker half. This freedom is to a certain extent a cultural phenomenon and the noble occupation of that fortunate Athenian who was not destined to become a slave. Only the man for whom another carries the burden of the earth can raise himself above nature.   [L, 62

Whoever is conscious of his guiding principle knows with what indisputable authority it rules his life. Generally, however, consciousness is too engrossed with the attainment of some beckoning goal ahead ever to take account of the nature of the spirit that determines its course.   [xix, 396 (G, 95 f)

There are many spirits, both bright and dark. One should therefore accept the view that spirit is something relative, not absolute, that calls for completion and embodiment in life.
                                             [xix, 398 (G, 97)
But just as there is a passion that strives for blind, unrestricted life, so there is also a passion that yearns to bring the whole of life as a sacrifice to the spirit, just because of its creative superiority. This passion makes of the spirit a malignant growth that senselessly destroys human life.   [xix, 399 f (G, 98)

Life is a test of the truth of the spirit. Spirit that drags a man away from all possibility of life, seeking fulfilment only in itself, is a false spirit—and the guilt rests also on the man, since he can choose whether he gives himself up to the spirit or not. Life and spirit are two powers, or necessities, between which man is placed. Spirit gives meaning to his life, and the possibility of the greatest development. But life is essential to spirit, since its truth is nothing if it cannot live.   [xix, 400 (G, 98)

Without the psyche, mind is as dead as matter, because both are artificial abstractions; to primordial intuitions, however, mind is a volatile body, and matter is not lacking in soul.
                                             [xiv, 69 (H, 131)
The cleft which Christianity has torn open between nature and Spirit enabled the human mind to think not only beyond

239

but even against nature, and thereby to prove its—I might say—
divine freedom. [L, 59

It would be a ridiculous and quite unjustified presumption
were we to imagine that we are more energetic or more intelligent than the ancients. Our fund of knowledge has increased
but not our intellectual capacity. Therefore we are just as narrow-minded and incapable of accepting new ideas as were the
men of the darkest ages of antiquity. We have become rich in
knowledge but not in wisdom. [IV, 21

At present we no longer know, or we do not yet know, to what
depths or to what extent the psyche is stirred up by a great
change in the times. Therefore the Holy Ghost appears to have
departed, without the answer being found to the question he
had put to humanity. [L, 50

Only a life lived in a certain spirit is worth while. It is a remarkable fact that a life lived entirely from the ego usually
strikes not only the person himself, but observers also, as being
dull. [XIX, 399 (G, 98)

The manifestations of the spirit are truly wondrous, and as
varied as creation itself. The living spirit grows and even out-
grows its earlier forms of expression; it freely chooses the men
in whom it lives and who proclaim it. This living spirit is eternally renewed and pursues its goal in manifold and inconceivable ways throughout the history of mankind. Measured against
it, the names and forms which men have given it mean little
enough; they are only the changing leaves and blossoms on the
stem of the eternal tree. [XXI, 30 (J, 282)

ON ULTIMATE THINGS

When to infinity the one thing
Self-repeating ever flows,
The thousandfold divided arches
Firmly fitting each in each,
Then streams life-joy from every object,
The smallest and the greatest star,
And every strife, and every conflict
Find eternal peace in God.
      —GOETHE, "Zahme Xenien" (VI)

Higher consciousness determines *Weltanschauung*.* Every increase in experience and knowledge means a further step in the development of *Weltanschauung*. And with the image the thinking man makes of the world, he also changes himself. The man whose sun still moves round the earth is essentially different from the man whose earth is a satellite of the sun. Not in vain was it that Giordano Bruno's immortal thought represents one of the most important beginnings of modern consciousness. The man whose cosmos hangs in the empyrean is different from one whose spirit is illuminated by Kepler's vision. The man who is still dubious about the sum of twice two is different from the thinker for whom nothing is less doubtful than the *a priori* truths of mathematics. To sum up—it is not immaterial what sort of *Weltanschauung* we possess; because it is not just a matter of our creating an image of the world, since retroactively it also changes us. [XIX, 301 f (G, 144 f)]

A science is never a *Weltanschauung;* it is merely the tool for one. Whether a man takes this tool in his hand or not is a question which depends entirely on the counter-question of what sort of *Weltanschauung* he already possesses. For no one is without a *Weltanschauung*. At worst he has at least that *Weltanschauung* which education and environment have forced upon him. If this *Weltanschauung* tells him, for instance, that "the sons of earth find greatest joy in personality alone," then he will unhesitatingly and willingly apply himself to science and its results, using this tool to build up a *Weltanschauung* and thereby also himself. But should his hereditary attitude tell him that science is no tool but an aim and end in itself, he will obey the watchword which, for the last one hundred and fifty years, has increasingly shown itself to be the valid, i.e., the actually decisive, one. A few individuals, it is true, have strug-

* [This word, now frequently used in English, means "rather general view of the world or of life"; it is also sometimes translated as "philosophy of life."—TRANSLATOR.]

gled desperately against this point of view, for their idea of completion and meaning culminated in the perfecting of human personality and not in the differentiation of technical means, which inevitably leads to a highly one-sided differentiation of one instinct, e.g., the urge for knowledge. If science is an end in itself, then mankind's *raison d'être* is merely to be an intellect. If art is an end in itself, then artistic ability is mankind's only value and the intellect disappears into the lumberroom. If money-making is an end in itself, then science and art can pack their bags and go. No one can deny that modern consciousness is hopelessly split up into all these "ends-in-themselves," and human beings are thereby "cultivated" as mere separate qualities, and have themselves become tools.

[xix, 328 f

The totality of the psyche can never be grasped by the intellect alone. Whether we wish it or no, we cannot escape the pressure of the present *Weltanschauung*, because the psyche craves an expression that will embrace its whole nature.

[li, 213 (d, 121)

Intellect is only one among several psychological functions, and therefore does not suffice to give a complete picture of the world. Feeling, for instance, which is another psychological function, sometimes arrives at different conclusions from those of the intellect, and we cannot always prove that the conclusions of feeling are necessarily inferior to those of the intellect.

[xiii, 224 (g, 269)

Although this fear of the other side is peculiar to us Western peoples, there is nevertheless something in it. For this fear is not wholly unjustified, quite apart from the fact that it is real. We understand at once the fear that children and primitives have of the great, unknown world. We have the same fear of our childish inner side, where we likewise touch a wide, unknown world. The affect, however, is all we have to go upon: we do not recognize it as a cosmic or world fear, because that world is invisible. Either we have purely theoretical prejudices about it, or superstitious ideas. There are actually numbers of educated people in whose presence one cannot even speak of the unconscious without being charged with mysticism. The fear is justified inasmuch as our rational *Weltanschauung*, with

its scientific and moral certainties so hotly believed in (because
so deeply dubious), is convulsed by data from the other side.

[XI, 143 f (D, 221 f)

The energy and the interest which we devote to science and
to technology the man of antiquity gave in great part to his
mythology. This explains the confusing changes, the kaleido-
scopic transformation and new syncretistic groupings and endless rejuvenations of the myths in the sphere of Greek culture.
Here we are moving in a world of fantasies which, little concerned with the outward march of events, flow from an inner
source, creating ever-changing figures, now plastic, now phan-
tom-like. This fantastical agency of the classical mind per-
formed the act of artistic creation par excellence. To grasp the
"how" of the actual world as objectively and exactly as possible
does not seem to have been the aim of this interest, but rather
to adapt the actual world aesthetically to subjective fantasies
and expectations. Only very few of the men of antiquity were
fated to suffer the disenchantment and disappointment which
Giordano Bruno's idea of infinity and Kepler's discoveries have
brought to modern men. The naïve man of that time saw the
sun as the great father of heaven and earth and the moon as the
fruitful, good mother. And every single thing had its daemon,
i.e., was animated and similar to man, or to his brother, the animal. Everything was pictured anthropomorphically or therio-
morphically, as man or as animal. Even the disc of sun was
given wings or four feet to illustrate its movement. Thus arose
a picture of the universe which was far removed from reality
but which wholly corresponded to the subjective fantasies.

[IV, 22

Freud was a great destroyer,* but the turn of the last century
was a time which offered so much opportunity for tearing down
that even a Nietzsche could not suffice. Freud dealt with what
was left, and thoroughly. He awakened a healthy distrust and
thereby indirectly sharpened our sense of true values. The illusion of the "good man," which befogged people's minds when
they were no longer able to understand the dogma of original
sin, was to no small extent dispelled by Freud. And whatever
is still left over will, it is to be hoped, be finally driven out by
the barbarism of the twentieth century.   [XLV

* [In the Nietzschean sense.—TRANSLATOR.]

245

I believe that history is capable of anything. There exists no folly that men have not tried out. And if anything can be made cheap, then those who would like to make it dear are to be counted among the very stupid.   [xxxi, 192 (f, 62)

In the last one hundred and fifty years we have experienced numerous kinds of *Weltanschauung*—a proof that *Weltanschauung* itself is discredited, for the more difficult an illness is to treat the more medicines there are for it; and the more medicines there are the less reputable is each one of them.   [xix, 329

The departing nineteenth century has left us a heritage of so many doubtful conceptions that doubt is not only possible, but also justified and even useful. For gold cannot be proved without the test of the flames.   [xlv

It seems to me that the fatal mistake of our *Weltanschauung* hitherto consists in the fact that it claims to be an objectively valid truth, and even, in the last resort, a sort of scientific evidence. This leads, for instance, to the intolerable result that the same God must help the Germans, the French, the English, the Turks, and the heathens, and finally each against each.
[xix, 329

If the image we make of the world did not have a retroactive effect upon ourselves, we could be content with any sort of beautiful or diverting sham. But such self-deception has its inevitable result, making us unreal, foolish, and incapable. Because we are fighting with a false image of the world, we are overcome by the superior power of reality.   [xix, 303 f (g, 146)

How directly a man's philosophy of life is connected with the well-being of the psyche can be seen from the fact that the nature of his conception of life, that is, his way of looking at things, is actually of supreme importance to him and to his mental health. This is so true that we might almost say things are not nearly so much how they are as how we see them. If, for instance, we have a disagreeable impression about a situation or thing, our pleasure in it is spoiled, and then it does in fact usually disagree with us. How much, on the contrary, becomes not only bearable, but often acceptable, if we can give up certain prejudices and change our point of view. Paracelsus, who was above all a physician of genius, stressed the fact that no one was a doctor who did not understand the art of "theorizing" [*Theoricieren*]. What he meant by this was that the doctor must not only himself attain, but must also convey to the patient, a mental attitude and a way of looking at the illness which would enable the doctor to cure and the patient to be cured, or at least to endure the illness. That is why he says, "Every illness is a purgatorial fire." He consciously recognized and made extensive use of the healing power of the mental attitude. [LIX, 8 (K, 23 f)

To have a *Weltanschauung* means to make an image of the world and of oneself, to know what the world is and who I am. Taken literally this would be too much. No one can know what the world is, and as little also can he know himself; but *cum grano salis,* it means the best possible knowledge—a knowledge that requires wisdom and the avoidance of unfounded assumptions, arbitrary assertions, and didactic opinions. For such knowledge one must seek the well-founded hypothesis, without forgetting that all knowledge is limited and subject to error.
[XIX, 303 (G, 146)

The world changes its face—*tempora mutantur et nos in illis*—for the world can only be grasped by us as a psychic image in ourselves, and it is not always easy to decide, when the image changes, whether the world or ourselves or both have changed. The image of the world can change at any time, just as our conception of ourselves can change. Every new discovery, every new thought, can put a new face on the world. We must be prepared for this, else we suddenly find ourselves in an antiquated world, a mere old-fashioned survival of a lower level of consciousness. Everyone sooner or later gets his dismissal from life, but our will to live would postpone this moment as long as possible, and to this end we must never allow the image of the world to become rigid. Every new thought must be tested to see whether it adds something to our world-image. [XIX, 304 (G, 146)

The fundamental error in every *Weltanschauung* is its pe-

247

culiar propensity to appear as the truth of the thing itself, whereas actually it is only a name which we give to things. Are we likely to make a scientific dispute out of the question whether the name of the planet Neptune corresponds to the nature of this celestial body and is consequently its only "right" name? Most definitely not—and that is the reason why science has a higher standing, for it only accepts working hypotheses. Only the primitive mind believes in the "right name." In the fairytale, you can blast Rumpelstiltskin into pieces if you can find his right name. The chieftain keeps his real name secret and takes an exoteric name for daily use, so that no one can bewitch him through knowing his real name. When the Egyptian Pharaoh was laid in his tomb, he was given the real names of the gods in word and image so that he might compel them through the knowledge of the real name. To the cabalist, the possession of the real name of God meant absolute magic power. In brief, in the primitive mind the name constitutes the thing itself.

[XIX, 330

If we do not wish to develop backwards, then a new *Weltanschauung* must discard all superstition regarding its objective validity, and must be able to admit that it is only a picture which we have painted for our own psyche and not a magic name with which we can create objective things. We have a *Weltanschauung* not for the world but for ourselves. If we do not create a picture of the world as a whole, then we do not see ourselves either, for we are just the faithful images of this world, and only in the mirror of our world-image can we see ourselves completely. Only in the image which we create do we ourselves appear. Only in our creative act do we step fully into the light and become recognizable to ourselves as a whole being. We never give the world any other face than our own, and this is just why we have to do so, i.e., in order to discover ourselves. For above science or art as ends in themselves stands man, the creator of his tools.

[XIX, 331 f

The world exists not merely in itself but also as it appears to me. Indeed, at bottom, we have absolutely no criterion that could help us to form a judgment of a world whose nature was unassimilable by the subject. If we were to ignore the subjective factor, it would mean a complete denial of the great doubt as to the possibility of absolute cognition. And this would mean sliding again into that stale and hollow positivism which disfigured the beginning of our epoch—an attitude of intellectual arrogance that is invariably accompanied by a crudeness of feeling, and an essential violation of life, as stupid as it is presumptuous. Through an over-valuation of the objective powers of cognition, we repress the importance of the subjective factor, which simply means the denial of the subject. But what is the subject? The subject is man—we are the subject. Only a sick mind could forget that cognition must have a subject, for there exists no knowledge and, therefore, for us, no world where "I know" has not been said, although with this statement one has already expressed the subjective limitation of all knowledge.

[IX, 537 (I, 472 f)

There are many scientists who avoid having a *Weltanschauung* because this is supposed not to be scientific. But it is manifestly not clear to these people what they are really doing. For what actually happens is this: by deliberately leaving themselves in the dark as to their guiding ideas they are clinging to a deeper, more primitive level of consciousness than would correspond to their full conscious capacities. A certain critical and sceptical attitude is by no means always the expression of intelligence; often it is just the reverse, especially when a man uses scepticism as a screen to cloak his lack of *Weltanschauung*. Not infrequently, it is a moral rather than an intellectual deficiency. Because to see the world also means seeing yourself, therefore *as* you see the world so you see yourself, and this demands much in labour and sincerity. Hence it is always fatal to have no *Weltanschauung*. [XIX, 302 f (G, 145 f)

If we were conscious of the spirit of the age, we should know why we are so inclined to account for everything on physical grounds; we should know that it is because, up till now, too much was accounted for in terms of the spirit. This realization would at once make us critical of our bias. We should say: most likely we are now making as serious an error on the other side. We delude ourselves with the thought that we know much more about matter than about a "metaphysical" mind, and so we overestimate physical causation and believe that it alone affords us a true explanation of life. But matter is just as inscrutable as mind. As to the ultimate we can know nothing, and only when we admit this do we return to a state of equilibrium.   [xxvii, 7 (j, 205)

Has mankind ever quite freed itself from the myth? Every man has eyes and all his senses to tell him that the world is dead, cold, and unending, and he has never yet seen a God nor claimed God's existence from empirical compulsion. On the contrary, it required an indestructible and fantastic optimism, opposed to all sense of reality, to see, for instance, such an experience as the shameful death of Christ as the highest salvation and redemption of the world. In the same way we can keep from a child all knowledge of earlier myths, but we cannot take from him the need for mythology. We might say that, were it possible to sweep away all the tradition in the world with one fell stroke, with the next generation the whole mythology and history of religion would begin all over again. Only a few individuals succeed in eliminating mythology in an epoch of a certain intellectual arrogance; the mass of the people never free themselves from it. All the rationalism in the world is of no avail; it only destroys a temporary form of manifestation but not the creative urge.   [iv, 26 f

There need be only conditions of some insecurity for the "magical formalities" to be brought to life again in a quite natural fashion. Through these ceremonies the deeper emotional forces are released; conviction becomes blind auto-suggestion and the psychic field of vision is narrowed to one fixed point, upon which the whole weight of the unconscious *vis a tergo* is concentrated. And it is an objective fact that success attends the sure rather than the unsure.   [xiii, 76 (c, 50)

The retarding ideal is always more primitive, more natural (in the good sense as in the bad), and more "moral" in that it keeps faith with law and tradition. The progressive ideal is always more abstract, more unnatural, and less "moral" in that it demands disloyalty to tradition. Progress enforced by will is always convulsive. Backwardness may be closer to naturalness, but in its turn it is always menaced by painful awakenings.
                                    [xlix, 121 (o, 114)

I know nothing of a super-reality: reality contains everything that one can know, for whatever works is real. If it does not work, then one does not notice it and can therefore know nothing about it. Consequently I can only speak about real things, but not about super-real or unreal or sub-real. This could only be possible if it had occurred to someone to limit the concept of reality in some way so that only a certain section of the world-reality could claim the attribute of "real." The way of thinking of the so-called healthy human mind and the usual mode of speech produce this limitation, this narrowing down to the so-called material or concrete reality of obvious objects, quite regardless of the fact that all sorts of things are in our mind which do not come from sensory data. In this sense everything is "real" which directly or indirectly arises or appears to arise from the world which can be grasped by the senses. This limitation of the world-image is a reflection of the one-sidedness of Western man. [XXII, 1

How totally different did the world appear to medieval man! For him the earth was eternally fixed and at rest in the centre of the universe, encircled by the course of a sun that solicitously bestowed its warmth. Men were all children of God under the loving care of the Most High, who prepared them for eternal blessedness; and all knew exactly what they should do and how they should conduct themselves in order to rise from a corruptible world to an incorruptible and joyous existence. Such a life no longer seems real to us, even in our dreams. Natural science has long ago torn this lovely veil to shreds. That age lies as far behind as childhood, when one's own father was unquestionably the handsomest and strongest man on earth. The modern man has lost all the metaphysical certainties of his medieval brother and set up in their place the ideals of material security, general welfare, and humaneness. But it takes more than an ordinary dose of optimism to make it appear that these ideals are still unshaken. [XIX, 412 f (J, 235)

Accordingly, primitive man, being closer to his instincts, like the animal, is characterized by his fear of novelty and adherence to tradition. To our way of thinking, he is painfully backward, whereas we exalt progress. But our progressiveness,

251

though it may result in a great many delightful wish-fulfilments, piles up an equally gigantic Promethean debt which has
to be paid off from time to time in the form of hideous catastrophes. For ages man has dreamed of flying, and all we have got
for it is saturation bombing! We smile today at the Christian
hope of a life beyond the grave, and yet we often fall into
chiliasms a hundred times more ridiculous than the notion of a
happy Hereafter.   [XLIX, 121 (o, 113)

Man is not a machine that one can reconstruct, as occasion
demands, upon other lines and for quite other ends, in the hope
that it will then proceed to function, in a totally different way,
just as normally as before. Man bears his age-long history with
him; in his very structure is written the history of mankind. The
historical factor represents a vital need, to which a wise econ-
omy must respond. Somehow the past must become vocal and
participate in the present. Complete assimilation to the object,
therefore, encounters the protest of the suppressed minority,
elements belonging to the past and existing from the beginning.
                                                  [IX, 484 f (I, 423)

A man is only half understood when we know whence everything in him came. If it were only a matter of that, he might just
as well have been dead long ago. This does not comprehend
the whole of him as a living being, for life has not only a yesterday and is not explained if the "today" is reduced to a "yesterday." Life has also a tomorrow, and the "today" can only be
understood if we are able to add to our knowledge of that which
was yesterday the tendencies for tomorrow. This is true of all
psychological expressions of life, even of pathological symptoms.   [LI, 83

Psychology teaches us that, in a certain sense, there is nothing in the psyche that is old; nothing that can really, definitively
die away. Even Paul was left with a sting in his flesh. Whoever
protects himself against what is new and strange, and thereby
regresses to the past, falls into the same neurotic condition as
the man who identifies himself with the new and runs away

from the past. The only difference is that the one has estranged himself from the past and the other from the future. In principle both are doing the same thing: they are salvaging a narrow state of consciousness. The alternative is to shatter it with the tension inherent in the play of opposites—in the dualistic stage —and thereby to build up a state of wider and higher consciousness. [XIX, 258 f (J, 117)

Is a thing beautiful because I attribute beauty to it? It is well known that great minds have wrestled with the question whether it is the glorious sun, or the human eye by virtue of its relation to the sun, that illumines the worlds. Archaic man believes it to be the sun, and civilized man believes it is the eye, so far, at any rate, as he reflects at all and does not suffer from the disease of poets. He must strip nature of psychic attributes in order to dominate it; to see his world objectively he must take back all his archaic projections. [XIX, 238 (J, 166)

Consciousness must have reason, first, in order to discover some system in the chaos of irregular, individual events occuring in the universe; and, second, at least in the domain of human affairs, in order to act. We have the praiseworthy and useful ambition to root out the chaos of the irrational within and without us as completely as possible, and have apparently advanced some distance in the achievement of this aim. A mental patient once said to me: "Doctor, I disinfected the whole heavens last night with corrosive sublimate, but have not discovered any God." Something of the same kind has happened to us.
[LI, 130 (D, 73 f)

And what kind of an answer did the next generation give to the individualism of Nietzsche's superman? It answered with a collectivism, a mass organization, a herding together of the mob, *tam ethice quam physice*, that made everything that went before look like a bad joke. Suffocation of the personality and an impotent Christianity that may well have received its death-wound—such is the unadorned balance-sheet of our time.
[LVIII, 641 (M, 559)

When something quite universal happens to a man and he supposes it to be an experience peculiar to himself, then his attitude is obviously wrong, that is, too personal, and it tends to exclude him from human society. We require not only a present-day personal consciousness but also a supra-personal consciousness which is open to the sense of historical continuity.

[xix, 104 (j, 76 f)

We are now reaping the fruit of nineteenth-century education. Throughout that period the Church preached to young people the merit of blind faith, while the universities inculcated an intellectual rationalism, with the result that today we plead in vain whether for faith or reason. Tired of this warfare of opinions, the modern man wishes to find out for himself how things are. And though this desire opens bar and bolt to the most dangerous possibilities, we cannot help seeing it as a courageous enterprise and giving it some measure of sympathy. It is no reckless adventure but an effort inspired by deep spiritual distress to bring meaning once more into life on the basis of fresh and unprejudiced experience.   [xxi, 23 f (j, 276)

Life *is* both nonsensical and significant. And when we do not laugh about one aspect and speculate about the other, life is exceedingly banal, and everything is of the smallest proportions; there is then only a tiny sense and a tiny nonsense. In the very first place, nothing signifies anything; for when as yet there were no thinking beings, no one was there to interpret manifestations. It is only for him who does not understand that things must be interpreted. Only the ununderstandable has significance. Man has awakened in a world that he does not understand, and this is why he tries to interpret it. For there is a cosmos in all chaos, secret order in all disorder, unfailing law in all contingency.   [xxxi, 213 (f, 81)

It all depends on how we look at things, and not on how they are in themselves. The least of things with a meaning is worth more in life than the greatest of things without it.

[xix, 102 (j, 75)

It is the East that has taught us another, wider, more profound, and higher understanding, that is, understanding through life. We know this way only vaguely, as a mere shad-

owy sentiment culled from religious terminology, and therefore we gladly dispose of Eastern "wisdom" in quotation marks,
and push it away into the obscure territory of faith and superstition. But in this way Eastern "realism" is completely misunderstood. It does not consist of sentimental, exaggeratedly
mystical intuitions bordering on the pathological and emanating
from ascetic recluses and cranks; the wisdom of the East is
based on practical knowledge coming from the flower of Chinese intelligence, which we have not the slightest justification
for undervaluing.   [xv, 531 (H, 78)

Every single thing needs for its existence its opposite, otherwise it must pale into non-existence. The ego needs the Self,
and vice versa. The changing relationship between these two
factors represents a field of experience which the introspective
knowledge of the East has exploited to an extent almost unattainable for Western man. The philosophy of the East, which
is so infinitely different from our own, means for us a supremely
valuable gift, which however we must "earn in order to possess."   [LVII, 21

Western man is held in thrall by the "ten thousand things";
he sees only particulars, is ego-bound and thing-bound and unaware of the deep root of all being. Eastern man on the other
hand experiences the world of particulars, and even his own
ego, like a dream; he is rooted essentially in the Ground, which
attracts him so powerfully that his relations with the world are
relativized to a degree that is often incomprehensible to us.
                                                    [LVIII, 19 f (M, 8)
The West is always seeking uplift, but the East seeks a sinking or deepening. The outer reality, its corporeality and weight,
appears to impress the European much more powerfully and
sharply than the Indian. Therefore the European seeks to raise
himself above the world, while the Indian likes to return into
the maternal depths of Nature.   [LIV, 47 (L, 176)

The Christian during contemplation, would never say, "I am
Christ," but with Paul he will confess, "I live; yet not I, but
Christ liveth in me" [Gal. 2:20]. Our Sutra, however, says,

"Thou wilt know that *thou* art Buddha." Fundamentally these confessions are identical, inasmuch as the Buddhist only attains this knowledge when he is without self, "anatman." But there exists an immense difference between the two formulations. The Christian attains his end in Christ, the Buddhist recognizes that he *is* Buddha. The Christian, starting from the transitory and egocentric world of his consciousness, dissolves in Christ, but the Buddhist *still* rests on the eternal foundation of inner nature, whose at-one-ness with the divinity, or with the universal Being, we meet in other Indian confessions as well.

[LIV, 53 (L, 179)

If the supreme value (Christ) and the supreme negation (sin) are outside, then the soul is void: its highest and lowest are missing. The Eastern attitude (more particularly the Indian) is the other way about: everything, highest and lowest, is in the (transcendental) Subject. Accordingly the significance of the Atman, the Self, is heightened beyond all bounds. But with Western man the value of the Self sinks to zero.   [LVIII, 20 f (M, 9)

Great as the value of Zen-Buddhism is for the understanding of the religious process of transformation, it is most improbable that it could ever be used by Western man. The preparatory spiritual training necessary for Zen-Buddhism is lacking in the West. Which of us would have implicit confidence in a superior master and his incomprehensible ways? This respect for the greater human personality is to be found only in the East. Who could boast of being ready to believe in the possibility of a transformation the result of which is paradoxical beyond all measure, and, moreover, to believe to the extent of sacrificing many years of his life to the laborious acquirement of such a goal? Who would really dare to assume the authority for an inner heterodox experience of transformation?—Unless it were the undertaking of a person unworthy of trust, someone who perhaps for pathological reasons wanted to boast. Just such a type would not need to complain of a lack of followers in the West either. But if the "Master" sets a difficult task, which demands more than parrot-like repetition, then the European is seized with doubt, for the steep path to the attainment of Self seems to him as sad and gloomy as Hades itself.   [XLII, 31

Buddhism itself was born out of the spirit of yoga, which is much older and more universal than the historical reformation of Buddha. Anyone who attempts to understand Indian art, philosophy, and ethics from the inside must of necessity befriend this spirit. Our habitual understanding from the outside breaks down here, because it is hopelessly inadequate and cannot grasp the essence of Indian spirituality.　[LIV, 45 (L, 175)

Western consciousness is by no means consciousness in general, but rather a historically conditioned and geographically limited factor, representative of only one part of humanity. The widening of our own consciousness ought not to proceed at the expense of other kinds of consciousness, but ought to take place through the development of those elements of our psyche which are analogous to those of a foreign psyche, just as the East cannot do without our technique, science, and industry. The European invasion of the East was a deed of violence on a great scale, and it has left us the duty—*noblesse oblige*—of understanding the mind of the East. This is perhaps more necessary than we realize at present.　[XIV, 75 (H, 136)

It is far from my wish to undervalue the tremendous differentiation of Western intellect, because, measured by it, Eastern intellect can be described as childish. (Obviously this has nothing to do with intelligence.) If we should succeed in bringing another, or still a third, function to the dignity accorded intellect, then the West could expect to surpass the East by a great deal.　[XV, 534 (H, 82)

When faced with this problem of grasping the ideas of the East, the usual mistake of the Western man is like that of the student in *Faust*. Ill-advised by the devil, he contemptuously turns his back on science, and, getting a whiff of Eastern ecstatics, takes over their yoga practices quite literally, only to become a pitiable imitator. (Theosophy is our best example of this mistake.) And so he abandons the one safe foundation of the Western mind, and loses himself in a mist of words and ideas which never would have originated in European brains and which can never be profitably grafted upon them.

[XV, 531 f (H, 78 f)

There could be no greater mistake than for a Westerner to take up the direct practice of Chinese yoga, for then it would still be a matter of his will and consciousness and would only strengthen the latter against the unconscious, bringing about the very effect which should have been avoided. The neurosis would then be increased. It cannot be emphasized strongly enough that we are not Orientals and therefore have an entirely different point of departure in these things.

[xv, 537 (H, 87)

Yoga has quite definite conceptions concerning what is to be achieved, and does everything to reach this anticipated goal. But with us, our intellectualism, rationalism, and our doctrine of free will are such dangerous psychic forces that, whenever possible, psychotherapy must avoid setting itself such goals.

[LVI, 18

If anyone should succeed in giving up Europe from every point of view, and actually be nothing else than a yogi, taking on all the ethical and practical consequences of sitting in the lotus position on a gazelle-skin under a dusty banyan tree, floating out of this world and closing his days in nameless non-being, to such a one I would have to admit that he understood yoga in the Indian sense. But whoever cannot do that should not behave as if he understood yoga. He neither can nor should give up his Western understanding, but on the contrary he should exert himself to apply his mind in an honest manner, without imitation or sentimentality, to understand as much of yoga as is possible to our understanding.   [LIV, 45 f (L, 175)

Western imitation of the East is doubly tragic in that it comes from a psychological misunderstanding as sterile as are the modern escapades in New Mexico, the blissful South Sea Islands, and Central Africa, where "primitivity" is being staged in all seriousness, in order that western civilized man may covertly slip out of his menacing duties, his *hic Rhodus hic salta*. It is not for us to imitate what is organically foreign or, worse still, to send out missionaries to foreign people; it is our task to build up our own Western culture, which sickens with a thousand ills. This has to be done on the spot, and into the work must be drawn the real European as he is in his Western commonplaceness, with his marriage problems, his neurosis, his so-

cial and political illusions, and his whole philosophical disorientation.   [xv, 532 (h, 80)

Sometimes it seems—especially in the light of a historical retrospect—as though the present had an analogue in certain epochs
of the past, in which great empires and cultures went beyond
their zenith and hurried irresistibly towards decay. But such
analogies are deceptive, since there are also renaissances. Something relatively clear seems to move into the foreground; and
this is the intermediate position occupied by Europe between
the Asiatic East and the Anglo-Saxon—or shall we say American?—West. Europe stands between two colossi, both immature
in their form and yet immeasurably opposed in their already
discernible nature. They are fundamentally divorced, both
racially and in their ideals. In the West there is as great freedom politically as there is a lack of it personally; whereas in the
East we find just the opposite. In the West there is the immense impetus of a technical and scientific culture-tendency;
whereas in the East there is an awakening of all those forces
which, in Europe, this cultural urge holds in check. The power
of the West is material, that of the East ideal.   [x, 8 f (g, 164 f)

The breathless striving for power, in the political, social, and
mental sense, which stirs the soul of the Westerner with apparently unquenchable passion is spreading irresistibly also in the
East and threatens to bring about unpredictable consequences.
Not only in India but also in China, much in which the soul
once lived and flourished has already vanished. The outward
trend of culture may well clear away many evils whose elimina-
tion appears to be highly desirable and advantageous, but at
the same time, as experience shows us, this progress is all too
dearly bought with a loss of psychic culture.   [lvii, 22

The wisdom and mysticism of the East have indeed very
much to give us even though they speak their own language
which is impossible to imitate. They should remind us of that
which is similar in our own culture and which we have already
forgotten, and should direct our attention to that which we
have pushed aside as insignificant, namely, the fate of our own
inner man.   [lvii, 23

The growing acquaintanceship with the spiritual East should mean to us only a symbolical expression of the fact that we are entering into connection with the strange elements in ourselves. Denial of our own historical premises would be sheer folly and would be the best way to bring about a second uprooting of consciousness. Only by standing firmly on our own soil can we assimilate the spirit of the East.   [xiv, 65 (h, 128)

The spirit of the age, which will not let itself be trifled with: it is a religion, or—even more—a creed which has absolutely no connection with reason, but whose significance lies in the unpleasant fact that it is taken as the absolute measure of all truth and is supposed always to have common sense upon its side.

[xxvii, 4 (j, 202)

The stages, as I said, are many, and there are greybeards who die as innocent as sucklings, and here, in the Year of Our Lord 1927, troglodytes are still being born. There are truths that are only true the day after tomorrow, truths that were still true yesterday—and truths that are never true.   [xi, 144 (d, 222)

There is, in fact, a quite substantial body of the population that only to a very limited extent lives in the present and participates in present-day problems. This is true of the overwhelming majority. We speak of the "battle of the mind," but how many are really occupied with it? And how many understanding, sympathetic onlookers does it enroll? Or the "woman's problem"—how many women have problems? In proportion to the sum total of European women, it is a dwindling minority of women who really live in the Europe of today; and these, moreover, are city dwellers and belong—I say it purposely—to complicated humanity. This must always be so, since it is only the few who express with any distinctness the spirit of a time.

[x, 9 f (g, 165)

The tasks of every age differ, and it is only in retrospect that we can discern with certainty what had to be and what should not have been. In the momentary present the conflict of convictions always predominates, for "war is the father of all."

History alone decides. Truth is not eternal—it is a programme. The more "eternal" a truth, the more is it lifeless and worthless; it tells us nothing more, because it is self-evident.

[IX, 85 (I, 78)

The new thing is always questionable and means something which must be tested. The new thing can just as well be an illness. Therefore true progress is only possible when there is a mature judgment. But a well-considered judgment requires a firm standpoint, which can only be based on thorough knowledge of what is already there. Whoever loses the bond with the past, unconscious of the historical connection, runs the risk of falling a victim to the power of suggestion and blinding fascination which all novelties radiate. [LIII, 8

Knowledge of the origins in the most general sense builds the bridge between the lost and forsaken world of the past and the coming and still incomprehensible world of the future. With what shall we grasp the future and how can we integrate it, if we do not possess that experience of mankind which the former ages have left us? But for this possession, we should be without root and without a point of view, and should fall defenceless victims to the future and to the new development. [LIII, 8

Those for whom the Middle Ages still offer adequate ways and possibilities demand nothing from the present and its experiments. But the man who belongs to the present—no matter why or how—cannot turn back again to the past without suffering essential loss. Often this turning back is altogether impossible, even when a man is prepared to make the sacrifice. The man of the present needs must work towards the future. He has to leave it to others to maintain the past. Hence, he is also a destroyer, not a builder only. To himself, both he and his world are questionable and ambiguous. The ways that the past shows him and the answers that it gives to his questions are insufficient for the needs of the present. Old and comfortable ways are blocked, new possibilities have been opened up, or new dangers have arisen of which the past knew nothing. It is proverbial, of course, that man never learns from history, and, as a rule, in respect to a problem of the present, it can teach us

261

simply nothing. The new way must be made through untrodden regions, without suppositions, and often, unfortunately, without piety also.   [x, 11 f (G, 166 f)

Contemporaries are always naïve and never know or understand that enthusiasm and apparently exaggerated exuberance are due much less to personal temperament than to the bubbling up of the source of a new age as yet unknown. People looked askance at Nietzsche's volcanic emotion, and yet how long in times to come will one still speak of him! Has not even Paracelsus been gratefully dug out of his grave after four hundred years, in an attempt to help his rebirth in the modern world?   [xxx, 4

I consider it the duty of everyone who takes a solitary path to share with society what he finds on his journey of discovery, be it refreshing water for the thirsty or a sandy desert of unfruitful error. The one aids, the other warns. Not the criticism of individual contemporaries will decide the truth or falsity of what has been discovered, but future generations and destiny. There are things that are not yet true today; perhaps we dare not find them true, but tomorrow they may be. So every man, whose fate it is to find his own individual way, must go with the bare hope and keen watchfulness of one who is conscious of the loneliness of his path and the danger of its mist-hung abysses.   [LI, 212 (D, 120)

New ideas which are not mere crazes usually need at least a generation to gain a footing, and new psychological ideas need much longer still, for especially in this field practically everyone believes himself to be an authority.   [LI, 11

Our modern attitude looks back proudly upon the mists of superstition and of medieval or primitive credulity and entirely forgets that it carries the whole living past in the lower stories of the skyscraper of rational consciousness. Without the lower stories our mind is suspended in mid air. No wonder that it gets nervous. The true history of the mind is not preserved in learned volumes but in the living mental organism of everyone.
                                   [XLVI, 64 f (B, 41)

Great innovations never come from above; they come invariably from below; just as trees never grow from the sky downward, but upward from the earth, however true it is that their seeds have fallen from above. The upheaval of our world and the upheaval in consciousness is one and the same. Everything becomes relative and therefore doubtful. And while man, hesitant and questioning, contemplates a world that is distracted with treaties of peace and pacts of friendship, democracy and dictatorship, capitalism and Bolshevism, his spirit yearns for an answer that will allay the turmoil of doubt and uncertainty. And it is just people of the lower social levels who follow the unconscious forces of the psyche; it is the much-derided, silent folk of the land—those who are less infected with academic prejudices than great celebrities are wont to be.

[xix, 421 f (j, 243)

To think differently from the accepted way of thinking always has the flavour of something illegitimate and disturbing; it is even somehow indecent, pathological, or blasphemous, and therefore socially dangerous for the individual. He is swimming nonsensically against the stream. [xxvii, 4

It is sheer juggling to look upon a denial of the past as the same thing as consciousness of the present. "Today" stands between "yesterday" and "tomorrow," and forms a link between past and future; it has no other meaning. The present represents a process of transition, and that man may account himself modern who is conscious of it in this sense. [xix, 405 (j, 229)

The so-called present is a thin surface-stratum that is produced in the great centres of mankind. But when too thin it is irrelevant. When, however, it has attained to a certain strength, we can speak of culture and progress, and then problems arise that are characteristic of an epoch. [x, 11 (g, 166)

What is a problem of the present day? If we speak of a general problem nowadays, it is because it exists in the heads of many people. These individual people are somehow chosen by fate and destined by their own natures to suffer under a gen-

erally unsatisfactory condition and to make it a problem. Therefore it is always individuals who are moved by the general
problem and who are called upon to respond and contribute to
the great solution of the problem, in that they tackle it in their
own lives and do not shirk it.   [xxxiv, 86

Who, if it comes to that, has finally and fully realized that
history, as an effective reality, is not contained in thick books,
but lives in our very blood?   [x, 40 (G, 184)

The age is as great as we see it, and man grows in accordance
with the greatness of the age.   [xxix

Life is a flux, a flowing into the future, and not a stoppage or
a backwash. It is therefore not surprising that so many of the
mythological *saviours* are child-gods.   [xlix, 122 (o, 115)

But it was of most profound psychological significance when
Christianity first discovered, in the orientation towards the future, a redeeming principle for mankind. In the past nothing
can be altered, and in the present little, but the future is ours
and capable of raising life's intensity to its highest pitch. A
little space of youth belongs to us, all the rest of life belongs to
our children.   [vii, 50 f (c, 277)

THE DEVELOPMENT OF THE PERSONALITY

The best cannot be told, anyhow, and the second best does not strike home. One must be able to let things happen. I have learned from the East what is meant by the phrase *Wu wei*: namely, "not-doing, letting be," which is quite different from doing nothing. Some Occidentals, also, have known what this not-doing means; for instance, Meister Eckhart, who speaks of *sich lassen*, "to let oneself be." The region of darkness into which one falls is not empty; it is the "lavishing mother" of Lao-tzu, the "images" and the "seed." When the surface has been cleared, things can grow out of the depths. People always suppose that they have lost their way, when they come up against these depths of experience. But if they do not know how to go on, the only answer, the only advice, that makes any sense is "Wait for what the unconscious has to say about the situation." A way is only *the* way when one finds it and follows it oneself. There is no general prescription for "how one should do it." [xxviii, 203 f (f, 31 f)

We must be able to let things happen in the psychic. For us, this becomes a real art of which few people know anything. Consciousness is forever interfering, helping, correcting, and negating, and never leaving the simple growth of the psychic processes in peace. It would be a simple enough thing to do, if only simplicity were not the most difficult of all things.
[xv, 539 (h, 90)

The public in general is possessed of the fundamental error that there are certain answers, "solutions," or attitudes of mind which need only be uttered in order to spread the necessary light. But the best of truths is of no use—as history has shown a thousand times—unless it has become the individual's most personal inner experience. Every equivocal, so-called "clear" answer mostly remains in the head and only finds its way down to the heart in the very rarest cases. Our need is not to "know" the truth, but to experience it. The great problem is not to have an intellectual view of things, but to find the way to the inner, perhaps inexpressible, irrational experience. Nothing is more fruitless than to speak of how things must and should be, and nothing is more important than to find the way which leads to these far-off goals.   [XIX, v f

It should never be forgotten that the world—and this above all—is also a subjective phenomenon. The experience of accidental impressions is also an achievement on our part. It is not as if the impressions pressed haphazard upon us, it is our own disposition which supplies the condition for the impression. A person with an already sensitive disposition will have a marked impression of an event which leaves a less sensitive nature quite cold.   [VI, 87

In face of the bewildering and impressive profusion of animated objects, the individual creates an abstraction, i.e., an abstract and general image, which conjures impressions into a law-abiding form. This image has the magical importance of a defence against the chaotic change of experience. He becomes so lost and submerged in this image that finally its abstract truth is set above the reality of life; and therewith life, which might disturb the enjoyment of abstract beauty, is wholly suppressed. He raises himself to an abstraction; he identifies himself with the eternal validity of his image and therein congeals, since it practically amounts to a redeeming formula. In this way he divests himself of his real self and transfers his life into his abstraction, in which it is, so to speak, crystallized. But since the feeling-into subject *feels* his activity, his life, *into* the object, he therewith also yields himself to the object, in so far as the felt-into content represents an essential part of the subject. He becomes the object; he identifies himself with it, and in this way gets rid of himself. Because he objectifies himself he, therefore, de-subjectifies himself.   [IX, 417 f (I, 368)

Is not every experience, even in the best of circumstances, to a large extent subjective interpretation? On the other hand, the subject also is an objective fact, a piece of the world. What issues from it comes, after all, from the universal soil, just as the rarest and strangest organism is none the less supported and

266

nourished by the earth which we all share in common. It is precisely the most subjective ideas which, being closest to nature and to the living being, deserve to be called the truest. But "what is truth?" [XIX, 75 (J, 133)

It may not be granted to many to see the world as a "given fact." Indeed it requires a great and self-sacrificing change of heart to see that the world is "given" through the nature of the psyche. It is so much more direct and striking, more impressive and therefore more convincing, to see how something happens to me, rather than to observe how I myself made it. The animal nature of man fights against the feeling that it is itself the maker of its given facts. Therefore attempts of this kind were always made the subject of secret initiations. [XXXII, 21

There are experiences which can only be experienced and for which reason can never be a substitute. Such experiences are often of inestimable value. [VI, 108

Human thought cannot conceive any system or final truth that could give the patient what he needs in order to live: that is, faith, hope, love, and insight. These four highest achievements of human effort are so many gifts of grace, which are neither to be taught nor learned, neither given nor taken, neither withheld nor earned, since they come through experience, which is something *given,* and therefore beyond the reach of human caprice. Experiences cannot be *made.* They happen —yet fortunately their independence of man's activity is not absolute but relative. We can draw closer to them—that much lies within our human reach. There are ways which bring us nearer to living experience, yet we should beware of calling these ways "methods." The very word has a deadening effect. The way to experience, moreover, is anything but a clever trick; it is rather a venture which requires us to commit ourselves with our whole being. [XXI, 8 f (J, 261)

Caution has its place, no doubt, but we cannot refuse our support to a serious venture which calls the whole of the personality into the field of action. If we oppose it, we are trying to suppress what is best in man—his daring and his aspiration.

And should we succeed, we should only have stood in the way of that invaluable experience which might have given a meaning to life. What would have happened if Paul had allowed himself to be talked out of his journey to Damascus?

[XXI, 24 (J, 276 f)

It is a matter of experience that the man whose interest is directed towards external things is never satisfied with the bare necessities but always aspires to still more and still better, which, true to his prejudice, he always seeks in outer things. He completely forgets that in spite of all outward success, he himself remains inwardly the same, and therefore complains of his poverty when he only owns one motor-car instead of two like most of his friends. In outer human life there is certainly room for many improvements and refinements, but these lose their meaning in proportion as the inner man does not keep pace with them. To be richly endowed with all the "necessities" of life is undoubtedly a source of happiness which is not to be underrated, but over and above this the inner man makes his claims which no outer worldly goods can satisfy. And the less this voice is heard, owing to the scramble for the good things of this world, the more the inner man becomes the source of inexplicable mishaps and incomprehensible unhappiness in the midst of outer conditions which would naturally lead one to expect a totally different state of things. This complete absorption in the external world becomes an incurable affliction, because no one can understand how one can possibly suffer from oneself. No one is surprised at his own insatiability, but regards it as his right and never stops to think that the one-sidedness of the psychic diet finally leads to the most serious disturbances of the equilibrium. Western man suffers from this disease, and he will not rest until he has infected the whole world with his restless greed. [LVII, 22 f

Too many people still search outwardly; some believe in the illusion of victory and victorious power; others in treaties and laws, and yet others in the destruction of the existing order. There are still too few who search inwardly, in their own selves, and too few who set themselves the question whether human society were not best served in the end were everyone to begin with himself and test all the break-up of the hitherto-existing order, all the laws and victories which he preaches at every street-corner, first and foremost and simply and solely on his own person and in his own inner state, instead of expecting his fellow men to try them. [LI, 10 f

Doubtless there are exceptional men who are able to sacrifice their entire life to one definite formula; but for most of us a permanent life of such exclusiveness is impossible.

[IX, 499 (I, 437)

It is through considering the demands of both worlds, the inner as well as the outer—or more accurately, through the conflict between these demands—that the possible and the necessary can be found. Unfortunately our Western mind, from a profound lack of culture in this relation to the soul, has never found a concept, not to mention a name, to represent that most fundamental mainspring of inner experience, namely, the union of the opposites in a middle way, which could in any way compare with the Chinese Tao. This conception is at the same time the most individual fact and the most universal and immutable significance of the living creature. [XI, 147 (D, 224 f)

We should do far better to realize that the tragic play of opposites between the inner and the outer (represented in the Book of Job and in *Faust* as the devil's wager with God) is fundamentally the dynamics of the life-process, the tension between the opposites, that is indispensable to self-regulation. However different in appearance and purpose these opposing forces may be, their fundamental meaning and will is the life of the individual. This is the centre of the balance which determines their every motion. Just because they are inseparably related through opposition, they also unite in a mediating meaning. This resultant is necessarily born out of the individual either willingly or unwillingly, and hence it is also discerned by him. He has a feeling of what should be, and also of what could be. To ignore or deny this intuition means going astray, making mistakes, and eventually neurosis. [XI, 131 (D, 212 f)

The man who is only wise and only holy interests me about as much as the skeleton of a saurian, which may be rare but does not move me to tears. On the other hand, the absurd contradiction between the being withdrawn from Maya into the cosmic Self and loving weakness that sinks its many roots fruitfully into the black earth, to repeat to all eternity the weaving and the tearing of the veil as India's eternal melody—this contradiction moves me; for how can one see light without shadow, or feel peace without noise, or achieve wisdom without foolishness? [LVII, 14

To become foolish is certainly not an art; but to draw wisdom out of foolishness is the whole of art. Foolishness is the mother of the wise, but never cleverness. [XLVIII, 164

The myth of the hero seems to us to be the myth of our own suffering unconscious, which has that unsatisfied yearning—which can rarely be appeased—for all the deep sources of its own being, for the body of the mother, and in it for communion with infinite life in the countless forms of existence. [IV, 198

In the same way as the unconscious world of mythological images speaks indirectly through experience of external things to him who gives himself entirely to the outer world, the actual outer world with its demands also speaks indirectly to him who gives himself entirely to the psyche, for no one can escape both realities. If a man turns only outwards, then he must live his myth; if he turns inwards, he must dream his outer so-called real life. [XLIII, 443

We know that there is no human foresight or wisdom of life which could enable us to give our lives a planned direction, except for short stretches of the way. This attitude applies, however, only to the "usual" type of life and not to the "heroic" type. The latter kind of life also exists, although it is undoubtedly much more rare than the former. Regarding this type of life, however, it cannot be said that it can hardly be directed, or only for short stretches. The heroic type of life is unconditional, that is, it is directed by fateful decisions whereby the resolve to follow a certain path may under certain circumstances last to the bitter end. [LI, 87

Although our intellect has developed almost to perfection the capacity of the bird of prey to see the smallest mouse from the greatest heights, yet if no longer seeking prey it turns at least one eye inwards to discover the one who searches, the weight of the earth holds it and the Sangskaras involve it in a world of startling images. Our intellect then falls into the throes of a demoniacal birth, where unknown terrors and dangers lurk and deceptive reflections and labyrinthian paths mislead. The worst fate awaits the venturous: abysmal, silent loneliness in a time which he calls his own. [XLII, 34

Our judgment of the inner voice varies between two extremes: it is regarded either as merest nonsense or else as the voice of God. That there might be a middle point worthy of consideration occurs to no one. [XLVII, 427

The greatest and most important problems of life are all fundamentally insoluble. They must be so, because they express the necessary polarity inherent in every self-regulating system. They can never be solved, but only outgrown. [xv, 538 (H, 89)

This "outgrowing," as I called it previously, revealed itself on further experience to be the raising of the level of consciousness. Some higher or wider interest arose on the person's horizon, and through this widening of his view, the insoluble problem lost its urgency. It was not solved logically in its own terms, but faded out in contrast to a new and stronger life-tendency. It was not repressed and made unconscious, but merely appeared in a different light, and so became different itself. What, on a lower level, had led to the wildest conflicts and to emotions full of panic, viewed from the higher level of the personality, now seemed like a storm in the valley seen from a high mountain top. This does not mean that the thunderstorm is robbed of its reality; it means that, instead of being in it, one is now above it. [XIV, 21 (H, 88)

The serious problems of life, however, are never fully solved. If it should for once appear that they are, this is the sign that something has been lost. The meaning and design of a problem seem not to lie in its solution but in our working at it incessantly. This alone preserves us from stultification and petrifaction. [xix, 259 f (j, 118 f)

A dissociation is not healed by repression but by a more complete tearing apart. All the healthy desire to be unified will resist the disintegration, and therewith he will realize the possibility of an inner integration which before he had always sought outside himself. He finds as his reward unity within himself. [xix, 287 (g, 198)

The urge and compulsion to self-realization is a law of nature and thus of invincible power, even though its effect, at the outset, is insignificant and improbable. [xlix, 131 (o, 124)

Nature is not only aristocratic; it is esoteric. Yet no man of understanding will thereby be induced to be silent about what he knows, for he realizes only too well that the secret of psychic development can never be betrayed, simply because that development is a question of individual capacity. [xix, 295 (g, 203)

Nature is aristocratic, but not in the sense of having reserved the possibility of differentiation exclusively for species high in the scale. Similarly the possibility of psychological development in human beings is not reserved for specially gifted individuals. In order to achieve a far-reaching psychological development, neither outstanding intelligence nor any other talent is necessary, since in this development moral qualities can make up for what the intellect fails to achieve. [li, 208 (d, 119)

Behind a man stands neither public opinion nor the general code of morals, but that personality which is still unconscious. Just as a man is always that which he once was, so is he also that which he is yet to become. Consciousness does not cover the whole of man, for this consists partly of his conscious contents and partly of his indefinitely wide unconscious, to which no limits can be assigned. Within this whole, consciousness is contained, as it were, like a smaller circle within a larger one.

272

Therefore there seems to be the possibility of making the "ego" the object, or rather the possibility that a wider personality may emerge step by step in the course of the development and take the former ego into its service. This growth of personality proceeds from the unconscious, whose frontiers cannot be defined. Therefore the scope of the personality which is gradually being realized is practically illimitable. [L, 136 f

To become a personality is not the absolute prerogative of the man of genius. He may even have genius without either having personality or being a personality. In so far as every individual has his own inborn law of life, it is theoretically possible for every man to follow this law before all others and so to become a personality—that is, to achieve completeness. But since life can only exist in the form of living units, which is to say, of individuals, the law of life in the last analysis always tends towards a life that is individually lived. [xxvii, 199 f (f, 296)

We know that the first impressions of childhood cannot be lost, but cling to the individual accompanying him throughout his whole life, and that certain educative influences which are equally indestructible are capable of restricting the individual within certain bounds for life. Under these conditions, it is no wonder and in fact even a frequent experience that conflicts break out between that personality which was shaped by education and other influences of the childhood's milieu and the true individual line of life. All people who are ordained to lead an independent, creative life must go through this conflict.

[vi, 48

I wish only to consider the conclusions to which we shall be led if we follow primitive man in supposing that all light comes from the sun, that things are beautiful in themselves and that a human part-soul is a leopard. In doing this we accept the primitive idea of "mana." According to this idea, the beautiful moves *us*, and it is not we who create beauty. A certain person *is* a devil—we have not projected our own evil upon him and in this way made a devil out of him. There are people—mana personalities—who are impressive in their own right, and in no way thanks to our imagination. [xix, 241 (j, 168 f)

I do not wish to deny the existence of real prophets in general, but for the sake of caution, I am inclined to doubt every individual case at first: for it is far too serious a matter to allow of any hasty decision to treat such a case straight-away as genuine. Every true prophet at first protests resolutely against the unconscious demands of this role. Therefore, wherever a prophet arises in the twinkling of an eye, it is wiser to suspect a psychic loss of equilibrium. [LI, 86

Exceptional individuals, carefully fenced off and enclosed, are always a gift of nature, which enriches us and enlarges the scope of our consciousness; but all this is only true so long as our reasoning faculties do not break down. The state of being seized and moved, almost possessed [*Ergriffenheit*], can be a real gift of the gods or a product of hell. With the lack of moderation which goes with this experience, crime begins, even when the accompanying confused state of consciousness makes the attainment of the highest aims seem close at hand. True and lasting gain is only an increased and widened self-possession.

[LVII, 20 f

Life that just happens in and for itself is not real life; it is only real when it is known. Only a unified personality can experience life, not that personality which is split up into partial aspects, that bundle of odds and ends which also calls itself "man." [LVIII, 122 (M, 105)

Self-realization or—what amounts to the same thing—the urge towards individuation gathers all that is scattered and multifarious and raises it to the original form of the One, the primordial man. The separate, individualized existence, i.e., the former state of imprisonment in the ego, is thereby superseded, the scope of consciousness is widened, and through the fact that the paradoxes have been made conscious the sources of conflict are dried up. [L, 146 f

---

To achieve a unity the participation of the whole is required. This demand cannot be undercut by anyone, and therefore there are no cheaper conditions, no substitutes and no compromises. But, when we consider that both *Faust* and *Zarathustra*, in spite of the high recognition they have received, are on the very boundary of European understanding, how can even an educated public that has only just begun to hear of the darkness of soul be expected to form any adequate conception of the psychic condition of a human being entangled in the perplexities of the process of individuation—as I have called the attaining of wholeness. People then turn to the vocabulary of pathology and comfort themselves with the terminology of neurosis and psychosis, or else they hint at the "creative mystery"—but what can a man "create" who happens to be no poet? Owing to this latter delusion, quite a number of people have felt compelled in recent times to call themselves "artists" of their own accord. As if "art" had nothing to do with "ability." If a man has nothing to "create," then perhaps he will create himself.

[xlii, 36

Complete persons are exceptions. It is true that an overwhelming majority of educated people are fragmentary personalities and have a lot of substitutes instead of the genuine goods.

[xlvi, 79 (b, 52)

The development of personality from its germinal state to full consciousness is at once a charism and a curse. Its first result is the conscious and unavoidable separation of the single being from the undifferentiated and unconscious herd. This means isolation, and there is no more comforting word for it. Neither family, nor society, nor position can save him from it, nor the most successful adaptation to actual surroundings, nor yet the most frictionless fitting in with them. The development of personality is a favour that must be paid for dearly.

[xxvii, 190 (f, 288)

No one develops his personality because someone told him it would be useful or advisable for him to do so. Nature has never yet allowed herself to be imposed upon by well-meaning advice. Only coercion working through casual connections moves nature, and human nature also. Nothing changes itself without need, and human personality least of all. It is immensely conservative, not to say inert. Only the sharpest need is able to rouse it. The development of personality obeys no wish, no command, and no insight, but only need; it wants the motivating coercion of inner or outer necessities. Any other development would be individualism. This is why the accusation of individualism is a cheap insult when it is raised against the natural development of personality.   [XXVII, 189 (F, 288)

No one can educate to personality who does not himself have it. And not the child but only the adult can attain personality as the mature fruit of an accomplishment of life that is directed to this end.   [XXVII, 186 (F, 286)

At the beginning, the personality is never that which it becomes later. Therefore, at least in the first half of life, there is the possibility of an increase in personality. This can happen as the result of addition from without, through new and vital contents streaming into the personality from without and being assimilated by the latter. In this way a considerable growth of personality can be experienced. Therefore we readily assume that this growth only comes from outside, and base on this the assumption that we can become a personality if we succeed in cramming in as much as possible from outside. But the more we follow this recipe, and the more we believe that all additional growth comes from without, the poorer we become inwardly. Therefore, when a great idea takes hold of us from without, we should realize that it only grips us because something within us comes to meet it half way and corresponds to it. The possession of psychic readiness is what signifies riches, not the piling up of hunting trophies. Everything which comes from without becomes our own only when we are capable of an inner spaciousness which corresponds to the size of the outer increase. The actual increase in personality is the becoming conscious of a widening, which flows from inner sources. Without the inner breadth we are never related to the size of our object. It is therefore right to say that a man grows with the size of his task. But he must have within him the ability to grow, otherwise the most difficult task will be no use to him; at the most he will break himself upon it.   [XLVII, 411

All beginnings are small. We should therefore not mind doing laborious but conscientious work with obscure individuals, even though the goal towards which we are striving seems to lie

276

at an unattainable distance. One goal is within our reach, and that is to develop and bring to maturity individual personalities. If we are convinced that the individual is the carrier of life, we have served the purpose of life when as a result of our efforts one tree at least bears fruit, even though a thousand others remain barren. But anyone who sets out to bring *everything* that wants to grow to the highest pitch of growth would soon find that the weeds, which always flourish best, had shot up above his head. I therefore consider it the highest task of psychotherapy today to pursue with singleness of purpose the goal of the development of the individual. [LIX, 18 (K, 35)

When we say "the animal in man," this always strikes us as something horrible. But this animal in man is not horrible, no more than animals are horrible, for they fulfil God's will most faithfully; they live to fulfil their Creator's purpose. We do not do this. We meddle with the work of the Creator, for we always want to be something different from what we are. Our ambition is not to be the whole of ourselves, for that would be unpleasant. But the animals are themselves and they fulfil the will of God that is within them in a true and faithful manner. [XXIV, 87

Consciousness guarded round about by psychic powers, or sustained or threatened or deluded by them, is the age-old experience of mankind. This experience has projected itself into the archetype of the child, which expresses man's wholeness. The "child" is all that is abandoned and exposed and at the same time divinely powerful; the insignificant, dubious beginning, and the triumphal end. The "eternal child" in man is an indescribable experience, an incongruity, a disadvantage, and a divine prerogative; an imponderable that determines the ultimate worth or worthlessness of a personality.

[XLIX, 141 (O, 135)

Personality is a germ in the child that can develop only by slow stages in and through life. No personality is manifested without definiteness, fulness, and maturity. These three characteristics do not, and should not, fit the child, for they would rob it of its childhood. [XXVII, 185 (F, 285)

In the adult there is hidden a child—an eternal child, something that is always becoming, is never completed, and that calls for unceasing care, attention, and fostering. This is the part of human personality that wishes to develop and to complete itself. But the human being of our time is as far from this completion as heaven is from earth. [xxvii, 184 (f, 284)

The feeling of bliss accompanies all those moments which have the character of flowing life, moments, therefore, or states, when what was dammed up can freely flow, when we have longer to satisfy this or that condition or seek around with conscious effort in order to find a way or effect a result. We have all known situations or moods "when it goes of itself," when there is no longer any need to manufacture all sorts of wearisome conditions by which joy or pleasure might be stimulated. The age of childhood is the unforgettable token of this joy, which, undismayed by things without, streams all-embracing from within. "Childlikeness" is therefore a symbol for the unique inner condition which accompanies blessedness. [ix, 349 (i, 308)

At a culminating point in life when the bud opens and from the smaller the greater being emerges, "one becomes two" and the greater being which one always was and which nevertheless had always remained invisible confronts the former man with the force of a revelation. The actual and hopelessly small being will always drag down the revelation of the greater into the realm of his smallness, and will never understand that for this smallness the day of judgment has dawned. But the inner great being knows that the long-expected "friend of the soul," the immortal being, has now actually come to "lead captivity captive" (Ephesians 4:8)—namely, himself to grasp the one who has always carried him and held him captive within him, and to allow this life to flow into his own: a moment of most deadly peril! [xlvii, 412

Only the man who is able *consciously* to affirm the power of the vocation confronting him from within becomes a personality; he who succumbs to it falls a prey to the blind flux of happening and is destroyed. The greatness and the liberating effect of all genuine personality consists in this, that it subjects itself of free choice to its vocation and consciously translates into its own individual reality what would lead only to ruin if it were lived unconsciously by the group. [xxvii, 200 f (f, 296)

The demand made by the *imitatio Christi*, i.e., to follow the ideal and seek to become like it, should have the result of developing and exalting the inner man. In actual fact, however, the ideal has been turned by superficial and mechanical-minded believers into an object of worship external to them, an outward show which, precisely because of the veneration accorded it, cannot reach down into the depth of the psyche and transform it into a wholeness harmonizing with that ideal. Accordingly the divine mediator stands outside as an image, while man remains fragmentary and untouched in the deepest part of him. Christ can indeed be imitated to the point of stigmatization without the imitator's even remotely approaching the ideal or heeding its meaning; the point here is not a mere imitation that leaves a man unchanged and makes him into an artifact—it is rather a matter of realizing the ideal on one's own account (*Deo concedente*) in the sphere of one's individual life. [lviii, 19 f (m, 7)

Everything good is costly, and the development of the personality is one of the most costly of all things. It is a question of yea-saying to oneself, of taking the self as the most serious of tasks, keeping conscious of everything done, and keeping it constantly before one's eyes in all its dubious aspects—truly a task that touches us to the core. [xiv, 26 (h, 92)

Personality can never develop itself unless the individual chooses his own way consciously and with conscious, moral decision. Not only the causal motive, the need, but a conscious, moral decision must lend its strength to the process of the development of personality. If the first, that is, need, is lacking, then the so-called development would be mere acrobatics of the will; if the latter is missing, that is, the conscious decision, then the development will come to rest in a stupefying, unconscious automatism. But a man can make a moral choice of his own way only when he holds it to be the best. If any other way were held to be better, then he would live and develop that other personality in place of his own. The other ways are the conventions of a moral, social, political, philosophic, or religious nature. The fact that the conventions always flourish in one form or another proves that the overwhelming majority of mankind chooses not its own way, but the conventions, and so does not develop itself, but a method and a collectivity at the cost of its own fulness.   [xxvii, 191 (F, 289 f)

Personality is the highest realization of the inborn distinctiveness of the particular living being. Personality is an act of the greatest courage in the face of life, and means unconditional affirmation of all that constitutes the individual, the most successful adaptation to the universal conditions of human existence, with the greatest possible freedom of personal decision.
[xxvii, 186 (F, 286)

In so far as a man is untrue to his own law and does not rise to personality, he has failed of the meaning of his life. Fortunately, in her kindness and patience, Nature has never put the fatal question as to the meaning of their lives into the mouths of most people. And where no one asks, no one needs to answer.
[xxvii, 206 (F, 301)

One meets among so-called "primitives" spiritual personalities for whom one feels the respect we instinctively accord to the fully matured products of an undisturbed destiny.
[xix, 288 (G, 198 f)

We may assume that human personality consists of two things: first, of consciousness and whatever this covers, and second, of an indefinitely large hinterland of unconscious psyche. So far as the former is concerned it can be more or less clearly defined and delimited, but so far as the sum total of human personality is concerned one has to admit the impossibility of a complete description or definition. In other words, there is unavoidably an illimitable and indefinable addition to every personality, because the latter consists of a conscious and observable part which does not contain certain factors whose existence, however, we are forced to assume in order to explain certain observable facts. The unknown factors form what we call the unconscious.   [xlvi, 74 (B, 47 f)

The purposive character of the Self which is *a priori* present, and the urge to realize this purpose, exist even without the participation of consciousness. They cannot be denied, but no more can ego-consciousness be dispensed with. It also states its demands imperatively, and very often in open or veiled opposition to the necessity of self-realization. In reality, apart from a few exceptional cases, the entelechy of the Self consists of a path of endless compromises, whereby ego and Self counterbalance each other with great effort if all is to go well. Too great a swing to one side or the other therefore often represents, in a deeper sense, no more than an example of how not to do it. This does not in the least mean that extremes which arise in a natural way are necessarily an evil. We can make good use of them, if we try to discover their meaning, for which they fortunately give us plenty of opportunity.   [XLVII, 20

What does "wholeness" mean? I feel that there is every reason here for some anxiety, since man as a whole being casts a shadow. The fourth was not separated from the three and banished to the kingdom of everlasting fire for nothing. But does not an uncanonical saying of our Lord declare, "Whoso is near unto me is near unto the fire"? Such dire ambiguities are not meant for grown-up children—which is why Heraclitus of old was named "the dark," because he spoke too plainly and called life itself an "ever-living fire." And that is why there are uncanonical sayings for those that have ears to hear.

[LVIII, 273 (M, 297)

There is no light without shadow and no psychic wholeness without imperfection. To round itself out, life calls not for perfection but for completeness; and for this the "thorn in the flesh" is needed, the suffering of defects without which there is no progress and no ascent.   [LVIII, 223 f (M, 208)

It is only the intervention of time and space here and now that makes reality. Wholeness is realized only in the moment—the moment that Faust was seeking all his life.

[LVIII, 294 (M, 321)

In the last analysis every life is the realization of a whole, that is, of a self, for which reason this realization can also be called "individuation." All life is bound to individual carriers who realize it and is simply inconceivable without them. But every carrier is charged with an individual destiny and destination, and the realization of these alone makes sense of life. True, the "sense" is often something that could just as well be called "nonsense," for there is a certain incommensurability between the mystery of existence and human understanding. "Sense" and "nonsense" are merely man-made labels which serve to give us a reasonably valid sense of direction.   [LVIII, 304 (M, 330)

FATE, DEATH, AND RENEWAL

What, in the last analysis, induces a man to choose his own way and so to climb out of unconscious identity with the mass as out of a fog bank? It cannot be necessity, for necessity comes to many and they all save themselves in convention. It cannot be moral choice, for as a rule a man decides for convention. What is it, then, that inexorably tilts the beam in favour of the *extraordinary?*—It is what is called vocation: an irrational factor that fatefully forces a man to emancipate himself from the herd and its trodden paths. True personality always has vocation and believes in it, has fidelity to it as to God, in spite of the fact that, as the ordinary man would say, it is only a feeling of individual vocation. But this vocation acts like a law of God from which there is no escape. That many go to ruin upon their own ways means nothing to him who has vocation. He must obey his own law, as if it were a demon that whisperingly indicated to him new and strange ways. Who has vocation hears the voice of the inner man; he is called.   [xxvii, 193 f (f, 291 f)

It is true that much can be attained by the will, but in view of the fate of certain especially strong-willed personalities, we must regard it as false in principle to seek to subdue our fate at all costs to our own will. Our will is a function directed by our reflective powers; thus it depends upon the quality of the superior part of our nature. This superior part, if true to itself, acts in accordance with reason or intellect. But has it ever been shown, or shall it ever be, that life and destiny harmonize with our human reason—that they, too, are rational? On the contrary, there is good ground for conjecturing that they are irrational, or rather, that in the last resort, their meaning lies beyond human reason.   [li, 88 f (d, 48)

We cannot rate reason highly enough, but there are times when we must ask ourselves: do we really know enough about the destinies of individuals to entitle us to give good advice under *all* circumstances? Certainly we must act according to

283

our best convictions, but are we so sure that our convictions are for the best as regards the other person? Very often we do not know what is best for ourselves, and in later years we may occasionally thank God from the bottom of our hearts that his kindly hand has preserved us from the "reasonableness" of our former plans. It is easy for the critic to say after the event, "Ah, but then it wasn't the right sort of reason!" Who can know with unassailable certainty when he has the right sort? Moreover, is it not essential to the true art of living, sometimes, in defiance of all reason and fitness, to include the unreasonable and the unfitting within the ambit of the possible?   [LX, 147 (N, 437)

Reason must always seek the solution upon rational, sequential, logical ways, in which it is certainly justified in all normal situations and problems; but in the greatest and really decisive questions the reason proves inadequate. It is incapable of creating the image, the symbol; for the symbol is irrational. When the rational way has become a *cul-de-sac*—which is its inevitable and constant tendency—then, from the side where one least expects it, the solution comes.   [IX, 364 f (I, 322)

It is a rational presupposition of ours that everything has a natural and perceptible cause. We distinctly resent the idea of invisible and arbitrary forces, for it is not so long ago that we made our escape from that frightening world of dreams and superstitions, and constructed for ourselves a picture of the cosmos worthy of rational consciousness—that latest and greatest achievement of man. We are now surrounded by a world that is obedient to rational laws. It is true that we do not know the causes of everything, but they will in time be discovered, and these discoveries will accord with our reasoned expectations. That is our hope, and we take it as much for granted as primitive man does his own assumptions. There are also chance occurrences, to be sure, but these are merely accidental, and we have granted them a causality of their own. Chance occurrences are repellent to the mind that loves order. They have a laughable and therefore irritating way of throwing out of gear the predictable course of events. We resent the idea of chance occurrences as much as that of invisible forces, for they remind us too much of Satanic imps or of the caprice of a *deus ex ma-*

china. They are the worst enemies of our careful calculations and a continual threat to all our undertakings. Being admittedly contrary to reason, they deserve contempt, and yet we should not fail to give them their due. The Arab shows them greater respect than we. He writes on every letter *"Insha-Allah,"* "If it please God," for only then will the letter arrive. In spite of our reluctance to admit chance, and in spite of the fact that events run true to general laws, it is undeniable that we are always and everywhere exposed to incalculable accidents. And what is more invisible and arbitrary than chance? What is more unavoidable and more annoying? [xix, 218 f (j, 149)

The effect of the unconscious images has something of fate in it. . . . Perhaps—who knows?—these eternal images may be the reality of what is called fate. [li, 195 f (d, 115)

Is it possible that there is something living and effective beyond the human day-world? Necessities and dangerous inevitabilities? More intentional things than electrons? Is it possible that we only think we possess and dominate our souls, while that which science calls the psyche and understands as a question mark shut in the capsule of the skull is in the end an open door through which, from time to time, there emerge unknown things working fearful effects, from out the non-human world and, on wings of night, removing man from humanity and leading him to a supra-personal serfdom and destiny? Yes, it almost seems as if the love-experience had sometimes acted only as a releasing factor, and as if the human-personal were merely the upward beat to the "divine comedy," which alone is essential. [xvi, 323

"In thine own breast dwell the stars of thy fate," says Seni to Wallenstein—a dictum that would do ample justice to all astrology, if we knew even a little something about this secret of the heart. But for this, so far, men have had little understanding. Nor do I dare to assert that the matter stands any better today. [xxxi, 183 f (f, 56)

It is dangerous to confess to spiritual poverty, for whoever is poor has cravings and whoever craves draws his fate upon himself. [xxxi, 193 (f, 63)

Whether primitive or not, mankind always stands upon the
verge of those actions that it performs itself but does not control. The whole world wants peace, and the whole world prepares for war, to give but one example. Mankind is powerless
against mankind, and gods, as they have ever done, show it the
ways of fate. Today we call the gods "factors," which comes
from *facere,* "to make." The makers stand behind the wings of
the world-theatre. It is in great things as in small. In the realm
of consciousness we are our own masters; we seem to be the
factors themselves. But if we step through the door of the
shadow we discover with fright that we are the objects of factors.   [xxxi, 302 (f, 71)

In our strength we are independent and isolated, there we
can forge our own fates; but in our weakness we are dependent
and therefore bound, and here we become, albeit unwillingly,
instruments of fate. For here it is not the individual will that
commands, but the will of the race.   [x, 35 (g, 181)

People often behave as if they did not rightly understand
what constitutes the destructive character of the creative force.
A woman who gives herself up to passion, particularly under
present-day civilized conditions, experiences this destructive
element all too soon. We must think a little beyond the framework of purely bourgeois moral conditions to understand the
feeling of boundless uncertainty which befalls the man who
gives himself over unconditionally to fate. Even to be fruitful
means to destroy oneself, for with the creation of a new generation the previous generation has passed beyond its climax. Our
offspring thus become our most dangerous enemies, with whom
we cannot get even, for they will survive us and so inevitably
will take the power out of our weakening hands. Fear of our
erotic fate is quite understandable, for there is something unpredictable about it.   [iv, 101 f

The more the ego seeks to secure every possible liberty, independence, superiority, and freedom from obligations, the
deeper does it fall into the slavery of objective facts. The subject's freedom of mind is chained to an ignominious financial
dependence, his unconcernedness of action suffers now and

again a distressing collapse in the face of public opinion, his moral superiority gets swamped in inferior relationships, and his desire to dominate ends in a pitiful craving to be loved.

[ix, 542 f (i, 478)

It is not I who create myself, but rather I happen to myself.

[l, 138

The great decisions of human life have as a rule far more to do with the instincts and other mysterious unconscious factors than with conscious will and well-meaning reasonableness. The shoe that fits one person pinches another; there is no recipe for living that suits all cases. Each of us carries his own life-form—an indeterminable form which cannot be superseded by any other.

[xix, 95 (j, 69)

Fate hides unknown dangers, and the constant hesitation of the neurotic to venture into life is easily explained by the desire to be allowed to stand aside and not to have to join in the dangerous battle of life. He who renounces the venture of experience must stifle within himself the desire for life, which is a form of suicide.

[(iv, 102)

That which happens in the secret hour of life's noonday is the reversal of the parable, the birth of death. Life in its second half is no longer an ascent, an unfolding, an increase, and an exuberance of life, but death; for its aim is the end. Not to want the climax of our life is the same as not to want our end. Both mean not wanting to live. Not wanting to live is synonymous with not wanting to die. Becoming and passing away are the same curve.

[xxvii, 216 f

As the arrow flies to the target, so life ends in death, which is the target of all life. Even the ascent and its climax are but steps and means to the end, to reach the target, death.

[xxvii, 218

Death is psychologically just as important as birth, and, like it, is an integral part of life.

[xiv, 61 (h, 124)

The birth of a human being is pregnant with meaning; then

287

why is this not true of death also? Twenty years or more of a young man's life are spent in preparation for the full unfolding of his individual existence; why then should he not spend twenty years or more preparing for his end?   [xxvii, 218 f

I am convinced that it is hygienic—if I may use the word—to discover in death a goal towards which one can strive, and that shrinking away from it is something unhealthy and abnormal which robs the second half of life of its purpose.

[xix, 272 (j, 129)

We know that when for one reason or another we are out of sorts, we are liable not only to make great or little blunders but also to do dangerous things which, given the psychologically appropriate moment, might even be fatal. There is a common saying, "So-and-so died at the right moment," which comes out of a correct appreciation of the secret psychological causality of the case.   [li, 205 (d, 118)

It is a well-known fact that the highest summit of life is expressed by the symbolism of death, for creation beyond oneself means one's own death. The coming generation is the end of the preceding one.   [iv, 275

The psyche pre-existent to consciousness (e. g., in the child) participates in the maternal psyche on the one hand, while on the other it reaches across to the daughter psyche. We could therefore say that every mother contains her daughter in herself and every daughter her mother, and that every woman extends backwards into her mother and forwards into her daughter. This participation and intermingling give rise to that peculiar uncertainty as regards *time:* a woman lives earlier as a mother, later as a daughter. The conscious experience of these ties produces the feeling that her life is spread out over generations—the first step towards the immediate experience and conviction of being outside time, which brings with it a feeling of immortality. The individual's life is elevated into a type, indeed it becomes the archetype of woman's fate in general. This leads to restoration, or "apocatastasis," of the lives of her ancestors, who now, through the bridge of the momentary individual, pass down into the generations of the future. An experience of this kind gives the individual a place and a meaning in the life of the generations, so that all unnecessary obstacles are cleared out of the way of the life-stream that is to flow through her. At the same time the individual is rescued from her isolation and restored to wholeness.   [XLIX, 224 f (o, 225 f)

Indeed our life is the same as it ever was. At all events, in our sense of the word it is not transitory; for the same physiological and psychological processes as have belonged to man for hundreds of thousands of years still endure and give to the inner feeling this profound intuition of the eternal continuity of the living process. But the Self, as an inclusive term embracing our whole living system, contains not only the deposit and the totality of all past life, but it is also a point of departure, the fertile soil from which all future life must spring. A certain premonition of this fact is clearly sensed by the inner feeling as is the historical aspect. From these psychological foundations the idea of immortality is legitimately derived.   [XI, 124 (D, 207)

For the man of today, the enlargement of life and its culmination are plausible goals; but the idea of life after death seems to him questionable or beyond belief. And yet life's cessation, that is, death, can only be accepted as a goal when existence is so wretched that we are glad for it to end, or when we are convinced that the sun strives to its setting—"to illumine distant races"—with the same perseverance it showed in rising to the zenith. But to believe has become today such a difficult art that people, and particularly the educated part of humanity, can hardly find their way there. They have become too accustomed to the thought that, with regard to immortality and such questions, there are many contradictory opinions and no convincing proofs. Since "science" has become the catchword which carries the weight of conviction in the contemporary world, we ask for "scientific" proofs. But educated people who can think know that proof of this kind is out of the question. We simply know nothing whatever about it.

[XIX, 270 f (J, 127 f)

It would all be so much simpler if we could only deny the existence of the psyche. But here we are with our immediate experiences of something that *is*—something that has taken root in the midst of our measurable, ponderable, three-dimensional reality, that differs bafflingly from this in every respect and in all its parts, and yet reflects it. The psyche may be regarded as a mathematical point and at the same time as a universe of fixed stars. It is small wonder, then, if, to the unsophisticated mind, such a paradoxical being borders on the divine. If it occupies no space, it has no body. Bodies die, but can something invisible and incorporeal disappear? What is more, life and psyche existed for me before I could say "I," and when this "I" disappears, as in sleep or unconsciousness, life and psyche still go on, as our observation of other people and our own dreams inform us. Why should the simple mind deny, in the face of such experiences, that the "soul" lives in a realm beyond the body? I must admit that I can see as little nonsense in this so-called superstition as in the findings of research regarding heredity or the basic instincts.　　　　　　　　　　　[xxvii, 16 f (j, 213)

Naturally the cult of the dead is based rationally on belief in the immortality of the soul, but irrationally it comes from a psychological need of the living to do something for the departed. It is a question of a quite elementary need which befalls even the most enlightened when faced with the death of relations and friends. Therefore we still have all manner of customs connected with death, in spite of all enlightenment. Even Lenin had to put up with being embalmed and with a pompous mausoleum like an Egyptian ruler, although certainly not because his followers believe in his bodily resurrection. Apart from the masses for the dead in the Catholic Church, our care for the departed is rudimentary and on the lowest level, not because we are not sufficiently convinced of the immortality of the soul, but because we have rationalized away the psychic need. We behave as if we did not feel this need, and because people cannot believe in survival after death, they therefore do nothing about it. But the more naïve feeling looks after itself and produces—as, for instance, in Italy—frightfully imposing tombstones. At a considerably higher level, there is the mass for the dead, which is meant expressly for the welfare of the souls of the dead and is not merely a consolation for the bereaved feeling. The greatest spiritual display for the sake of

the departed is to be found in the teaching of the Tibetan Book
of the Dead, the *Bardo Thödol*.   [XXXII, 33

Nothing makes us more painfully conscious of fleeting time
and the terrible transitoriness of all blossoms than an idle and
empty life. Idle dreaming is the mother of the fear of death,
the sentimental bewailing of the past and a futile putting back
of the clock. Even if we can forget that the wheel is turning by
preserving the feeling of youth for a long time, perhaps too
long, in a dreamlike state of memories obstinately clung to,
our grey hair, our sagging skin, and the wrinkles on our face
soon ruthlessly show us that, even without exposing our body
to the destructive force of the whole battle of life, the poison
of the stealthily slithering snake of time has been gnawing our
(ah, so dearly loved) body. It avails us nothing to cry out, like
the tragic hero Chiwantopel, "I have kept my body inviolate";
the flight from life does not free us from the law of advancing
age and death. The neurotic who tries to escape from the necessity of life gains nothing and only takes upon his shoulders the
fearful burden of age and death tasted in advance, which must
be especially cruel because of the total emptiness and pointless-
ness of his life. When the libido is denied a progressive life
which also desires all dangers and decay, then it follows the
other road and buries itself in its own depths, digging down to
the ancient feeling of the immortality of all life and to a longing
for rebirth.   [IV, 372 f

Man leaves the mother, the source of libido, and is driven by
an eternal thirst to find her again and to drink renewal from
her; thus he completes his cycle and returns again to the
mother's womb. Every obstacle which obstructs the path of
his life and threatens his ascent bears the shadowy features of
the "terrible mother," who paralyses his courage for life with
the consuming poison of a secret, retrospective longing. In
every victory he wins back the smiling, loving, life-giving
mother. Both of the images are part of the intuitive depths of
human feeling, but their features have been twisted out of all
recognition by the progressive development of the surface of the
human mind. The hard necessity of adaptation works incessantly to eradicate the last traces of those original memorials

of the period which saw the birth of the human mind, and to replace them by features which are intended to denote with ever increasing clarity the nature of real objects. Only the overcoming of the obstacles in the outer world can bring liberation from the mother, who is a constant and inexhaustible source of life to the creative human being, but death to the cowardly, timorous, and lazy. [IV, 368

By acknowledging the reality of the psyche and making it a codetermining ethical factor in our lives, we offend against the spirit of convention which for centuries has regulated spiritual life from outside by means of institutions as well as by reason. Not that unreasoning instinct rebels of itself against firmly established order—by the strict logic of its own inner laws it is itself of the firmest structure imaginable and, in addition, the creative foundation of all binding order. But just because this foundation is creative, all order which proceeds from it—even in its most "divine" form—is a phase, a stepping-stone. Despite appearances to the contrary, the establishment of order and the dissolution of what has been established are at bottom beyond human control. The secret is that only what can destroy itself is truly alive. [LVIII, 110 f (M, 93)

The highest value bestowing life and meaning has been lost; this process is a typical, i.e., frequently repeated, experience, and therefore it found its central expression in the Christian mystery. This death or loss must always repeat itself; Christ forever dies, as he is always born again. For the psychic life of the archetype is beyond time compared with our individual dependence on time. By what laws first one and then another aspect of the archetype comes into effective action is beyond my knowledge. I only know—and thereby I express the knowledge of countless people—that at present we are living in an age of God's death and disappearance. The myth says: He will not be found where His body was laid. The "body" means the outer, visible form, the previous but transitory conception of the highest value. The myth says further that the value will arise again in a miraculous manner but transformed.

[XLVI, 162 f

The descent into hell during the three days of death describes the sinking of the lost value into the unconscious where —through victory over the power of darkness—it brings about a new order, and from whence it rises again to the height of heaven, i.e., to the height of fullest consciousness. Since only a few saw the Resurrected One, it means that the difficulties of again finding and recognizing the transformed value are not inconsiderable. [XLVI, 163

When the libido leaves the upper world of light, whether by individual decision, or owing to the decline of vital energy, it sinks back into its own depths, into the source from which it once flowed out, and returns to the point of cleavage, the navel, through which it once entered our body. This point of cleavage it called the "mother," for it is from her that the source of the libido came to us. Therefore, when there is any great work to be done, from which the weak human being shrinks, doubting his own strength, his libido streams back to that source—and that is the dangerous moment, the moment of decision between destruction and new life. If the libido remains caught in the wonderland of the inner world, the human being becomes a mere shadow in the upper world: he is no better than a dead man or a seriously ill one. But if the libido succeeds in tearing itself free and struggling up to the upper world again, then a miracle occurs, for this descent to the underworld has been a rejuvenation for the libido, and from its apparent death a new fruitfulness has awakened. [IV, 283 f

The birth of the deliverer is equivalent to a great catastrophe, since a new and powerful life issues forth just where no life or force or new development was anticipated. It streams forth out of the unconscious, i.e., from that part of the psyche which, whether we desire it or not, is unknown and therefore treated as nothing by all rationalists. From this discredited and rejected region comes the new tributary of energy, the revivification of life. But what is this discredited and despised region? It is the sum of all those psychic contents which are repressed on account of their incompatability with conscious values, hence the ugly, immoral, wrong, irrelevant, useless, etc., which means everything that at one time appeared so to the individual in question. Now herein lies the danger that the very force with which these things reappear, as well as their new and wonderful brilliance, may so intrigue the individual that he either forgets or repudiates all former values. What he formerly despised is now a supreme principle, and what was formerly truth now becomes error. This reversal of values is tantamount to a destruction of previously accepted values; hence it resembles the devastation of a country by floods.   [IX, 371 f (I, 328)

If the old were not ripe for death, nothing new would appear; and, if the old were not injuriously blocking the way for the new, it could not and need not be rooted out.   [IX, 370 (I, 327)

In the initiation of the living, the "beyond" is primarily by no means the realm of the dead, but a reversal of attitude, i.e., a psychological "beyond" or, in Christian terms, a "redemption" from the bonds of the world and of sin. Redemption is a release and a liberation from an earlier state of darkness and unconsciousness and the attainment of a state of enlightenment, of detachment, of victory, and of triumph over "given facts."

[XXXII, 21

The fact that men speak of rebirth and that there is such a conception at all means that a psychic state which is so described also exists. What this state consists of we can only conclude from the assertions concerning it. We must therefore set up a "cross-examination" with world history as to what it describes as rebirth if we wish to know what rebirth is.

[XLVII, 405

"Rebirth" is an assertion which belongs to the primordial assertions of mankind.   [XLVII, 405

Out of the unfolding embrace, the enveloping womb of the sea, the sun tears itself free and rises victoriously, and then, leaving the heights of noonday and all its glorious works behind it, sinks back into the maternal sea, into the night which hides all and gives new birth to all. This image was the first to become—and with the most profound justification—the symbolic bearer of human destiny: in the morning of life, man painfully tears himself away from the mother, from the home-hearth, and fights his way up to his full heights, not seeing his worst enemy before him but carrying him within him as a deadly longing for his own abyss, a yearning to drown in his own source, to be engulfed in the mother. His life is a constant battle with death, a violent and transitory liberation from the ever-threatening night. This death is no outer enemy, but his own inner longing for the silence and deep peace of non-existence, that dreamless sleep in the sea of all birth and death. Even in his highest strivings for harmony and balance, for philosophical depths and artistic "possession," he seeks death, immobility, satiety, and peace. If, like Peirithous, he stays too long in the place of rest and peace, he becomes torpid and the poison of the snake has paralysed him for ever. If he is to live, he must fight, and must sacrifice his longing for the past in order to climb up to his own heights. And when once he has reached the noonday heights, he must also sacrifice his love for his own achievement, for there can be no standing still. The sun also sacrifices its greatest strength to hasten forward to the fruits of autumn, which are seeds of immortality: in children, in works, in fame, in a new order of things, which in their turn begin and complete the sun's course over again.   [IV, 335

In life we are so beset by a multitude of pressing, pushing things, that we never get the time—on account of so many "given facts"—to think about who really "gave" them.

[XXXII, 20

If I know and admit that I give myself or give up myself and do not wish to be paid for it, then I have sacrificed my claim, i.e., a part of myself. Therefore every act of giving free from any claim, i.e., giving *à fond perdu* in every respect, means an act of self-sacrifice. The usual giving which is not paid back is felt to be a loss. But a sacrifice should be like a loss, so that the egoistical claim can definitely no longer exist. The gift should therefore be made as if it had been destroyed. But, inasmuch as the gift represents myself, I have destroyed myself with it, i.e., I have given myself away without any expectation of return. Seen from another point of view, however, this intentional loss is no real loss, but on the contrary a gain, for to be able to sacrifice oneself proves that one possesses oneself. No one can give who does not possess.   [L, 136

Through the sacrifice of ourselves we gain ourselves, *the* Self; for we only have what we give. [L, 143

The fear of self-sacrifice lurks in and behind every ego; for this fear is the claim of unconscious powers to come into full effect, and is often restrained only with difficulty. No process of individuation is ever spared this dangerous stage, for to the totality of the Self also belongs that which is feared, the underworld or overworld of psychic dominants, from which the ego has once painfully—and only to a certain extent—emancipated itself, attaining a more or less illusory freedom. This liberation is certainly a necessary heroic undertaking; but it is not a final achievement, for it is only the making of a subject which, in order to be fulfilled, must encounter an object. This object seems at first sight to be the world, which is indeed magnified through projection for this purpose. We seek and find our difficulties, we seek and find our enemy, we seek and find that which is beloved and precious; and it is a satisfaction to know that all evil and all good are outside us in a visible object, where they can be overcome, punished, destroyed, or blessed. But, in the long run, nature herself will not always allow this paradisial, innocent condition of the subject to continue undisturbed. There are people, as there always have been, who cannot avoid the insight that the world and experience of the world are essentially in the nature of a parable and really illustrate something which lies hidden deep down in the subject itself, in its own trans-subjective reality. [XXXII, 29 f

———————

For the experience of wholeness, there can be no question of anything cheaper or less than just the whole. What this means psychologically can easily be grasped through the simple realization that consciousness is always only a part of the psyche and therefore never capable of being the psychic whole: the indeterminable extension of the unconscious must be added to it as well. But this can neither be captured with clever formulas, nor spellbound by scientific theorems, for there is something fateful about it, indeed it is at times fate itself. [XLII, 36

I have been deeply impressed with the fact that the new thing prepared by fate seldom or never corresponds to conscious expectation. It is a still more remarkable fact that, though the new thing contradicts deeply rooted instincts as we know them, yet it is a singularly appropriate expression of the total personality, an expression which one could not imagine in a more complete form. [xv, 539 (H, 90)

If you sum up what people tell you about their experience, you can formulate it in about this way: they came to themselves, they could accept themselves, they were able to become reconciled to adverse circumstances and events. This is much like what was formerly expressed by saying: he has made his peace with God, he has sacrificed his own will, he has submitted himself to the will of God. [XLVI, 147 (B, 99)

When I examined the way of development of those persons who, quietly, and as if unconsciously, grew beyond themselves, I saw that their fates had something in common. Whether arising from without or within, the new thing came to all those persons from a dark field of possibilities; they accepted it and developed further by means of it. It seemed to me typical that in some cases the new thing was found outside themselves and in others within; or rather, that it grew into some persons from without and into others from within. But it was never something that came exclusively either from within or from without. If it came from outside the individual, it became an inner experience; if it came from within, it was changed into an outer event. But in no case was it conjured into existence through purpose and conscious willing, but rather seemed to flow out of the stream of time. [xv, 539 (H, 89)

THE WAY TO GOD

The spirit of mankind has been concerned with the suffering soul for thousands of years, perhaps even earlier than with the suffering body. The "salvation" of the soul, the "propitiation of the gods," and the "perils of the soul" are by no means recent problems. Religions are psychotherapeutic systems in the most actual meaning of the word, and in the widest measure. They express the scope of the soul's problems in mighty images. They are the acknowledgment and recognition of the soul, and at the same time the revelation and manifestation of the nature of the soul. No human soul is separated from this universal basis; only an individual consciousness which has lost the connection with the whole soul is caught in the illusion that the soul is a tiny, circumscribable region, suitable as the object of some "scientific" theory. The loss of the wider connection is the fundamental evil of neurosis, and therefore the path of the neurotic strays into the smallest side-streets of doubtful reputation, for whoever denies the big things must look for the blame in the smallest things. [XXVI, 15

The religious statements are the most improbable of all and yet they have been maintained over thousands of years. (The boldness, indeed the danger, of this Tertullian-like argument* is undeniable, but is no proof against its psychological truth.) The fact that their vitality so far exceeds what might be expected points to the existence of an adequate cause, the scientific recognition of which has as yet escaped the human mind. [L, 126

The ways and customs of his childhood, once so sublimely good, can barely lay man aside even when their harmfulness has long since been proved. The same, only on a gigantic scale, is the case with historical changes of attitude. A general attitude

* [Tertullian said (*De Carne Christi,* 5): "And the Son of God died; this is therefore credible, just because it is absurd. And He rose again from the tomb; this is certain, because it is impossible." Cf. Jung, *Psychological Types* (London, 1923), p. 21.—TRANSLATOR.]

corresponds with a religion, and changes of religion belong to the most painful moments in the world's history. In this respect our age has a blindness without parallel. We think we have only to declare an acknowledged form of faith to be incorrect or invalid in order to become psychologically free of all the traditional effects of the Christian or Judaic religion. We believe in enlightenment, as if an intellectual change of opinion had somehow a deeper influence on emotional processes, or indeed upon the unconscious! We entirely forget that the religion of the last two thousand years is a psychological attitude, a definite form and manner of adaptation to inner and outer experience, which moulds a definite form of civilization; it has, thereby, created an atmosphere which remains wholly uninfluenced by any intellectual disavowal.   [IX, 264 (I, 229 f)

Religions, in my opinion, with all which they are and assert, are so near to the human soul that psychology least of all can afford to overlook them.   [L, 33

It would be a regrettable mistake if anybody should understand my observations to be a kind of proof of the existence of God. They prove only the existence of an archetypal image of the Deity, which to my mind is the most we can assert psychologically about God.   [XLVI, 108 (B, 73)

The competence of psychology as an empirical science only goes so far as to establish, on the basis of comparative research, whether for instance the imprint found in the psyche can or cannot reasonably be termed a "God-image." Nothing positive or negative has thus been asserted about the possible existence of God, any more than the archetype of the "hero" proves the actual existence of a hero.   [LVIII, 28 (M, 15)

It is in the inward experience that the connection between the psyche and the outward image or creed is first revealed as a relationship or correspondence like that of *sponsus* and *sponsa*. Accordingly when I say as a psychologist that God is an archetype, I mean by that the "type" in the psyche. The

word "type" is, as we know, derived from the Greek *typos,*
"blow" or "imprint"; thus an "archetype" presupposes an im-
printer.   [LVIII, 27 f (M, 15)

The ideas of moral law and of the Godhead are part of the indestructible constituents of the human soul. Therefore every
honest psychology which is not blinded by a narrow-minded
conceit of enlightenment, must come to terms with these facts.
They cannot be explained away, or dismissed, with irony. In
physics we can dispense with a concept of God, but in psychology the concept of God is a definite entity, which must be
reckoned with, just as much as with "affect," "instinct,"
"mother," etc. It is naturally due to the perpetual confusion
between object and image that we are unable to imagine a difference between "God" and the "imago of God," and that therefore we suppose that we are speaking of God and giving a
"theological" explanation when we are really speaking of the
"idea of God." It is not for psychology as a science to hyposta-
size the imago of God; psychology has only to reckon with the
function of an image of God, in accordance with the actual
facts.   [XIII, 180 f

If a blind man can gradually be helped to see, it is not to be
expected that he will at once discern new truths with an eagle
eye. One must be glad if he sees anything at all and if he begins
to understand what he sees. Psychology is concerned with the
act of seeing and not with the construction of new religious
truths, when even the existing teachings have not yet been
perceived and understood. In religious matters it is a well-
known fact that we cannot understand a thing until we have
experienced it inwardly.   [LVIII, 27 (M, 15)

I use the standpoint of philosophy, of the science of religion,
of history, and of natural science exclusively to describe psychic connections. If in so doing I use a concept of God or an
equally metaphysical concept of energy, I am bound to because
these are things which have been in the human soul from the
beginning. I have constantly to repeat that neither the moral
law nor the concept of God nor any religion has ever fallen
down from outside, so to speak from heaven, upon mankind,

but man has all this within him from the beginning and therefore he creates it out of himself. Hence it is just an idle thought
that only enlightenment is required to drive out these ghosts.
[XIII, 180

The concept of God is simply a necessary psychological
function of an irrational character which has nothing to do
with the question of the existence of God. The human intellect
can never answer this question, and still less can it give any
proof of God. Furthermore, such proof is altogether superfluous,
for the idea of an all-powerful divine being is present everywhere, if not consciously recognized, then unconsciously accepted, because it is an archetype.   [LI, 128 f (D, 73)

A definition is an image which does not raise the unknown
facts it describes into the sphere of comprehensibility, otherwise we would be able to say we had created a God. The "Lord"
whom we have chosen is not identical with the image which we
have drawn of Him in time and space. He works within us as
of old, as an unknowable power in the depths of the soul. We
do not even know the nature of simple thought, not to speak
of the ultimate principles of the psyche. Besides, we have no
control whatsoever over the inner life of the soul. But because
it is beyond our free will and purpose, and is free in relation to
us, it can happen that the chosen living power described in our
definition may, even against our will, step out of the frame of
the picture painted by human hand. Then we might perhaps
say with Nietzsche, "God is dead." But it would be more correct to say, "He has rejected our image, and where shall we
find Him again?" The interregnum is fraught with danger, for
the facts of nature will raise their claims in the form of various
isms, and nothing but anarchy and destruction come of it; because, as a result of inflation, the human hubris elects the ego
in its ridiculous poverty to be Lord of the Universe.   [XLVI, 158

In the trinitarian life process of the Deity, man is at first
necessarily excluded. However we cannot, for instance, imagine
this process other than as a pictorial process in the human
mind—somewhat in the sense of St. Augustine, who says, "Dictum est, tres personae, non ut illud diceretur, sed ne taceretur"

301

("It is said, three persons, not in order that it should be said, but that it should not be passed over in silence")—in other words, as a Platonic eidolon which is related to an eternal *eidos*, whereby this eidolon does not assert anything in any way binding, or posit that which is fundamental to it. For this foundation, namely God, is unknowable, or at least can only be recognized by that which is akin to it.   [L, 43

If we take into consideration the fact that the idea of God is an "unscientific" hypothesis, we can easily explain why people have forgotten to think along such lines. And even if they cherish a certain belief in God they would be deterred from the idea of God within by their religious education, which always depreciated this idea as "mystical." Yet it is precisely this "mystical" idea which is enforced by the natural tendencies of the unconscious mind.   [XLVI, 107 (B, 72)

At first the materialistic error seems to be inevitable. Since the throne of God could not be discovered among the galactic systems, the inference was that God had never existed. The second inevitable mistake is psychologism: if God is anything, He must be an illusion derived from certain motives, from fear, for instance, from will to power, or from repressed sexuality. These arguments are not new. Similar things have already been said by the Christian missionaries who overthrew the idols of the pagan gods. But whereas the early missionaries were conscious of serving a new God by combatting the old ones, modern iconoclasts are unconscious of the one in whose name they are destroying old values.   [XLVI, 154 (B, 103)

We always think that Christianity consists of a certain confession of faith and of belonging to a Church. No, Christianity is our world. Everything we think is the fruit of the Middle Ages and indeed of the Christian Middle Ages. Our whole science, everything that passes through our head, has inevitably gone through this history. The latter lives in us and has left its stamp upon us for all time and will always form a vital layer of our psyche, just like any phylogenetic traces in our body. The whole character of our mentality, the way in which we look at things, is also the result of the Christian Middle Ages; whether we know it or not is quite immaterial. The age of rational enlightenment has eradicated nothing. Even our method of rational enlightenment is Christian. The Christian *Weltanschauung* is therefore a psychological fact which does not allow of any further rationalization; it is something which has happened, which is present. We are inevitably stamped as Christians; but we are also stamped by that which existed before Christianity. Christianity is now about nineteen hundred years old, but that is but a quarter-hour of the world's history, and before that came untold thousands of years when everything was quite different: infinitely much longer periods which were quite different. All of us who have had a religious education are most deeply impressed by the fact that Christianity entered into history without an historical past, like a stroke of lightning out of a clear sky. This attitude was necessary, but I am convinced that it is not true; for everything has its history, everything has "grown"; and Christianity, which is supposed to have appeared suddenly as a unique revelation from Heaven, undoubtedly also has its history. Moreover, how it began is as clear as daylight. I need not speak of the rites of the mass and of certain peculiarities of the priests' clothing which are borrowed from pagan times, for the fundamental ideas of the Christian Church can also be traced to predecessors. But a certain break in continuity has occurred, owing to the fact that we are all overcome by the impression of the uniqueness of Christianity. It is exactly as if we had built a cathedral over a pagan temple, and no longer knew that it is still there underneath; that is, the inner correspondence of the outer image of God is undeveloped through lack of psychic culture, and has therefore remained caught in paganism.   [xxxiv, 84

The great events of our world as planned and executed by man do not breathe the spirit of Christianity, but rather of unadorned paganism. These things originate in a psychic condition that has remained archaic and has not been even remotely touched by Christianity. The Church assumes, not altogether without reason, that the fact of *semel credidisse* ("having once believed") leaves certain traces behind it; but of these traces nothing is to be seen in the march of events. Christian civilization has proved hollow to a terrifying degree: it is all veneer, but the inner man has remained untouched and therefore unchanged. His soul is out of key with his external beliefs; in his soul the Christian has not kept pace with external developments. Yes, everything is to be found outside—in image and in word, in Church and Bible—but never inside. Inside reign the archaic gods, supreme as of old. [LVIII, 24 (M, 12)

Between the religion of a people and its actual mode of life there always exists a compensatory relation; if this were not so, religion would have no practical significance at all. Beginning with the sublime moral religion of the Persians co-existing with the notorious dubiousness—even in antiquity—of the Persian manner of life, right down to our "Christian" epoch, where the religion of love assisted in the greatest butchery of the world's history: wherever we turn we find evidence of this rule.

[IX, 198 (I, 174)

The more passionately modern consciousness is concerned with things of a totally different nature from religion, the more religion and its object, elementary sin, have been thrust aside, i.e., to a great extent into the unconscious. Therefore nowadays man believes neither the one nor the other. Consequently the Freudian school is reproached with having an impure phantasy, when even a fleeting glance at the history of religion and morals in antiquity would convince us of the demons which the human soul harbours. Disbelief in the power of religion is bound up with this disbelief in the crudeness of human nature. The phenomenon, well known to every psychoanalyst, of the unconscious transformation of an erotic conflict into religious activity is something ethically wholly worthless and nothing but hysterical acting. But on the other hand, whoever can just as consciously confront his conscious sin with religion does something which, from the point of view of history, cannot be denied the quality of greatness. This is sound religion. But the unconscious transformation of the erotic element into religion deserves the reproach of being a sentimental and ethically worthless pose.

[IV, 71

For it should not be forgotten that, in the same measure as the conscious attitude has a real claim to a certain Godlikeness by reason of its lofty and absolute standpoint, an unconscious attitude also develops whose Godlikeness is orientated downwards towards an archaic god whose nature is sensual and brutal. The enantiodromia of Heraclitus forebodes the time when this *deus absconditus* shall also rise to the surface and press the God of our ideals to the wall.   [ix, 137 (i, 123)

The very earliest intuition of mankind personified these powers as gods, and described them fully and carefully according to their various characters, in the myths. This was all the more possible because it is a question of basic and permanent types or images which are inherent in the unconscious of many nations. The behaviour of the nation takes on its specific character from its underlying images, and therefore we may speak of an archetype "Wotan." As an autonomous psychic factor, Wotan produces effects in the collective life of the people, and thus also reveals his own character. For Wotan has a peculiar biology of his own, quite apart from the nature of man. It is only from time to time that individuals fall under the irresistible influence of this unconscious factor. When it is quiescent, one is no more aware of the archetype Wotan than of a latent epilepsy.
[xxxvi, 664 (k, 10)

The gigantic catastrophes that threaten *us* are not elemental happenings of a physical or biological kind, but are psychic events. We are threatened in a fearful way by wars and revolutions that are nothing else than psychic epidemics. At any moment a few million people may be seized by a madness, and then we have another world war or a devastating revolution. Instead of being exposed to wild beasts, tumbling rocks, and inundating waters, man is exposed today to the elemental forces of his own psyche. Psychic life is a world-power that exceeds by many times all the powers of the earth. The Enlightenment, which stripped nature and human institutions of gods, overlooked the one god of fear who dwells in the psyche. Fear of God is in place, if anywhere, before the dominating power of psychic life.   [xxvii, 196 f (f, 293 f)

The Dionysian element has to do with emotions and effects which have found no suitable religious outlet in the predominantly Apollonian cult and ethos of Christianity. The medieval carnivals and *jeux de paume* in the Church were abolished relatively early; consequently the carnival became secularized and with it divine intoxication vanished from the sacred precincts. Mourning, earnestness, severity, and well-tempered spiritual joy remained. But intoxication, that most direct and dangerous form of possession, turned away from the gods and enveloped the human world with its ebullience and pathos. The pagan religions met this danger by giving drunken ecstasy a place within their cult. Heraclitus doubtless saw what was at the back of it when he said, "It is to Hades that they rave and celebrate their feasts." For this very reason orgies were granted religious licence, so as to exorcise the danger that threatened from Hades. Our solution, however, has served to throw the gates of hell wide open.   [I.VIII, 201 f (M, 182)

At a time when a great part of mankind is beginning to lay aside Christianity, it is worth while to realize clearly why it was ever actually accepted. It was accepted in order to escape at last from the brutality of antiquity. If we put Christianity aside, then that wantonness appears again of which life in our great modern cities gives us an impressive foretaste. This step is not progress but regression. It is like the case of an individual who lays aside some form of transference and has no new form; he will unfailingly regress to the old path of transference, to his own great detriment, for the surrounding world will have changed considerably in the meantime.   [IV, 222

The tremendous urge of conscience towards good, the powerful moral strength of Christianity, is not merely an argument in favour of Christianity; it also proves the strength of the suppressed and repressed opposite, the anti-Christian, barbaric element. Therefore I look upon the fact that there still is something in us which can take hold of us as not merely a dangerous but also a valuable characteristic. For it is the expression of a possession as yet untouched, a youthfulness, a treasure of unused strength, a promise of rebirth.   [VIII, 472

The Church presents a high spiritual surrogate for the merely natural or "carnal" tie to the parents. The individual is thus freed from an unconscious relation that, strictly speaking, is no relation, but a condition of primordial unconscious identity which, on account of its unconsciousness, has an extraordinary inertia and offers the greatest resistance to every higher spiritual development. It is hard to know wherein such a condition can be distinguished from that of an animal. To promote and make possible the liberation of the individual from his original, animal-like condition is by no means the special prerogative of the Christian Church. The role played by the latter is merely the modern, more especially the Western, form of an instinctive striving that is probably as old as mankind itself.

[LI, 188 (D, 109 f)

Accordingly, if I am treating practising Catholics, my duty as a doctor allows me, when faced with the transference problem, to step aside and guide the problem over to the Church. If, however, I am treating a non-Catholic, this way out is barred to me, and my duty as a doctor does not allow me to step aside, for there is as a rule no one and nothing to which I could appropriately lead over the father-imago. I can of course get the patient to recognize with his reason that I am not the father. But in that case I become the reasonable father—and in spite of everything still the father. Not only Nature but the patient too abhors a vacuum. He has an instinctive revulsion from letting the parental imagos and his childhood soul fall into the nothingness of a hopeless past without a future. His instinct tells him that if he is to be a complete person, these things must remain alive in some form or other. He knows that a complete withdrawal of the projection will be followed by what seems to be an endless isolation within the ego, which is all the more obtrusive because he has so little love for it. He found that state unbearable before, and it is not very likely that he will be able to endure it now simply out of pure reasonableness. Thus at this stage the Catholic who has been freed from an excessively personal tie to the parents can easily return to the mysteries of the Church, which he is now in a position to understand better and more deeply. There are some Protestants too who are able to find in one of the newer variants of Protestantism a meaning

307

which appeals to them, and thus attain once more to a genuine religious attitude. All other cases—unless there is a violent solution which is often injurious—will, as the saying goes, remain "stuck" in the transference situation, and so subject both themselves and the doctor to a severe trial of patience.

[LIX, 8 f (K, 24 f)

With the methods employed hitherto we have not succeeded in Christianizing the soul to the point where even the most elementary demands of Christian ethics can exert any decisive influence on the main concerns of the Christian European. The Christian missionary may preach the gospel to the poor naked heathen, but the spiritual heathen who infest Europe have as yet heard nothing of Christianity.   [LVIII, 25 (M, 13)

Christian education has done all that is humanly possible; but it has not been enough. Too few people have experienced the divine image as the innermost possession of their own souls.

[LVIII, 25 (M, 12)

Nobody can know what the ultimate things are. We must, therefore, take them as we experience them. And if such experience helps to make your life healthier, more beautiful, more complete, and more satisfactory to yourself and to those you love, you may safely say, "This was the grace of God." No proof of any superior truth is implied by this, and we must confess in all humility that the religious experience is *extra ecclesiam,* subjective, and open to the danger of unlimited error.

[XLVI, 190 (B, 114)

Religious symbols are life-phenomena, plain facts and not opinions. If the Church clung for so long to the idea that the sun rotates round the earth, and then abandoned this contention in the nineteenth century, she can always appeal to the psychological truth that for millions of people the sun did revolve round the earth and that it was only in the nineteenth century that any major portion of mankind became sufficiently sure of the intellectual function to grasp the proofs of the earth's planetary nature. Unfortunately there is no "truth" unless there are people to understand it.   [LVIII, 181 (M, 166)

This symbol function, existing since the most ancient times, is still present today, in spite of the fact that for many centuries the tendency of mental development has been toward the forcible suppression of individual symbols. One of the first steps in this direction was the establishing of an official state religion, a further step was the rooting out of polytheism, the first beginnings of which is to be found in the attempt of Amenophis IV. We know how much the Christian era has achieved in the suppression of individual symbol-making. As the intensity of the Christian idea begins to pale, we may anticipate a corresponding renewal of individual symbol-formation. The prodigious increase of Christian sects since the eighteenth century, the century of "enlightenment," is already a speaking witness to this anticipation. The great spread of "Christian Science," theosophy, anthroposophy, and modern Mazdaism are further steps along the same path. [XIII, 82 f (G, 55)

The history of the development of Protestantism is one of chronic iconoclasm. One wall after another fell. And the work of destruction was not too difficult, either, when once the authority of the Church had been shattered. We all know how, in large things as in small, in general as well as in particular, place after place collapsed, and how the alarming impoverishment of symbolism that is now the condition of our life came about. The power of the Church has gone with that loss of symbolism, too— a fortress that has been robbed of its bastions and casemates, a house whose walls have been plucked away, that is exposed to all the winds of the world and to all dangers. Though properly speaking it is a pitiful collapse which offends our sense of history, the disintegration of Protestantism into nearly four hundred denominations is yet an infallible sign of life, and shows that the restlessness is growing. The Protestant with nothing left but the historical figure of Christ, a much-debated idea of God, and a compulsive faith, in which—Heaven knows!—he has very poor success, is actually thrust forth into a state of defencelessness at which men must shudder who live close to nature and to the past. [XXXI, 189 f (F, 61)

The iconoclasm of the Reformation, however, quite literally

309

made a breach in the bulwarks of the holy pictures and, ever since, one after another has crumbled away. They became dubious, for they collided with awakening reason. Besides, people had long since forgotten what they meant. Or had they really forgotten? Could it be that men had never really known what they meant, and that it first occurred to Protestant mankind in recent times that we actually have no conception of what it means to believe in the virgin birth or in the complexities of the Trinity? It almost seems as if these images had just lived, and as if their living existence had simply been accepted without question and without reflection, much as everyone decorates Christmas trees and hides Easter eggs without ever knowing what these customs mean. The fact is that archetypal images are so significant in themselves that people never think of asking what they mean. That the gods die from time to time is due to man's discovery that they do not mean anything, that they are good-for-nothings made by human hands, fashioned out of wood and stone. In reality, man has thus discovered only this: that up till then he had not achieved one thought concerning these images. [xxxi, 189 (f, 60)]

As soon as the dogmatic fence was broken down and as soon as the ritual had lost the authority of its efficiency, man was confronted with an inner experience, without the protection and the guidance of a dogma and a ritual which are the unparalleled quintessence of Christian as well as of pagan religious experience. Protestantism has, in the main, lost all the finer shades of the dogma: the mass, the confession, the greater part of the liturgy, and the sacrificial importance of priesthood. I must emphasize the point that this statement is not a judgment of values and has no intention of being one. I merely state the facts. Protestantism has, however, intensified the authority of the Bible as a substitute for the lost authority of the Church. But as history has shown, one can interpret certain biblical texts in many ways. Nor has the scientific criticism of the New Testament been very helpful in enhancing the divine character of the holy writings. It is also a fact that under the influence of a so-called scientific enlightenment great masses of educated people have either left the church or have become profoundly indifferent to it. If they were all dull rationalists or neurotic intellectuals the loss would not be regrettable. But many of them are religious people, only incapable of agreeing with the actually existing forms of creed. If this were not so, one could hardly explain the remarkable effect of the Buchman movement on the more or less educated Protestant classes. The Catholic who has turned his back on the Church usually develops a secret or manifest inclination toward atheism, whereas the Protestant follows, if possible, a sectarian movement. The absolutism of the Catholic Church seems to demand an equally absolute negation, while Protestant relativism permits variations. [XLVI, 36 f (B, 22 f)

The Protestant has lost the sacred images expressive of important unconscious factors, together with the ritual, which, since time immemorial, has been a safe way of dealing with the unaccountable forces of the unconscious mind. A great amount of energy thus became liberated and went instantly into the old channels of curiosity and acquisitiveness, by which Europe became the mother of dragons that devoured the greater part of the earth.—Since those days Protestantism has become a hotbed of schisms and, at the same time, of a rapid increase of science and technics which attracted human consciousness to such an extent that it forgot the unaccountable forces of the unconscious mind. [XLVI, 86 f (B, 58)

This whole development is fate. I would not blame Protestantism or the Renaissance for it. But one thing is certain: that modern man, Protestant or not, has lost the protection of the ecclesiastical walls carefully erected and reinforced since Roman days, and on account of that loss has approached the zone of world-destroying and world-creating fire. Life has become quickened and intensified. Our world is permeated by waves of restlessness and fear. [XLVI, 88 (B, 59)

The Reformation in a great measure did away with the Church as the intermediary and dispenser of salvation, and established once again the personal relation with God. This was the culminating point in the objectification of the idea of God, and from this point the concept of God again became increasingly subjective. The logical result of this subjectifying process is a splitting up into sects, and its most extreme outcome is individualism, representing a new form of "remoteness."

[IX, 360 f (I, 318)

As the Christian vow of worldly poverty turned the senses from the good things of the world, so spiritual poverty seeks to renounce the false riches of the spirit. It wishes to retreat not only from the sorry remnants of a great past that call themselves today the Protestant Church but also from all the allurements of exotic reputation, in order to dwell with itself where, in the cold light of consciousness, the barrenness of the world extends even to the stars.   [XXXI, 193 (F, 64)

I must admit that I belong to those who suffer from convictions. Thus, for example, I am convinced that Protestant man has not in vain been despoiled by his own development and made to go naked. This development has an inner consistency. Everything that presented him with no thought-content has been torn from him. If now he should go and cover his nakedness with the gorgeous dress of the Orient, like the theosophists, he would be untrue to his own history. A man does not work his way down to beggarhood and then pose as an Indian king on the stage.   [XXXI, 192 (F, 63)

Since Protestantism has become the creed of the adventurous Germanic tribes with their characteristic curiosity, acquisitiveness, and recklessness, it seems to be possible that their peculiar character could not quite agree with the peace of the church, at least not for any length of time. It looks as if they were not quite prepared to have a process of salvation happen to them and for a submission to a deity crystallized in the magnificent structure of the Church. There was, perhaps, too much of the Imperium Romanum or of the Pax Romana in the Church, too much, at least, for their energies that were and are still insufficiently domesticated. It is quite likely that they were in need of an unmitigated and less controlled experience of God, as often happens to adventurous and restless people, too youthful for any form of conservatism or resignation. They removed therefore the intercession of the Church between God and man, some more and some less.   [XLVI, 86 (B, 57 f)

312

Protestantism was, and still is, a great risk and at the same time a great opportunity. If it keeps on disintegrating as a church, it succeeds in depriving man of all his spiritual safeguards and means of defence against the immediate experience of the forces waiting for liberation in the unconscious mind.

[XLVI, 88 (B, 59 f)

The Protestant has to digest his sins alone and he is not too sure of divine grace, which has become unattainable through lack of a suitable ritual. Owing to this fact the Protestant conscience has become wakeful, and this bad conscience has acquired a disagreeable tendency to linger and to make people uncomfortable. But through this the Protestant has a unique chance to realize sin to a degree hardly attainable by Catholic mentality, for confession and absolution are always ready to relieve too much tension. But the Protestant is left to his tension, which can continue to sharpen his conscience.

[XLVI, 90 (B, 61)

Dissension, as a world disease, is also a healing process, or better still the culmination of a pregnancy which represents the pangs of birth. A time of disruption, like that of Imperial Rome, is also an epoch of birth. The fact that we date our era from the time of Augustus Caesar is not without its significance, for it was in his epoch that the birth of the symbolic figure of Christ occurred, which was invoked by the ancient Christians as the Fish, i.e., as the Lord of the world-month of the Fish which had just begun, and which rose to be the leading spirit of an era which lasted two thousand years. He rose, so to speak, from out of the sea, like the legendary teacher of wisdom of the Babylonians, Oannes, as the primordial night swelled up and a whole era began to break up. He said "I came not to send peace, but a sword"; but that which brings dissension creates relatedness. Therefore his teaching was that of all-uniting love. [XXVII, 43 f

---

Religious sentimentality instead of the numinosum of divine experience: this is the well-known characteristic of a religion that has lost the living mystery. It is easily understandable that such a religion is incapable of giving help or of having any other moral effect. [XLVI, 59 (B, 37)

"God" is a primordial experience of man, and since time immemorial, mankind has taken the most inconceivable pains to describe this incomprehensible experience by interpretation, and either to assimilate it by means of speculation and dogma or to deny it altogether. And again and again the same thing has happened and is still happening, i.e., we know too much about the "good" God and know him too well, so that we confuse him with our own conceptions and regard these as holy because they can claim to be over a thousand years old; but this is a superstition and an idolatry which is just as bad as the crazy illusion that "God" could be "educated away."

[xxiv, 227

The primitive mentality does not invent myths, it experiences them. Myths are original revelations of the preconscious psyche, involuntary statements about unconscious psychic happenings, and anything but allegories of physical processes. Such allegories would be an idle amusement for an unscientific intellect. Myths, on the contrary, have a vital meaning. Not merely do they represent, they *are* the mental life of the primitive tribe, which immediately falls to pieces and decays when it loses its mythological heritage, like a man who has lost his soul. A tribe's mythology is its living religion, whose loss is always and everywhere, even among the civilized, a moral catastrophe. But religion is a vital link with psychic processes independent of and beyond consciousness, in the dark hinterland of the psyche. [xlix, 109 (o, 101 f)

If we were still living in a medieval setting where there was not much doubt about the ultimate things and where every history of the world began with Genesis, we could easily brush aside dreams and the like. Unfortunately we live in a modern setting, where the ultimate things are doubtful, where there is a prehistory of enormous extension, and where people are fully aware of the fact that if there is any numinous experience at all, it is the experience of the psyche. We can no longer imagine an empyrean world revolving round the throne of God, and we would not dream of seeking for Him somewhere behind the galactic systems. But the human soul seems to harbour mysteries, since to an empiricist all religious experience boils down to a peculiar condition of the mind. [xlvi, 113 f (b, 75)

Religious experience is absolute. It is indisputable. You can only say that you have never had such an experience, and your opponent will say, "Sorry, I have." And there your discussion will come to an end. [xlvi, 188 (b, 113)

No matter what the world thinks about religious experience, the one who has it possesses the great treasure of a thing that has provided him with a source of life, meaning, and beauty and that has given a new splendour to the world and to mankind. He has *pistis* and peace. Where is the criterion by which you could say that such a life is not legitimate, that such experience is not valid and that such *pistis* is mere illusion? Is there, as a matter of fact, any better truth about ultimate things than the one that helps you to live? [xlvi, 188 f (b, 113 f)

So long as religion is only faith and outward form, and the religious function is not experienced in our own souls, nothing of any importance has happened. It has yet to be understood that the *mysterium magnum* is not only an actuality but is first and foremost rooted in the human psyche. The man who does not know this from his own experience may be a most learned theologian, but he has no idea of religion and still less of education. [lviii, 25 (m, 13)

Every tribal teaching is sacred-dangerous, and therefore absolute. All esoteric teachings try to grasp the unseen happening of the psyche, and all assert their own final validity. Whatever is true of this primitive lore is even more unconditionally true of the ruling world religions. They contain what was originally the hidden knowledge of revelation and have set forth the secrets of the psyche in glorious images. Their temples and their sacred writings proclaim in image and word the prescript hallowed from of old and accessible to every believing disposition, every receptive outlook, and every last elaboration of thought. Indeed, we are forced to say that the more beautiful, the more grandiose, the more comprehensive is the image that has come into being and been handed on, so much the further is it removed from our experience. Nowadays we can feel our way into it and perceive something of it, but the original experience is lost. [xxxi, 174 (f, 56)

315

What is usually and generally called "religion" is to such an amazing degree a substitute that I ask myself seriously whether this kind of "religion," which I prefer to call a creed, has not an important function in human society. The substitution has the obvious purpose of replacing immediate experience by a choice of suitable symbols invested in a solidly organized dogma and ritual. The Catholic Church maintains them by her indisputable authority, the Protestant church (if this term is still applicable) by insistence upon faith and the evangelical message. As long as those two principles work, people are effectively defended and shielded against immediate religious experience. Even if something of the sort should happen to them, they can refer to the church, for it would know whether the experience came from God or from the devil, whether it was to be accepted or to be rejected. [XLVI, 79 f (B, 52 f)

Theology does not help those who are looking for the key, because theology demands faith, and faith cannot be made: it is in the truest sense a gift of grace. We moderns are faced with the necessity of rediscovering the life of the spirit; we must experience it anew for ourselves. It is the only way in which we can break the spell that binds us to the cycle of biological events. [XIX, 83 (J, 140)

We always hear of the pious man who goes through life firmly secure and serene with his faith in God unshaken, but I have never yet seen this Chidher. The wish is probably father to the figure. The general rule among believers is rather great uncertainty, which they drown in themselves and in others with fanatical protests; furthermore they suffer from doubts in the matter of faith, moral uncertainty, doubts concerning their own personality, feelings of guilt and at the bottom of all the great fear of the totally different other side of reality, against which even highly intelligent people struggle with all their might. This other side is the devil, the adversary or, in modern terms, the stern hand of reality which corrects the infantile picture of a world made palatable by the prevailing principle of pleasure. But the world is not a garden of God the Father; it is also a place of horror. Not only is heaven no father and earth no mother and men not brothers, but they represent as many hostile destructive forces to which we are the more surely delivered over the more confidently and thoughtlessly we entrust ourselves to the so-called fatherly hand of God.   [IV, 224

But God Himself cannot thrive in a humanity that is psychically undernourished.   [X, 45 (G, 188)

The man who is morally and spiritually more highly developed no longer wishes to follow a faith or a rigid dogma. He wants to understand. It is no wonder that he throws everything which he cannot understand aside, and the religious symbol is among those things which are not easily accessible to understanding. Therefore religion usually goes over board first of all. The *sacrificium intellectus,* which a positive faith demands, is an act of violence against which the conscience of the more highly developed man protests.   [VI, 102

But the individual's decision not to belong to a Church does not necessarily denote an anti-Christian attitude; it may mean exactly the reverse: a reconsidering of the kingdom of God in the human heart where, in the words of St. Augustine, the *mysterium paschale* is accomplished *in interioribus ac superioribus suis.* The ancient and long obsolete idea of man as a microcosm contains a supreme psychological truth that has yet to be discovered. In former times this truth was projected upon the body, just as alchemy projected the unconscious psyche upon chemical substances. But it is altogether different when the microcosm is understood as the interior world of the inward nature which is fleetingly glimpsed in the unconscious.
[LX, 54 (N, 372)

The "World of the Son" is the world of moral dissension, without which human consciousness could hardly have achieved the progress in intellectual differentiation which it has actually made. The fact that we are not wholly delighted with this progress nowadays is evidenced by the doubt which besets modern consciousness.   [L, 58

The more unconscious the religious problem of the future remains, the greater is the danger that man will misuse the di-

317

vine spark within him for a ridiculous or demoniacal self-glorification, instead of remaining conscious that he is, for instance, no more than the stable in which the Lord is born.　　　[L, 64

To be truly human also implies an extreme remoteness and difference from God. *De profundis clamavi ad te, Domine—* this confession shows both the farness and the nearness to God, the most extreme darkness and at the same time the flash of the divine spark. God in His human form is so far from Himself, that He must seek Himself again with the most complete surrender. Where would the wholeness of God be if He were not also able to be "quite different"?　　　[L, 127

The man who merely believes and does not think always forgets that he is the one who is constantly exposed to his most innate enemy, which is doubt. For wherever faith prevails, there doubt is always lurking. But to the thinking man doubt is welcome, for it serves him as a valuable step towards a better knowledge. People who can believe should be more patient with their fellow men who can only think. Faith has flown over the peak, which thought hopes to reach by toilsome climbing. The believer should not project his habitual enemy, doubt, on to the thinker and thus suspect him of destructive intentions.
　　　[L, 32

But dogmatism and fanaticism are always compensations for hidden doubt. Religious persecutions take place only where heresy is a menace. There is no instinct in man that is not balanced by another instinct.　　　[XL, 32 (G, 343)

Although the actual moment of a conversion often seems quite sudden and unexpected, yet we know from experience that such a fundamental occurence always has a long period of unconscious incubation. It is only when the preparation is complete, that is to say, when the individual is ready to be converted, that the new view breaks forth with great emotion. St. Paul had already been a Christian for a long time, only unconsciously; hence his fanatical resistance to the Christians, because fanaticism is only found in individuals who are compensating secret doubts. Therefore converts are always the worst fanatics.
　　　[XIII, 210 (G, 257)

People have dwelt far too long on the fundamentally sterile question of whether the assertions of faith are true or not. Quite apart from the impossibility of ever proving or refuting the truth of a metaphysical assertion, the very existence of the assertion is a self-evident fact that needs no further proof, and when a *consensus gentium* allies itself thereto, then the validity of the statement is proved to just that extent. The only thing about it that we can understand is the psychological phenomenon, which is incommensurable with the category of objective rightness or truth. No phenomenon can ever be disposed of by rational criticism, and in religious life we have to deal with phenomena and facts and not with arguable hypotheses.

[LVIII, 50 (M, 35)

But this objectivity is just what my psychology is most blamed for: it is said not to decide in favour of this or that religious doctrine. Without anticipating my own subjective convictions I should like to raise the question: is it not thinkable that when one refrains from setting oneself up as an *arbiter mundi* and, deliberately renouncing all subjectivism, fosters on the contrary the belief, for instance, that God has expressed himself in many languages and appeared in diverse forms and that all these statements are *true*—is it not thinkable, I say, that this too is a decision? The objection raised, more particularly by Christians, that it is impossible for contradictory statements to be true, must permit itself to be politely asked: Does one equal three? How can three be one? Can a mother be a virgin? And so on. Has it not yet been observed that all religious statements contain logical contradictions and assertions that are impossible in principle, that this is in fact the very essence of religious assertion? [LVIII, 29 f (M, 18)

Speaking for instance of the motive of the virgin birth, psychology is only concerned with the fact that there is such an idea, but it is not concerned with the question whether such an idea is true or false in any other sense. It is psychologically true inasmuch as it exists. [XLVI, 11 (B, 3)

Oddly enough, the paradox is one of our most valued spiritual possessions, while uniformity of meaning is a sign of weakness.

319

Hence a religion becomes inwardly impoverished when it loses or reduces its paradoxes; but their multiplication enriches, because only the paradox comes anywhere near to comprehending the fullness of life. Non-ambiguity and non-contradiction are one-sided and thus unsuited to express the incomprehensible.

[LVIII, 30 (M, 18)

The mystery of the virgin birth, or of the oneness of the Son with the Father, or of the Trinity which is no triad, no longer lends wings to any philosophical fantasy. They have become mere objects of belief. It is not surprising that the religious need, the believing mind, and the philosophical speculation of the cultured European feel themselves attracted to the symbols of the East—the grandiose conceptions of divinity in India and the abysms of Taoistic philosophy in China—just as once before the heart and mind of the Greco-Roman were gripped by Christian ideas. There are many Europeans who surrendered so completely to the influence of the Christian symbol that they were enmeshed in the neurosis of a Kierkegaard; and others, again, whose relation to God, owing to a progressive impoverishment of symbolism, developed into an unbearably refined I = you relation. It is not surprising that such persons later succumbed to the magic of the fresh strangeness of Eastern symbols. This surrender is no defeat, but rather bears witness to the receptiveness and vitality of the religious sense. We can observe the same thing in the Oriental man of education, who not seldom feels himself drawn in the same way to the Christian symbol, and even develops an enviable understanding of it. That people succumb to these eternal images is an entirely normal matter. It is for this very purpose that the images came into being. They are intended to attract, to convince, fascinate, and overpower. They are created out of the primal stuff of revelation, and portray the first-hand experience of divinity that every revelation contains.   [XXXI, 185 (F, 57)

Since the only salutary powers visible in the world today are the great "psychotherapeutic" systems which we call the religions and from which we expect the soul's salvation, it is quite natural that many people should make the justifiable and often successful attempt to find a niche for themselves in one of the

320

existing faiths and to acquire a deeper insight into the meaning of the traditional saving verities. This solution is normal and satisfying in that the dogmatically formulated truths of the Christian Church express, almost perfectly, the nature of psychic experience. They are the repositories of the secrets of the soul, and this matchless knowledge is set forth in grand symbolical images. The unconscious thus possesses a natural affinity with the spiritual values of the Church, particularly in their dogmatic form, which owes its special character to centuries of theological controversy—absurd as this seemed in the eyes of later generations—and to the passionate efforts of many great men.   [LX, 48 (N, 365 f)

In itself any scientific theory, no matter how subtle, has, I think, less value from the standpoint of psychological truth than the religious dogma, for the simple reason that a theory is necessarily highly abstract and exclusively rational, whereas the dogma expresses an irrational entity through the image. This method guarantees a much better rendering of an irrational fact such as the psyche. Moreover, the dogma owes its existence and form, on the one hand, to so-called "revealed" immediate experiences, such as the God-Man, the Cross, the Virgin Birth, the Immaculate Conception, the Trinity, and so on, and, on the other hand, to the ceaseless collaboration of many minds and many centuries. It is perhaps not quite clear why I call certain dogmas "immediate experiences," since a dogma is in itself the very thing which excludes immediate experience. Yet the Christian dogmas which I mentioned are not peculiar to Christianity alone. They occur just as often in pagan religions, and moreover, they can reappear spontaneously as psychical phenomena in all kinds of variations, as they have, in a remote past, originated from visions, dreams, or trances. Such ideas were never invented. They came into existence when mankind had not yet learned to use the mind as a purposeful activity. Before people learned to produce thoughts, the thought came to them. They did not think but perceived their mental function. The dogma is like a dream, reflecting the spontaneous and autonomous activity of the objective psyche, the unconscious. Such an expression of the unconscious is a much more efficient means of defense against further immediate experiences than a scientific theory. The theory has to disregard the emotional values of the experience. The dogma, on the contrary, is most expressive in this respect. A scientific theory is soon superseded by another. The dogma lasts for untold centuries.　　　　　　　　[XLVI, 84 f (B, 56 f)

The spiritual adventure of our time is the surrender of human consciousness to what is undetermined and undeterminable, even if it seems to us that in the infinite, those psychical laws also rule which no man invented but knowledge of which was given him through "gnosis" in the symbolism of Christian dogma, which only reckless madmen wish to shake, but never the true lover of the human soul.　　　　　　　　[XLVI, 190

A creed is always the result and fruit of many minds and many centuries, purified from all the oddities, shortcomings, and flaws of individual experience. But for all that, the individual experience, with its very poverty, is immediate life, it is the warm red blood pulsating today. It is more convincing to a seeker after truth than the best tradition.　　[XLVI, 92 (B, 63)

If the theologian really believes in the almighty power of God on the one hand and in the validity of dogma on the other, why then does he not trust God to speak in the soul? Why this fear of psychology? Or is, in complete contradiction to dogma, the soul itself a hell from which only demons gibber? Even if this were really so it would not be any the less convincing; for as we all know the horrified perception of the reality of evil has led to at least as many conversions as the experience of good.
　　　　　　　　　　　　　　　　[LVIII, 32 (M, 19)

Scarcely any other field shows the self-glorification of the "human-all-too-human" spirit more than does the history of dogma. Psychology therefore can hardly be said to encroach when it enters into the discussion, and puts the question as to the human being who devises the dogmas and as to the reasons which might lead him to do so.　　　　　　　　　[L, 44

Whence should religious renewal come if our much-praised

mind—which wants to understand everything and to reserve to itself an attitude towards everything, and even feels itself to be ethically responsible—cannot die? This spirit has become human spirit, fallible and limited; it is in need of "death" in order to become new—which it cannot do of its own power. What does the power of the *forces telluriques* mean but that the "spirit" has once again become senile and weak through being too much humanized? [xxix, 78

The Christian is a morally suffering man who in his suffering needs the "Comforter," the Paraclete. Man cannot overcome the conflict by his own strength, just as he also did not invent it. He is dependent upon divine consolation and reconciliation, i.e., upon the spontaneous revelation of the spirit which does not obey the human will but comes and goes as it wills. This spirit is an autonomous psychic happening, peace after the storm, a reconciling light in the darkness of the human mind and the secret order in our psychic chaos. The Holy Ghost is a comforter like the Father, a silent, eternal, abysmal "One" in which the love and the wrath of God are melted together into a wordless unity. And just therein is the primordial meaning of the still meaningless world of the Father re-established in the realm of human experience and reflection. The Holy Ghost is a reconciliation of opposites in a quaternary aspect and thus the answer to that suffering in the Deity which Christ personifies. [L, 58

For thousands of years, rites of initiation have been teaching spiritual rebirth; yet, strangely enough, man forgets again and again the meaning of divine procreation. This is surely no evidence of a strong life of the spirit; and yet the penalty of misunderstanding is heavy, for it is nothing less than neurotic decay, embitterment, atrophy, and sterility. It is easy enough to drive the spirit out of the door, but when we have done so the salt of life grows flat—it loses its savour. Fortunately, we have proof that the spirit always renews its strength in the fact that the central teaching of the ancient initiations is handed on from generation to generation. Ever and again human beings arise who understand what is meant by the fact that God is our father. The equal balance of the flesh and the spirit is not lost to the world. [XIX, 85 (J, 142)

The "bright God" crosses the bridge, "man," from the daylight side, but the "shadow of God" from the night side. Who will decide in this terrible dilemma which threatens to break the miserable vessel with terrors and intoxications such as have never been known before? It can only be the revelation of a Holy Spirit out of man himself. Once man was revealed out of God, and it may be that, when the circle closes, God will also be revealed out of man. [L, 63

The mass is a living example of the mystery drama which represents the permanence and transformation of life. If we watch the congregation during the holy service, we can observe every grade of attitude, from indifferent, mere presence to the deepest emotional participation [Ergriffensein]. The groups of men who stand together near the exit during the mass, talking of worldly things and making the sign of the cross and bending one knee quite mechanically, have, in spite of their lack of attention, nevertheless some share in the holy act, through their mere presence in the space filled with grace. In the mass, Christ is killed and sacrificed as an act beyond the world and outside time, and He rises again in the transformed substances. The ritual sacrificial death is not a repetition of the historical event, but the first, unique, and eternal process. Experience of the mass is therefore a participation in a transcendence of life overcoming all limitations of space and time. It is a moment of eternity within time. [XLVII, 407

Christ, the fulfilment of prophecy, put an end to the fear of God and taught mankind that the true relation to the Godhead is "love." Thus he destroyed the ceremonial constraint of the Law and gave the example of a personal, loving relationship to God. The later imperfect sublimation of the Christian mass leads again to the ceremonial of the Church from which occasionally the minds capable of sublimation among the saints and reformers have been able to free themselves. Not without cause therefore does modern theology speak of "inner" or "personal" experiences as having great enfranchising power, for always the ardour of love transmutes the dread and constraint into a higher, freer type of feeling.   [I, 171 (C, 173 f)

I wish everybody could be freed from the burden of their sins by the Church. But those to whom she cannot render this service must bend very low in the imitation of Christ in order to take the burden of their cross upon themselves. The ancients could get along with the Greek wisdom of the ages: "Exaggerate nothing, all good lies in right measure." But what an abyss still separates us from reason!   [LVIII, 54 (M, 37)

What the Christian sacrament of baptism purports to do is of the greatest importance for the psychic development of mankind. Baptism endows the human being with a unique soul. I do not mean, of course, the baptismal rite in itself as a magical act that is effective at one performance. I mean that the idea of baptism lifts a man out of his archaic identification with the world and changes him into a being who stands above it. The fact that mankind has risen to the level of this idea is baptism in the deepest sense, for it means the birth of spiritual man who transcends nature.   [XIX, 238 (J, 166 f)

If God wishes to be born as man and to unite mankind in the fellowship of the Holy Ghost, He suffers the terrible torment of having to bear the world in its reality. It is a crux, indeed, He Himself is His own cross. The world is God's suffering, and every individual human being who wishes even to approach his own wholeness knows very well that this means bearing his own cross. But the eternal promise for him who bears his own cross is the Paraclete.   [L, 62 f

KEY TO SOURCES

KEY TO SOURCES

Works in German

The references in the text give page numbers in the editions listed here; many of the works, however, have appeared in several editions. The annotations below cite translations; the capital letters refer to the list of works in English which follows the German list. Noted are, wherever possible, translations now available, in addition to the English originals or new translations in the *Collected Works of C. G. Jung*. The latter is a systematic edition being published, with new translations by R. F. C. Hull, simultaneously by Pantheon Books, Inc., for the Bollingen Foundation, Inc., in New York, and by Routledge and Kegan Paul, Ltd., in London.

I. "Die Bedeutung des Vaters für das Schicksal des Einzelnen," *Jahrbuch für psychoanalytische und psychopathologische Forschungen,* I (1909). Leipzig and Vienna: Deuticke.

"The Significance of the Father in the Destiny of the Individual" (trans. M. D. Eder) in C, pp. 156–75. *Coll. Works,* Vol. 4.

II. "Über Konflikte der kindlichen Seele," ibid., II (1910).

"Experiences Concerning the Psychic Life of the Child," *Coll. Works,* Vol. 17 (based on a later version in *Psychologie und Erziehung,* Zurich: Rascher, 1946).

III. "Randbemerkungen zu Wittels' *Die sexuelle Not,*" ibid., II (1910).

"Notes on Wittels' *Die sexuelle Not,*" *Coll. Works,* final vol.

IV. *Wandlungen und Symbole der Libido.* Leipzig and Vienna: Deuticke, 1912.

The Psychology of the Unconscious (trans. Beatrice Hinkle), New York, 1915; London, 1919. Greatly revised as *Symbols of Transformation, Coll. Works,* Vol. 5.

V. "Neue Bahnen der Psychologie," *Raschers Jahrbuch für Schweizer Art und Kunst.* Zurich: Rascher, 1912.

"New Paths in Psychology," appendix to *Coll. Works,* Vol. 7.

Originally first in English as "The Psychology of the Unconscious Processes" (trans. Dora Hecht) in C, pp. 352–444; later revised as "The Unconscious in the Normal and Pathological Mind" in D. For ultimate revision, see LI, below.

VI. "Versuch einer Darstellung der psychoanalytischen Theorie," *Jahrbuch für psychoanalytische und psychopathologische Forschungen,* V (1913). Leipzig and Vienna: Deuticke.

The Theory of Psychoanalysis, Nervous and Mental Disease Series 19, New York, 1915. *Coll. Works,* Vol. 4.

VII. *Psychotherapeutische Zeitfragen.* Leipzig and Vienna: Deuticke, 1914.

(A correspondence in 1913 between Professor Jung and Dr. R. Loÿ.) "On Some Crucial Points in Psychoanalysis" (trans. Mrs. Edith Eder) in C, pp. 236–77. *Coll. Works,* Vol. 4.

VIII. "Über das Unbewusste," *Schweizerland,* IV, 9–10 (June–July, 1918).

"The Role of the Unconscious," *Coll. Works,* Vol. 10.

IX. *Psychologische Typen,* Zurich: Rascher, 1921.

See I, *Psychological Types. Coll. Works,* Vol. 6.

X. "Die Frau in Europa," *Europäische Revue,* III, 7 (Oct., 1927): 481–99. (In book form: Zurich: Verlag der Neuen Schweizer Rundschau, 1929; Rascher, 1932.)

"Woman in Europe" in G, pp. 164–88. *Coll. Works,* Vol. 11.

XI. *Die Beziehungen zwischen dem Ich und dem Unbewussten.* Darmstadt: Reichl, 1928.

"The Relations between the Ego and the Unconscious" in D. Revised in *Coll. Works,* Vol. 7.

XII. "Die schweizerische Linie im Spektrum Europas," *Neue Schweizer Rundschau,* XXI, 6 (June, 1928): 469–79.

"The Swiss Line in the European Spectrum," *Coll. Works,* Vol. 10.

XIII. *Über die Energetik der Seele und andere psychologische Abhandlungen.* Zurich: Rascher, 1928.

CONTENTS AND TRANSLATIONS

7–111: "Über die Energetik der Seele."—"On Psychical Energy" in G, pp. 1–76. *Coll. Works,* Vol. 8 (based on a later version in *Über psychische Energetik und das Wesen der Träume,* Zurich: Rascher, 1948).

112–84: "Allgemeine Gesichtspunkte zur Psychologie des Traumes."—Pp. 112–30 as "The Psychology of Dreams" in C, pp. 299–311. "General Aspects of Dream Psychology," *Coll. Works,* Vol. 8.

185–99: "Instinkt und Unbewusstes."—"Instinct and Unconscious" in G, pp. 270–81. *Coll. Works,* Vol. 8.

200–224: "Die psychologischen Grundlagen des Geisterglaubens." —"The Psychological Foundations of Belief in Spirits" in G, pp. 250–69. *Coll. Works,* Vol. 8.

XIV. European commentary to: *Das Geheimnis der goldenen Blüte.* Translated from the Chinese by Richard Wilhelm. Munich: Dorn-Verlag, 1929.

See H, *The Secret of The Golden Flower.* Jung's commentary in *Coll. Works,* Vol. 13; obituary of Wilhelm Vol. 15.

XV. Introduction (with R. Wilhelm) to: Tschang Scheng Schu. "Die Kunst das menschliche Leben zu verlängern," *Europäische Revue,* V, 8 (Nov., 1929): 530–56.

Contained essentially in XIV, above.

XVI. "Psychologie und Dichtung," in *Die Philosophie der Literaturwissenschaft,* edited by Emil Ermatinger. Berlin: Junker and Dünnhaupt, 1930.

See E, "Psychology and Poetry"; also "Psychology and Literature" in J. *Coll. Works,* Vol. 15 (based on a later version in *Gestaltungen des Unbewussten,* Zurich: Rascher, 1950).

XVII. Introduction to: Wolfgang Müller Kranefeldt. *Die Psychoanalyse.* Berlin: W. de Gruyter ("Sammlung Göschen"), 1930.

Coll. Works, Vol. 4.

XVIII. Introduction to: Frances G. Wickes. *Analyse der Kinderseele.* Stuttgart: Julius Hoffman, 1931.

Coll. Works, Vol. 17.

XIX. *Seelenprobleme der Gegenwart.* Zurich: Rascher, 1931.

CONTENTS AND TRANSLATIONS

1–39: "Probleme der modernen Psychotherapie."—"Problems of Modern Psychotherapy" in J, pp. 32–62. *Coll. Works,* Vol. 16,

40–73: "Über die Beziehungen der analytischen Psychologie zum dichterischen Kunstwerk."—"On the Relation of Analytical Psychology to Poetic Art" in G, pp. 225–49. *Coll. Works,* Vol. 15.

74–86: "Der Gegensatz Freud und Jung."—"Freud and Jung—Contrasts" in J, pp. 132–42. *Coll. Works,* Vol. 4.

87–114: "Ziele der Psychotherapie."—"Aims of Modern Psychotherapy" in J, pp. 63–84. *Coll. Works,* Vol. 16.

115–43: "Psychologische Typologie."—"A Psychological Theory of Types" in J, pp. 85–108. *Coll. Works,* Vol. 6.

144–75: "Die Struktur der Seele."—"The Structure of the Psyche," *Coll. Works,* Vol. 8.

176–210: "Seele und Erde."—"Mind and Earth" in G, pp. 99–140. *Coll. Works,* Vol. 10.

211–47: "Der archaische Mensch."—"Archaic Man" in J, pp. 143–74. *Coll. Works,* Vol. 10.

248–74: "Die Lebenswende."—"The Stages of Life" in J, pp. 109–31. *Coll. Works,* Vol. 8.

275–95: "Die Ehe als psychologische Beziehung."—"Marriage as a Psychological Relationship" in G, pp. 189–203. *Coll. Works,* Vol. 17.

296–335: "Analytische Psychologie und Weltanschauung."—"Analytical Psychology and Weltanschauung" in G, pp. 141–63. *Coll. Works,* Vol. 8.

369–400: "Geist und Leben."—"Spirit and Life" in G, pp. 77–98. *Coll. Works,* Vol. 8.

401–35: "Das Seelenproblem des modernen Menschen."—"The Spiritual Problem of Modern Man" in J, pp. 226–54. *Coll. Works,* Vol. 10.

XX. Foreword to: O. A. Schmitz. *Märchen aus dem Unbewussten.* Munich: Hanser, 1932.

Coll. Works, final vol.

XXI. *Die Beziehungen der Psychotherapie zur Seelsorge.* Zurich: Rascher, 1932.

"Psychotherapists or the Clergy—a Dilemma" in J, pp. 255 ff. *Coll. Works,* Vol. 11.

XXII. "Wirklichkeit und Überwirklichkeit," *Querschnitt,* XII, 12 (Dec., 1933): 844–45.

"The Real and the Surreal," *Coll. Works,* Vol. 8.

XXIII. "Über Psychologie," *Neue Schweizer Rundschau* (N.S.), I, 1–2 (May–June, 1933): 21–28, 98–106.

(Lecture in the Zurich town hall.) "The Meaning of Psychology for Modern Man," *Coll. Works*, Vol. 10 (based on a later version, "Die Bedeutung der Psychologie für die Gegenwart" in XXVII, below).

XXIV. "Bruder Klaus," ibid., I, 4 (Aug., 1933): 223–29.

"Brother Klaus" (trans. Horace Gray), *Journal of Nervous and Mental Diseases*, CIII, 4 (Apr., 1946). *Coll. Works*, Vol. 11.

XXV. Review of G. R. Heyer, *Organismus der Seele. Europäische Revue*, IX, 10 (Oct., 1933): 639.

XXVI. "Zur gegenwärtigen Lage der Psychotherapie," *Zentralblatt für Psychotherapie und ihre Grenzgebiete*, VII (1934), 2.

"The State of Psychotherapy Today," *Coll. Works*, Vol. 10.

XXVII. *Wirklichkeit der Seele.* Zurich: Rascher, 1934.

CONTENTS AND TRANSLATIONS

1–31: "Das Grundproblem der gegenwärtigen Psychologie."—"Basic Postulates of Analytical Psychology" in J, pp. 200–225. *Coll. Works*, Vol. 8.

32–67: "Die Bedeutung der Psychologie für die Gegenwart."—"The Meaning of Psychology for Modern Man," *Coll. Works*, Vol. 10.

68–103: "Die praktische Verwendbarkeit der Traumanalyse."—"Dream Analysis in Its Practical Application" in J, pp. 1–31. *Coll. Works*, Vol. 16.

104–18: "Paracelsus."—*Coll. Works*, Vol. 15.

119–31: "Sigmund Freud als kulturhistorische Erscheinung."—"Sigmund Freud in His Historical Setting" in *Character and Personality*, I (1932), 1:48–55. "Sigmund Freud—a Cultural Phenomenon," *Coll. Works*, Vol. 15.

132–69: "Ulysses."—*Coll. Works*, Vol. 15.

170–79: "Picasso."—*Coll. Works*, Vol. 15.

180–211: "Vom Werden der Persönlichkeit."—"The Development of Personality" in F, pp. 281 ff. *Coll. Works*, Vol. 17.

212–230: "Seele und Tod."—"The Soul and Death," *Coll. Works*, Vol. 8.

XXVIII. "Zur Empirie des Individuationsprozesses," *Eranos-Jahrbuch* 1933. Zurich: Rhein-Verlag, 1934.

"A Study in the Process of Individuation" in F, pp. 30–51. *Coll. Works*, Vol. 9 (based on a later version in *Gestaltung des Unbewussten*, Zurich: Rascher, 1950).

XXIX. Review of H. A. Keyserling, *La Révolution Mondiale. Basler Nachrichten*, XXVII, 19 (May 13, 1934).

Coll. Works, Vol. 10.

XXX. Foreword to: K. L. Schleich. *Die Wunder der Seele.* Berlin: S. Fischer, 1934.

Coll. Works, final vol.

XXXI. "Über die Archetypen des kollektiven Unbewussten," *Eranos-Jahrbuch* 1934. Zurich: Rhein-Verlag, 1935.

"Archetypes of the Collective Unconscious" in F, pp. 52–95. *Coll. Works*, Vol. 9.

XXXII. Foreword and commentary to: *Bardo Thödol: Das Tibetanische Totenbuch.* Edited by W. Y. Evans-Wentz; translated with an introduction by Louise Göpfert-March. Zurich: Rascher, 1935.

Coll. Works, final vol.

XXXIII. Introduction to: M. Esther Harding. *Der Weg der Frau.* Zurich: Rhein-Verlag, 1935.

See A, *The Way of All Women. Coll. Works*, final vol.

XXXIV. Seminar, Basel, October, 1934. Basel (privately printed), 1935.

XXXV. "Psychologische Typologie," *Süddeutsche Monatshefte*, XXXIII, 5 (Feb., 1936): 264–72.

"Type Psychology," *Coll. Works*, Vol. 6.

XXXVI. "Wotan," *Neue Schweizer Rundschau* (N.S.), III, 11 (Mar., 1936): 657–69.

In K (trans. Barbara Hannah), pp. 1–16. *Coll. Works*, Vol. 10.

XXXVII. Review of G. R. Heyer, *Praktische Seelenheilkunde. Zentralblatt für Psychotherapie*, IX (1936), 3: 184–87.

Coll. Works, final vol.

XXXVIII. "Traumsymbole des Individuationsprozesses," *Eranos-Jahrbuch* 1935. Zurich: Rhein-Verlag, 1936.

"Dream Symbols of the Process of Individuation" in F, pp. 96–204.

"Individual Dream Symbolism in Relation to Alchemy" in M (*Coll. Works*, Vol. 12).

XXXIX. "Über den Archetypus, mit besonderer Berücksichtigung des Animabegriffes," *Zentralblatt für Psychotherapie*, IX (1936), 5.

"Concerning the Archetypes, with Special Reference to the Anima Concept," *Coll. Works*, Vol. 9.

XL. *Analytische Psychologie und Erziehung*. Heidelberg: Kampmann, 1926.

(Three lectures given in London in May, 1924.) "Analytical Psychology and Education" in G, pp. 313–82. *Coll. Works*, Vol. 17 (based on a later version in *Psychologie und Erziehung*, Zurich: Rascher, 1946).

XLI. "Die Erlösungsvorstellungen in der Alchemie," *Eranos-Jahrbuch* 1936. Zurich: Rhein-Verlag, 1937.

"The Idea of Redemption in Alchemy" in F, pp. 205–80. "Religious Ideas in Alchemy" in M (*Coll. Works*, Vol. 12).

XLII. Foreword to: D. T. Suzuki. *Die grosse Befreiung*. Leipzig: Curt Weller and Co., 1939.

Foreword to: Suzuki, *An Introduction to Zen Buddhism*, London: Rider and Co., and New York: Philosophical Library, 1950. *Coll. Works*, Vol. 11.

XLIII. "Die psychologischen Aspekte des Mutterarchetypus," *Eranos-Jahrbuch* 1938. Zurich: Rhein-Verlag, 1939.

"Psychological Aspects of the Mother Archetype," *Coll. Works*, Vol. 9.

XLIV. "Bewusstsein, Unbewusstes und Individuation," *Zentralblatt für Psychotherapie*, XI (1939), 5.

"The Conscious Mind, the Unconscious, and the Individuation," *Coll. Works*, Vol. 9.

XLV. "Sigmund Freud, ein Nachruf," *Basler Nachrichten*, XXXIII, 40 (Oct. 1, 1939).

"Sigmund Freud, an Obituary," *Coll. Works*, Vol. 15.

XLVI. *Psychologie und Religion*. Zurich: Rascher, 1940.

See B, *Psychology and Religion*, which was the original of this work; the version in *Coll. Works*, Vol. 11, is based on the somewhat enlarged 1940 edition in German.

XLVII. "Die verschiedenen Aspekte der Wiedergeburt," *Eranos-Jahrbuch* 1939. Zurich: Rhein-Verlag, 1940.

"Concerning Rebirth," *Coll. Works*, Vol. 9 (based on a later version in *Gestaltungen des Unbewussten*, Zurich: Rascher, 1950).

XLVIII. *Paracelsica.* Zurich and Leipzig: Rascher, 1942.

"Paracelsus as a Spiritual Phenomenon," *Coll. Works*, Vol. 13, and "Paracelsus the Physician," *Coll. Works*, Vol. 15.

XLIX. With K. Kerényi. *Einführung in das Wesen der Mythologie.* "Das göttliche Kind" and "Das göttliche Mädchen." Amsterdam and Leipzig: Pantheon, 1942.

See O, *Essays on a Science of Mythology. Coll. Works*, Vol. 9.

L. [a] "Zur Psychologie der Trinitätsidee" and [b] "Das Wandlungssymbol in der Messe," *Eranos-Jahrbuch* 1940/1941. Zurich: Rhein-Verlag, 1942.

[a] "A Psychological Approach to the Dogma of the Trinity," *Coll. Works*, Vol. 11 (based on an expanded version in *Symbolik des Geistes*, Zurich: Rascher, 1948). [b] "Transubstantiation Symbolism in the Mass," *Coll. Works*, Vol. 11 (based on an unpublished expanded version).

LI. *Über die Psychologie des Unbewussten.* Zurich: Rascher, 1943.

"The Psychology of the Unconscious," *Coll. Works*, Vol. 7. (A revised and expanded version of V, above; an earlier trans. was in D, below.)

LII. "Der Geist Mercurius," *Eranos-Jahrbuch* 1942. Zurich: Rhein-Verlag, 1943.

"The Spirit Mercurius," *Coll. Works*, Vol. 13 (based on a later version in *Symbolik des Geistes*, Zurich: Rascher, 1948).

LIII. "Der Begabte," *Schweizer Erziehungs-Rundschau*, XVI, 1 (Apr., 1943).

"The Gifted Child," *Coll. Works*, Vol. 17.

LIV. "Zur Psychologie östlicher Meditation," *Mitteilungen der schweizerischen Gesellschaft der Freunde ostasiatischer Kultur*, V (1943): 33–53.

See L, "The Psychology of Eastern Meditation." *Coll. Works*, Vol. 11.

LV. "Psychotherapie und Weltanschauung," *Schweizerische Zeitschrift für Psychologie und ihre Anwendungen,* I (1943), 3.

"Psychotherapy and Philosophy of Life" (trans. M. Briner) in K, pp. 36–44. *Coll. Works,* Vol. 16.

LVI. "Tiefenpsychologie und Selbsterkenntnis," *Du,* III, 9 (Sept., 1943).

(An interview with Professor Jung in a Swiss magazine.)

LVII. "Über den indischen Heiligen," foreword to: Heinrich Zimmer, *Der Weg zum Selbst.* Edited by C. G. Jung. Zurich: Rascher, 1944.

"The Holy Men of India," *Coll. Works,* Vol. 11.

LVIII. *Psychologie und Alchemie.* Zurich: Rascher, 1944.

See M, *Psychology and Alchemy (Coll. Works,* Vol. 12).

LIX. "Die Psychotherapie in der Gegenwart," *Schweizerische Zeitschrift für Psychologie und ihre Anwendungen,* IV (1945), 1.

"Psychotherapy Today" (trans. M. Briner) in K, pp. 17–35. *Coll. Works,* Vol. 16.

LX. *Die Psychologie der Übertragung.* Zurich: Rascher, 1946. See N, *The Psychology of the Transference (Coll. Works,* Vol. 16).

Works in English

Following is a list of those English translations and works in English of Jung that are drawn upon in this volume (aside from translations prepared by Mrs. Verzar and Miss Welsh). Text references indicate page numbers in the editions cited here. The annotations give the volumes of the *Collected Works* that are to contain the material (in some cases, revised by the author).

A. Introduction to: M. Esther Harding. *The Way of All Women; a Psychological Interpretation.* London and New York: Longmans, Green and Co., 1933.*

Coll. Works, final vol.

* Written by Professor Jung in English.

B. *Psychology and Religion.* The Terry Lectures, 1937. New Haven: Yale University Press, and London: H. Milford, Oxford University Press, 1938.*

Coll. *Works,* Vol. 11.

C. *Collected Papers on Analytical Psychology.* Authorized translation edited by Dr. Constance E. Long. London: Baillière, Tindall and Cox, 1916; 2nd edition, 1917; New York: Moffatt, Yard and Co., 1920.

Coll. *Works,* Vols. 1–4, 6, 7.

D. *Two Essays on Analytical Psychology.* Authorized translation by H. G. and C. F. Baynes. London: Baillière, Tindall and Cox, and New York: Dodd, Mead and Co., 1928.

Coll. *Works,* Vol. 7.

E. "Psychology and Poetry." Translated by Eugene Jolas. *Transition, an International Quarterly for Creative Experiment,* 19–20 (June, 1930): 23–45.

Coll. *Works,* Vol. 15.

F. *The Integration of the Personality.* Translated by Stanley M. Dell. New York: Farrar and Rinehart, 1939; London: Kegan Paul, 1940.

Coll. *Works,* Vols. 9, 12, 17.

G. *Contributions to Analytical Psychology.* Translated by H. G. and Cary F. Baynes. London: Kegan Paul, Trench, Trübner and Co., and New York: Harcourt, Brace and Co., 1928.

Coll. *Works,* Vols. 6, 8, 10, 15–17.

H. *The Secret of the Golden Flower.* Translated and explained by Richard Wilhelm, with a European commentary by C. G. Jung. Authorized English translation by Cary F. Baynes. London: Kegan Paul, Trench, Trübner and Co., and New York: Harcourt, Brace and Co., 1931.

Jung's commentary in Coll. *Works,* Vol. 13; obituary of Wilhelm in Vol. 15.

I. *Psychological Types; or, The Psychology of Individuation.* Translated by H. Godwin Baynes. London: Kegan Paul, Trench,

* Written by Professor Jung in English.

Trübner and Co., and New York: Harcourt, Brace and Co., 1923.

Coll. Works, Vol. 6.

J. *Modern Man in Search of a Soul*. Translated by W. S. Dell and Cary F. Baynes. London: Kegan Paul, Trench, Trübner and Co., and New York: Harcourt, Brace and Co., 1933.

Coll. Works, Vols. 4, 6, 8, 10, 11, 13, 16.

K. *Essays on Contemporary Events*. Translated by Elizabeth Welsh, Barbara Hannah, and Mary Briner. London: Kegan Paul, 1947.

Coll. Works, Vols. 10, 16.

L. "On the Psychology of Eastern Meditation." Translated by Carol Baumann. In *Art and Thought* (issued in honour of Dr. Ananda K. Coomaraswamy), edited by K. Bharatha Iyer, London: Luzac and Co., 1947, pp. 169–79.

Coll. Works, Vol. 11.

M. *Psychology and Alchemy*. Translated by R. F. C. Hull. *Collected Works of C. G. Jung*, Vol. 12. New York: Pantheon Books (Bollingen Series XX, 12), and London: Routledge and Kegan Paul, 1953.*

N. *The Practice of Psychotherapy*. Essays on the Psychology of the Transference and Other Subjects. Translated by R. F. C. Hull. *Collected Works of C. G. Jung*, Vol. 16. New York: Pantheon Books (Bollingen Series XX, 16), and London: Routledge and Kegan Paul, 1953.*

O. C. G. Jung and C. Kerényi. *Essays on a Science of Mythology*. The Myth of the Divine Child and the Mysteries of Eleusis. Translated by R. F. C. Hull. New York: Pantheon Books (Bollingen Series XXII), 1949; London (entitled *Introduction to a Science of Mythology*): Routledge and Kegan Paul, 1950.

* In the *Coll. Works*, reference is by paragraph number rather than by page.

Mottoes

COLLECTED WORKS OF C. G. JUNG

The publication of the first complete collected edition, in English, of the works of C. G. Jung has been undertaken by Routledge and Kegan Paul, Ltd., in England and by Pantheon Books, Inc., for the Bollingen Foundation, Inc., in the United States. The edition contains revised versions of works previously published, such as *The Psychology of the Unconscious* (*Wandlungen und Symbole*), now to be titled *Symbols of Transformation;* works originally published in English, such as *Psychology and Religion;* and, in general, new translations of the major body of Professor Jung's writings. The author has supervised the textual revision, which in some cases is extensive. Sir Herbert Read, Michael Fordham, M.D., and Gerhard Adler, Ph.D., compose the Editorial Committee; the translator is R. F. C. Hull.

The volumes are not published in numerical order, but, generally speaking, new works of which translations are lacking are given precedence. The published or projected volumes of the *Collected Works* are as follows:

1. PSYCHIATRIC STUDIES

2. EXPERIMENTAL RESEARCHES
    In two parts; includes "Studies in Word Association"

3. PSYCHOGENESIS IN MENTAL DISEASE

4. FREUD AND PSYCHOANALYSIS

5. SYMBOLS OF TRANSFORMATION
    In two parts

6. PSYCHOLOGICAL TYPES
    In two parts

7. TWO ESSAYS ON ANALYTICAL PSYCHOLOGY

8. ON PSYCHIC ENERGY

9. ARCHETYPES AND THE COLLECTIVE UNCONSCIOUS
   In two parts: includes "Contributions to the Symbolism of the Self," from "Aion"

10. CIVILIZATION IN TRANSITION

11. PSYCHOLOGY AND RELIGION
    Contains the work of that title and related short works

12. PSYCHOLOGY AND ALCHEMY

13. ALCHEMICAL STUDIES
    Includes "Paracelsus as a Spiritual Phenomenon"

14. MYSTERIUM CONIUNCTIONIS

15. THE SPIRIT IN MAN, ART, AND LITERATURE

16. THE PRACTICE OF PSYCHOTHERAPY
    Includes "Psychology of the Transference"

17. THE DEVELOPMENT OF PERSONALITY

Final volume. MISCELLANEOUS WORKS, BIBLIOGRAPHY, AND GENERAL INDEX